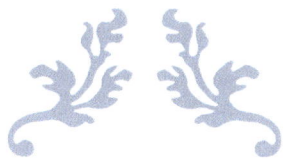

SCHIFF BASE METAL COMPLEXES: SYNTHESIS, STRUCTURE, AND THERAPEUTIC APPLICATIONS

Dr. Shuhua Zhang.

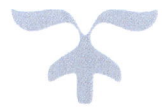

Copyright © 2023

All rights reserved. No part of this publication may be reproduced, distributed, or transmitted in any form or by any means, including photocopying, recording, or other electronic or mechanical methods, without the prior written permission of the AUTHOR, except in the case of brief quotations embodied in critical reviews and certain other non-commercial uses permitted by copyright law. For permission requests, write to the author, addressed "Attention: Permissions Coordinator," at the address below.

Index of Sciences Ltd.

Kemp House,

160 City Road, London.

www.indexofsciences.com

Ordering Information:

Quantity sales. Special discounts are available on quantity purchases by corporations, associations, and others. For details, contact the publisher at the address above.

Printed in the United Kingdom

ISBN: 9-798-86565962-4

Preface

In this erudite volume, "Schiff Base Metal Complexes: Synthesis, Structure, and Therapeutic Applications," we are privileged to journey through the intricate universe of inorganic chemistry, guided by the renowned scholar, Shu-Hua Zhang. Dr. Zhang, a distinguished Figure in the field, offers a comprehensive and systematic exploration of Schiff base metal complexes, encompassing years of expertise, research, and passionate inquiry.

A seasoned scholar, Dr. Zhang's contributions to the discipline of Inorganic Chemistry are formidable, marked by a relentless pursuit of knowledge and a commitment to scientific excellence. He has presided over a number of projects from the National Natural Science Foundation of China and more than 10 provincial and ministerial-level projects. He has published more than 230 papers in *Advanced Functional Materials*, *Small*, *Inorg. Chem. Front.*, *Int. J. Biol. Macromol.*, *European Journal of Medicinal Chemistry*, *Journal of Materials Chemistry A*, et al. He has obtained more than 50 invention patents authorized by China, and transferred some of them to Chinalco Guangxi Nonferrous Rare Earth Development Co., LTD., Guangxi Baoli Star Lighting Technology Co., LTD., and other enterprises.

He was awarded the Best Innovation Award of the 2022 International New Scientific Invention Research Award by the Father of Science. He won the third prize of Guangxi Science and Technology Progress Award and the third prize of Guangxi Natural Science Award. He won the special prize, second prize and third prize of Guangxi Teaching Achievement Award. He is the chief editor of the digital courses of General Chemistry and General Chemistry, and the deputy chief editor of the Diagram of Modern Fine Chemical Production Process Process. His writings consistently embody meticulous detail, depth of understanding, and an exceptional capacity to connect theoretical principles to real-world applications.

He is the director of Guangxi Chemical and Chemical Industry Society, editorial board of synthetic chemistry, editorial board of Frontiers in Chemistry, member of Chinese Chemical Society, evaluation expert of National Teaching Achievement Award, evaluation expert of Distinguished Professor of Changjiang, etc.

The opening chapter, "Introduction to Schiff Base and Metal Complexes," initiates readers into the subject, conveying the core tenets of Schiff base metal complexes with clarity and accessibility. This foundation allows the uninitiated to grasp the fundamentals of a complex field, demonstrating Dr. Zhang's prowess as both a scholar and an educator.

As we delve deeper into the text, chapters such as "Synthesis of Schiff Base Metal Complexes" and "Structural Characterization Techniques" embody Dr. Zhang's gift for distilling complex procedures into digestible, comprehensive narratives. His approachability and keen attention to detail ensure these pivotal aspects of the discipline are well within the reader's grasp.

Chapters on "Catalytic Applications of Schiff Base Metal Complexes" and "Biological Activities and Therapeutic Applications" expertly bridge the gap between theoretical chemistry and practical application. By weaving together these threads, Dr. Zhang underscores the immense potential of Schiff base metal complexes within diverse areas such as medicine and environmental science.

The concluding chapter, "Recent Advances and Future Directions," exemplifies Dr. Zhang's forward-thinking mindset. By shedding light on recent innovations and speculating on potential trajectories, this chapter not only concludes a thorough exploration of the subject matter but also excites curiosity about the field's future.

The appendices, detailing experimental procedures and spectroscopic data, solidify the book's standing as an invaluable reference tool. With these additions, the text serves dual purposes, catering both to those engaged in cutting-edge research and to those seeking a robust educational resource.

"Schiff Base Metal Complexes: Synthesis, Structure, and Therapeutic Applications" is a manifestation of Dr. Shu-Hua Zhang's expertise, scholarly rigor, and deep-rooted passion for his field. It illuminates the complexities of inorganic chemistry in an accessible manner, setting the stage for the continued exploration of this fascinating field. A must-read for both experienced scholars and budding scientists alike, it exemplifies how knowledge and research can drive progress, paving the way for innovative solutions.

About the Author

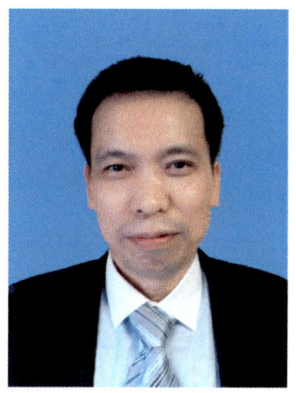

Shuhua Zhang is a distinguished Professor and Doctor at Guangdong University of Petrochemical Technology. A recognized high-level talent in his field, Dr. Zhang holds a Doctorate in Science from Nanjing University, which he earned in 2009. His scholarly pursuits have led him to esteemed institutions like Middlesex University and San Jose State University as a visiting scholar.

With a commendable track record in research, Dr. Zhang has spearheaded numerous projects under the National Natural Science Foundation of China and has been at the helm of over ten provincial and ministerial-level initiatives. He is credited with publishing an impressive 230+ papers in renowned journals such as Advanced Functional Materials, Small, European Journal of Medicinal Chemistry, and many more. His innovative contributions have been recognized with over 50 invention patents in China, with some being transferred to prominent corporations like Chinalco Guangxi Nonferrous Rare Earth Development Co., LTD. and Guangxi Baoli Star Lighting Technology Co., LTD.

In recognition of his outstanding work, Dr. Zhang was honored with the Best Innovation Award at the 2022 International New Scientific Invention Research Award by the Father of Science. Additionally, he has received accolades like the Guangxi Science and Technology Progress Award and the Guangxi Natural Science Award. As a contributor to education, he has secured awards for teaching achievements in Guangxi and is the chief editor for digital courses on General Chemistry. Dr. Zhang's writings reflect his acute attention to detail, profound understanding, and the rare ability to bridge theoretical concepts with practical applications.

On the professional front, he is the director of Guangxi Chemical and Chemical Industry Society and holds esteemed positions on the editorial boards of Synthetic Chemistry and Frontiers in Chemistry. He is also a proud member of the Chinese Chemical Society and serves as an evaluation expert for the National Teaching Achievement Award and the Distinguished Professor of Changjiang, among other roles.

Contents

Chapter 1 7

Mononuclear Schiff-base metal complexes: synthesis, characterization, and anticancer activity 7

Chapter 2 25

4-amino-1,2,4-Triazole Schiff Base Two-Dimensional Zn/Cd Coordination Polymers and their Electrochemiluminescent Efficiency 25

Chapter 3 39

Five novel dinuclear copper (II) complexes: Crystal structures, properties, Hirshfeld surface analysis, and vitro antitumor activity study 39

Chapter 4 53

Syntheses, Crystal structures, and Magnetic Properties of a Novel Decanuclear Copper Cluster Based on 3- amino-1,2,4 triazole Schiff Base at Room Temperature .. 53

Chapter 5 67

Synthesis, Structures, and Properties of Heterometallic One-Dimensional Tetranuclear Cu–Na Cluster-Based Polymers at Room Temperature 67

Chapter 6 79

Analysis of the synthesis, crystal structures, fluorescence, electrochemiluminescent properties, and Hirshfeld surface of four Cu/Mn Schiff-basecomplexes 79

Chapter 7 96

Synthesis, crystal structures, and investigation of the magnetic and electrochemiluminescent properties of three manganese (II) complexes 96

Chapter 8 111

Synthesis, characterization, and anticancer evaluation of hydrazylpyridine salicylaldehyde-copper(II)-1,10-phenanthroline complexes as possible anticancer agents 111

Chapter 9 136

Syntheses, crystal structures and biological evaluation of two new Cu(II) and Co(II) complexes based on (E)-2-(((4H-1,2,4-triazol-4-yl)imino)methyl)-6 methoxyphenol .. 136

Chapter 10 151

Manganese trinuclear clusters based on schiff base: Synthesis, characterization, magnetic and electrochemiluminescence properties 151

Chapter 1

Mononuclear Schiff-base metal complexes: synthesis, characterization, and anticancer activity

Cancer stands as the primary cause of mortality on a global scale. Over the past two decades, there has been a notable proliferation of chemotherapy and anticancer medications.[1] Currently, the administration of cisplatin and other chemotherapy medicines remains the most efficacious approach for the clinical management of cancer.[2-5] The prolongation of treatment duration is anticipated to result in significant adverse effects, including heightened toxicity, intensified drug resistance, and compromised biological dispersion. At now, the limitations associated with chemotherapy medications have spurred scientific researchers to explore alternative anticancer treatments that exhibit enhanced efficacy against cancer cells while minimizing adverse effects.[6-10] Schiff bases represent a significant category of biologically relevant ligands, owing to their potential for favorable biological effects when utilized in conjunction with metal complexes.[11-12] These effects encompass a wide range of applications, such as anticancer, antimalarial, antibacterial, antifungal, and antiviral properties. Schiff-base ligands have been found to exhibit high efficiency as chelating agents in the context of simple metal-organic hybrid materials.[13] Chelation typically induces alterations in the pharmacological characteristics of both ligands and metals.[14] Chelation therapy has been implicated as both a potential etiological factor and a therapeutic approach for several disorders, including cancers. Schiff-base ligands possess a notable propensity to effectively coordinate with diverse metals, hence facilitating the formation of complex compounds. In addition, these medications are employed in the management of diabetes and AIDS.[15]

The Schiff ligands and their corresponding metal complexes exhibit notable efficacy in suppressing the growth of human cancer cells, therefore demonstrating potent anticancer properties.[16,17] The anticancer action exhibited by Schiff-bases can be attributed to their capacity to break DNA and intercalate between DNA base pairs, therefore rendering them promising candidates for anticancer therapeutics.[18] Moreover, Schiff-bases represent a highly prevalent category of ligands in the field of metal coordination chemistry. These ligands offer a broad range of applications due to their adaptability and versatility, enabling the formation of diverse metal complexes.[19] Consequently, these complexes exhibit shared structural characteristics and features.[20-25] Hence, it is anticipated that Schiff-bases will serve as a primary ligand in the strategic development of new metal complexes possessing potential anticancer properties. In recent studies, it has been demonstrated that Zinc(II) ions and complexes play a significant role in various cellular processes, including catalytic functions, DNA/RNA expression, DNA synthesis, protein stability, and apoptosis.[26-38] These findings have revealed the remarkable efficacy of Zinc(II) ions and complexes in combating a wide range of tumor types. Simultaneously, Nickel serves as a crucial constituent in hydrogenase, urease, and carbon monoxide dehydrogenase.[39] Several potential therapeutic targets for Ni(II)-based drugs have been identified.[39-43] These targets include the triggering of phosphorylation of mixed-lineage kinase domain-like protein, induction of apoptosis pathways through reactive oxygen species (ROS)-dependent mitochondrial signaling, induction of DNA damage, stabilization of oncogene promoter G-quadruplex DNA, and enhancement of protein and enzyme binding interactions.[39,44-49] Nevertheless, there is currently a lack of clinically authorized chemotherapeutic agents that possess the ability to specifically target and eliminate A549/DDP tumor cells.[39-52]

This study aimed to assess the anti-tumor efficacy of nine complexes on several cell lines, including HepG2, NCI-H460, MGC80-3, BEL-7404, and HL-7702. The present study investigated the correlation between Schiff-base complexes and their potential as antitumor agents using the MTT method. This approach offers a theoretical foundation for the further identification of Schiff-base complexes that exhibit superior efficacy, minimal toxicity, and remarkable selectivity in terms of their anticancer activities. The experiment yielded results indicating that complexes **chapt1-1-chapt1-9** had notable anticancer efficacy against the specific tumor cells under investigation. Additionally, the toxicity of complexes **chapt1-1-chapt1-9** towards normal human liver cells was observed to be lower than that of cisplatin.

Experimental

Materials

All of the chemicals and solvents utilized in the synthesis process were of reagent grade quality. The solvents and chemicals included in the experiment were procured from Xilong Chemical Factory and utilized without undergoing additional purification.

Physical techniques

The materials, procedures, and apparatus utilized in this study were procured from commercial sources. The collection of microanalytical data (C, H, and N) was conducted using a Perkin-Elmer 240 Q elemental analyzer. The Fourier-transform infrared (FT-IR) spectra were obtained using a Nicolet Nexus 470 FT-IR instrument. The spectra were recorded within the wavenumber range of 4000–400 cm^{-1}, with the samples prepared as potassium bromide (KBr) pellets. The collection of powder X-ray diffraction (PXRD) curves was conducted using an X'Pert3 Powder XRD Commander diffractometer under ambient conditions.

Synthesis

Synthesis of ligands H_2L^i-H_2L^v

The ligands were synthesized in accordance with the existing scientific literature. The provided diagram illustrates the structural arrangement of the ligand H_2L^i-H_2L^v employed in the conducted experiment.

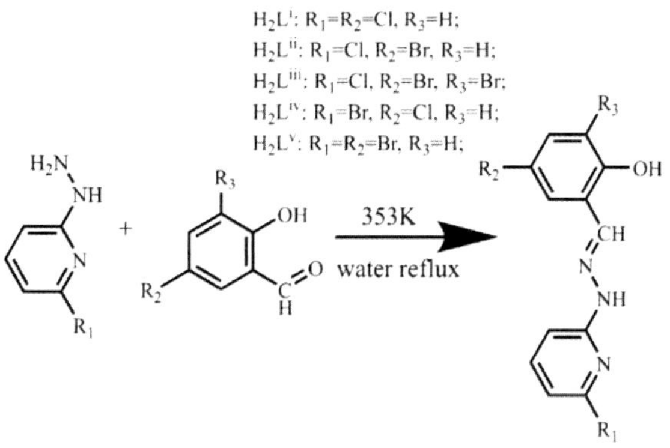

Scheme1-1. Synthesis of substances The H$_2$L^i-H$_2$L^v

Synthesis of complexes chapt1-1-chapt1-9

The synthesis of the complex Ni(HL^i)$_2$·0.5(H$_2$O) (**chapt1-1**) was performed. The compound denoted as "**chapt1-1**" was produced by a solvothermal process. A solution containing Ni(NO$_3$)$_2$·6H$_2$O (0.14540 g, 0.5 mmol), H$_2$L^i (0.14106 g, 0.5 mmol), DMF (5 mL), and Ethanol (5 mL) was prepared and transferred into a 20 ml stainless-steel vessel. The combination was then agitated for a duration of five minutes and thereafter subjected to thermal treatment at a temperature of 80°C for a period of three days. Following a gradual cooling process over a period of 12 hours to reach room temperature, a substantial quantity of green block-shaped crystals precipitated onto the inner surface of the reaction vessel. The green block crystals of compound **chapt1-1** were obtained through the process of filtration, followed by washing with ethanol and subsequent air drying. The resulting yield was determined to be 0.0991 g, approximately 63.0% based on the amount of H$_2$L^i present. The analysis is a crucial component of this study. The compound denoted as **chapt1-1** is referred to as C$_{24}$H$_{17}$Cl$_4$N$_6$NiO$_{2.5}$, with a molar mass of 629.93 g/mol. The elemental composition of the compound is as follows: carbon (C) at 45.76%, hydrogen (H) at 2.72%, and nitrogen (N) at 13.33%. The elemental composition of the sample was determined to be as follows: carbon (C) at a concentration of 46.31%, hydrogen (H) at a concentration of 2.73%, and nitrogen (N) at a concentration of 13.51%. The infrared spectrum (KBr, Figure S1) displays peaks at the following wavenumbers: 3460 w, 1674 s, 1617 w, 1528 w, 1461 w, 1388 m, 1346 s, 1321 s, 1289 m, 1248 s, 1213 s, 1170 m, 1135 s, 991 s, 814 s, 774 s, 724 s, 686 s, 449 s, and 413 w.

The compound Zn(HL^i)$_2$·0.5(H$_2$O) (**chapt1-2**) was synthesized. The compound **chapt1-2** was produced by a solvothermal synthesis procedure. A solution containing Zn(NO$_3$)$_2$·6H$_2$O (0.14874 g, 0.5 mmol), H$_2$L^i (0.14106 g, 0.5 mmol), DMF (5 mL), and H$_2$O (5 mL) was prepared. The solution was transferred into a 20 ml stainless-steel vessel and subjected to stirring for a duration of five minutes. Subsequently, the vessel was sealed and placed in an oven set at a temperature of 120°C for a period of three days. Upon gradual cooling to ambient temperature over a period of 12 hours, a substantial quantity of yellow block-shaped crystals precipitated over the inner surface of the reaction vessel. The yellow block crystals of compound **chapt1-2** were obtained through the process of filtration, followed by washing with water and subsequent air drying. The resulting yield was determined to be 0.0882 g, approximately 55.4% based on the amount of H$_2$L^i present. The analysis of the subject matter is of utmost importance. The compound denoted as **chapt1-2** is referred to as $C_{24}H_{17}Cl_4N_6ZnO_{2.5}$, with a molar mass of 636.63 g/mol. The elemental composition of the compound under consideration is as follows: carbon (C) accounts for 45.28%, hydrogen (H) accounts for 2.69%, and nitrogen (N) accounts for 13.19%. The elemental composition of the sample was determined to be as follows: carbon (C) at 44.59%, hydrogen (H) at 2.72%, and nitrogen (N) at 13.38%. The infrared spectrum (KBr) has several characteristic peaks at the following wavenumbers: 3460 w, 1674 m, 1617 w, 1528 w, 1461 w, 1388 m, 1346 s, 1321 s, 1289 s, 1248 s, 1170 m, 1135 s, 774 s, 686 s, 449 s, and 413 w.

The compound Ni(HL^{ii})$_2$·0.5(H$_2$O) (**chapt1-3**) was synthesized. The synthetic procedure employed for complex **chapt1-3** closely resembled that of complex **chapt1-1**, with the sole difference being the substitution of the ligand H$_2$L^i with the ligand H$_2$L^{ii}. The resulting yield was 0.1011g, or 56.3% based on H$_2$L^{ii}. The elemental analysis for compound **chapt1-3**, $C_{24}H_{17}Br_2Cl_2N_6NiO_{2.5}$ (molecular weight = 718.83 g/mol), yielded the following percentages: carbon (C) 40.10%, hydrogen (H) 2.38%, and nitrogen (N) 11.86%. The elemental composition of the sample was determined to be as follows: carbon (C) at a concentration of 40.17%, hydrogen (H) at a concentration of 2.43%, and nitrogen (N) at a concentration of 11.83%. The infrared (IR) spectrum of the sample (KBr) is shown in Figure S2. The observed wavenumbers are as follows: 2607 cm^{-1}, 1666 cm^{-1}, 1526 cm^{-1}, 1461 cm^{-1}, 1172 cm^{-1}, 995 cm^{-1}, 947 cm^{-1}, 869 cm^{-1} (sharp), 782 cm^{-1}, 695 cm^{-1}, 639 cm^{-1} (medium), 639 cm^{-1} (medium), and 463 cm^{-1} (sharp).

The present study focuses on the synthesis of a complicated compound, specifically [Zn(HL^{ii})$_2$]. The expression "0.25(H$_2$O) (**chapt1-4**)" refers to a chemical formula or equation involving water. The synthesis procedure employed for complex **chapt1-4** closely resembled that of complex **chapt1-2**, with the sole distinction being the substitution of ligand H$_2$L^i with ligand H$_2$L^{ii}. The yield obtained was approximately 0.1002 grams, corresponding to approximately 55.4% based on the H$_2$L^{ii} compound. The elemental composition of the compound with the molecular formula $C_{24}H_{16.5}Br_2Cl_2N_6ZnO_{2.25}$ (molar mass = 721.02 g/mol) is as follows: carbon (C) 39.98%, hydrogen (H) 2.31%, and nitrogen (N) 11.65%. The elemental composition of the sample was determined to be as follows: carbon (C) at a concentration of 40.16%, hydrogen (H) at a concentration of 2.23%, and nitrogen (N) at a concentration of 11.72%. The infrared spectrum (KBr) exhibits several prominent peaks at the following wavenumbers: 2607 w, 1666 w, 1526 w, 1461 w, 1172 w, 995 w, 947 w, 869 s, 782 w, 695 w, 639 m, 639 m, 463 s.

The synthesis of the complex [Zn(HL^{iii})$_2$] is being discussed. The synthesis procedure for complex **chapt1-5** closely resembled that of complex **chapt1-2**, with the exception that the ligand H$_2$L^{ii} was substituted with the ligand H$_2$L^{iii}. The yield obtained from the reaction, based on H$_2$L^{iii}, was approximately 0.1643 g, corresponding to a percentage yield of approximately 68.1%. The elemental analysis for compound **chapt1-5**, with the molecular formula $C_{27}H_{23}Br_4Cl_2N_7O_4Zn$ and a molar mass of 965.43 g/mol, is as follows: carbon (C) 33.59%, hydrogen (H) 2.40%, and nitrogen (N) 10.15%. The elemental composition of the sample was determined to be as follows: carbon (C) at a concentration of 33.50%, hydrogen (H) at a concentration of 2.48%, and nitrogen (N) at a concentration of 10.24%. The infrared (IR) spectrum of potassium bromide (KBr) was obtained and analyzed. The spectrum exhibited several characteristic peaks at specific wavenumbers. The observed wavenumbers were as follows: 3420 s, 2928 s, 1657 s, 1617 m, 1581 s, 1534 s, 1461 s, 1417 s, 1383 s, 1303 s, 1215 s, 1170 m, 1147 m, 998 s, 777 s, 724 s, 453 s.

The present study focuses on the synthesis of complex Ni((HL^{iv})$_2$], with an emphasis on its structural and chemical properties. The molar concentration of ethanol (C$_2$H$_5$OH) is 0.5 M with a coefficient of **chapt1-6**. The synthetic procedure employed for the production of complex **chapt1-6** exhibited similarities to that of complex **chapt1-3**, with the sole distinction being the substitution of the ligand H$_2$L^{ii} with the ligand H$_2$L^{iv}. The yield obtained from the reaction was around 0.105 g, which corresponds to approximately 56.0% based on the H$_2$L^{iv}. The elemental analysis for compound **chapt1-6**, with the molecular formula C$_{25}$H$_{19}$Br$_2$C$_{l2}$NiN$_6$O$_{2.5}$ and a molar mass of 732.85 g/mol, reveals the following percentages: carbon (C) 40.97%, hydrogen (H) 2.61%, and nitrogen (N) 11.46%. The elemental composition of the sample was determined to be as follows: carbon (C) at 41.27%, hydrogen (H) at 2.68%, and nitrogen (N) at 11.51%. The infrared (IR) spectrum of potassium bromide (KBr) was obtained and analyzed. The observed peaks in the spectrum were found at the following wavenumbers: 3420 s, 2928 s, 1657 s, 1617 w, 1581 w, 1534 w, 1461 w, 1417 w, 1388 w, 1303 s, 1255 s, 1215 m, 1170 w, 1147 w, 998 s, 777 s, 724 w, 453 s.

The synthesis of the complex Zn(HL^{iv})$_2$·0.5(H$_2$O) (**chapt1-7**) was performed. The synthetic procedure employed for complex **chapt1-7** closely resembled that of complex **chapt1-4**, with the sole distinction being the substitution of ligand H$_2$L^{ii} with ligand H$_2$L^{iv}. The yield obtained from the reaction was determined to be 0.1252 grams, approximately 58.0 % based on the theoretical yield calculated using the stoichiometry of H$_2$L^{iv}. The elemental analysis for compound **chapt1-7**, with the molecular formula C$_{24}$H$_{17}$Br$_2$C$_{l2}$ZnN$_6$O$_{2.5}$ and a molar mass of 725.53 g/mol, yielded the following percentages: carbon (C) 39.73%, hydrogen (H) 2.36%, and nitrogen (N) 11.76%. The elemental composition of the sample was determined to be as follows: carbon (C) at a concentration of 40.05%, hydrogen (H) at a concentration of 2.43%, and nitrogen (N) at a concentration of 11.74%. The infrared spectrum (KBr, Figure S4) has several characteristic peaks at the following wavenumbers: 3420 s, 2928 s, 1657 s, 1617 w, 1581 w, 1534 w, 1461 w, 1417 w, 1388 w, 1303 s, 1255 s, 1215 m, 1170 w, 1147 w, 998 s, 777 s, 724 w, 453 s.

The present study focuses on the synthesis of a complex, specifically [Ni(HL^{v})$_2$], where HL^{v} represents a ligand. The given expression, 0.25(H$_2$O) (**chapt1-8**), represents a mathematical equation. The synthetic procedure employed for complex **chapt1-8** closely resembled that used for complex **chapt1-6**, with the sole distinction being the substitution of the ligand H$_2$L^{iv} with the ligand H$_2$L^{v}. The yield obtained was around 0.1141 grams, which corresponds to a percentage yield of approximately 56.8% based on the theoretical yield calculated from the amount of H$_2$L^{v}. The elemental analysis results for compound **chapt1-8**, C$_{24}$H$_{16.5}$Br$_4$NiN$_6$O$_{2.25}$ (molecular weight = 803.22 g/mol), are as follows: carbon (C) content is 35.88%, hydrogen (H) content is 2.07%, and nitrogen (N) content is 10.46%. The elemental composition of the sample was determined to be as follows: carbon (C) at a mass percentage of 36.05%, hydrogen (H) at a mass percentage of 2.00%, and nitrogen (N) at a mass percentage of 10.52%. Infrared spectroscopy was performed on the sample using potassium bromide (KBr) as the medium. The resulting spectrum displayed several peaks at different wavenumbers. The observed peaks were located at 3420 s, 2928 s, 1657 s, 1617 w, 1581 w, 1534 w, 1461 w, 1417 w, 1388 w, 1303 s, 1255 s, 1215 m, 1170 w, 1147 w, 998 s, 777 s, 724 w, 453 s.

The synthesis procedure for complex **chapt1-9** closely resembled that of complex **chapt1-7**, with the only difference being the substitution of the ligand H_2L^{iv} with the ligand H_2L^{v}. The obtained yield was determined to be around 0.1393 grams, corresponding to a percentage yield of approximately 69.2% based on the theoretical yield calculated from the amount of H_2L^{v}. The elemental analysis results for compound **chapt1-9**, with the molecular formula $C_{24}H_{16}Br_4ZnN_6O_2$ and a molar mass of 805.44 g/mol, are as follows: carbon (C) 35.79%, hydrogen (H) 2.00%, and nitrogen (N) 10.43%. The elemental composition of the sample was determined to be as follows: carbon (C) at a mass fraction of 35.76%, hydrogen (H) at a mass fraction of 1.99%, and nitrogen (N) at a mass fraction of 10.49%. The observed peaks are located at the following wavenumbers: 1657 s, 1617 w, 1581 w, 1534 w, 1461 w, 1417 w, 1388 w, 1303 s, 1255 s, 1215 m, 1170 w, 1147 w, 998 s, 777 s, 724 w, 453 s.

Crystallographic data collection

The data for all compounds were obtained using single-crystal X-ray diffraction using a CrysAlis PRO CCD diffractometer (Agilent, 2014). The diffraction was performed with graphite-monochromatic Mo-Kα radiation ($\lambda = 0.71073$ Å) in the ω scan mode at a temperature of 298(2) K. The raw frame data were processed and combined with the SAINT tool.[53] The structures **chapt1-1-chapt1-9** were solved using direct methods with the SHELXT software[53] and subsequently revised using full-matrix least-squares on F^2 with the OLEX2 software.[54] The application of an empirical absorption correction was carried out using spherical harmonics, which was performed within the SCALE3 ABSPACK scaling method. Anisotropic refinement was performed on all atoms except for hydrogen. The hydrogen atoms were arranged in a geometric manner and subjected to refinement using a riding model. Table 1-1 presents the crystallographic data.

Anticancer activity evaluation

The proliferation of the test cells was assessed in this experiment using the MTT technique. The assessment of activity screening aimed at reducing cell growth in vitro and the measurement of IC_{50} values were conducted at Guangxi Normal University, which served as the collaborating institution for this project. The molecules that were examined in this study encompassed complexes **chapt1-1-chapt1-9**, along with ligands H_2L^i-H_2L^v. The cell lines utilized in this experimental study to assess their potential for reducing cell proliferation in vitro included the HepG2 cancer cell line, NCI-H460 cancer cell line, MGC80-3 cancer cell line, BEL-7404 cancer cell line, and HL-7702 normal liver cell line. The cell lines that were chosen for the experiment were cultivated in incubators set at a temperature of 37 °C and an atmosphere of 5% CO_2. The culture medium used for the cells consisted of either DMEM or RPMI-1640 medium, supplemented with 10 % neonatal bovine serum and 100 U/mL penicillin-streptomycin. An inverted microscope can be employed to view the cellular growth, digestion, and passage processes facilitated by 0.25% trypsin during the inoculation phase.

Furthermore, cells in the logarithmic growth phase can be specifically chosen for the cytotoxicity test.

Tumor cells were introduced into a culture medium consisting of 10% newborn calf serum PPMI1640. The cells were then incubated in a controlled environment at a temperature of 37 °C, with a humidity level saturated with 5% CO_2. The culture medium was refreshed 2 to 3 times each week, and the cells were subcultured every 6 to 7 days. The cells were introduced into a 96-well cell culture plate containing a culture medium at a concentration of 2×104 cells/mL. Each well was filled with 190 μL of the cell suspension. The plate was then incubated at a temperature of 37 °C and a CO_2 concentration of 5% for a duration of one day. Following cell adhesion, 10 μL of test complexes at varying concentrations were introduced into each well, ensuring that the content of dimethyl sulfoxide (DMSO) did not exceed 1%. Simultaneously, a matching negative control group was established in which no medication was added to the culture media. This control group consisted just of the test cells and an equivalent quantity of DMSO. In the in-well experiments, there were six wells replicated within each sample. Following a two-day culture period, an MTT reagent with a concentration of 5 mg/mL was introduced into each well, using a volume of 10 μL. The cells were then allowed to continue cultivating for a duration of 4 hours. Subsequently, the supernatant was aspirated. Subsequently, a volume of 150 μL of dimethyl sulfoxide (DMSO) was introduced into each well, followed by the measurement of the optical density (OD) at 490 nm using a microplate analyzer. The calculation of the inhibition rate of cell proliferation was performed using the following formula: inhibition rate (%) = (OD of control group - OD of sample group / OD of control group) × 100%. The IC_{50} values were determined individually using the Bliss method. The experiments were replicated three times and the mean value was computed.

Outcomes and Analysis
Crystal structures of complexes chapt1-1-chapt1-9
The results obtained from the single-crystal X-ray diffraction investigations indicate that the structures of complexes **chapt1-1-chapt1-9** exhibit a remarkable similarity, as depicted in Figure 1-1. The only discernible difference among these complexes is the presence of distinct halogen substituents on the Schiff-base HL^n ligands. Hence, the analysis in this study is focused just on complex **chapt1-1**.

Figure 1-1 illustrates the crystal structure of $Ni(HL^i)_2$. The central Ni^{II} ion is controlled by a pair of symmetrical H_2L^i ligands. The coordination structure of nickel ions involves the coordination of four nitrogen atoms (N1, N3, N4, N6) and two oxygen atoms (O1, O2) from two distinct ligands, H_2L^i. This results in the formation of a twisted octahedral coordination structure with NiN_4O_2 coordination. The points Ni1, N1, and O1 lie in the same plane, which can be represented by the equation $-0.678\,z + 0.702\,x + 0.220\,y = -7.612$. The lengths of the coordination bonds in the compound are as follows: Ni1−O1 with a length of 2.051 (4) Å, Ni1−N1 with a length of 2.005 (5) Å, and Ni1−N3 with a length of 2.188 (5) Å. Complex **chapt1-1** was seen to undergo N-H···O hydrogen bonding interactions (N5···O1iii, 2.693(7) Å, N2···O2ii, 2.704(8), symmetry codes: (ii) 2 − x, 2 − y, 1 − z; (iii) 2 - x, 1 - y, 1 - z), resulting in the formation of a one-dimensional supramolecular chain. The supramolecular chain in one dimension is extended to form a three-dimensional network through Cl···Cl interactions

(Cl3⋯Cl2^{iii}, with a distance of 3.445 Å, symmetry code: (iii) 1 + x, y, z − 1) and C−H⋯Cl hydrogen bonds (C20−H20⋯Cl4^{iv}, with a distance of 3.805 Å, symmetry code: (iv) x, y, z − 1).

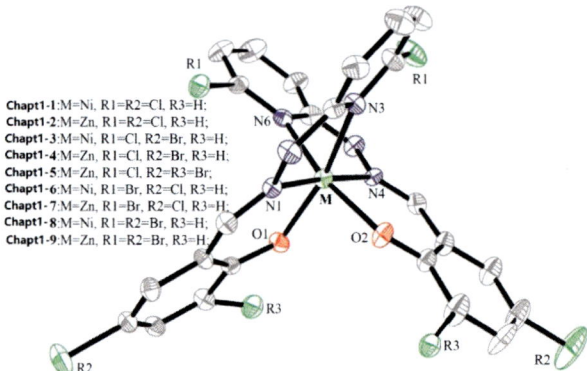

Figure 1-1. Molecule structure of chapt1-1-chapt1-9

Table 1-1 presents the crystal data and structure refinement results for the compounds chapt1-1-chapt1-9.

Complex	chapt1-1	chapt1-2	chapt1-3	chapt1-4	chapt1-5	chapt1-6	chapt1-7	chapt1-8	chapt1-9
Formula	C$_{24}$H$_{17}$Cl$_4$N$_6$NiO$_{2.5}$	C$_{24}$H$_{17}$Cl$_4$N$_6$O$_{2.5}$Zn	C$_{24}$H$_{17}$Br$_2$Cl$_2$N$_6$NiO$_{2.5}$	C$_{24}$H$_{16.5}$Br$_2$Cl$_2$N$_6$O$_{2.25}$Zn	C$_{27}$H$_{23}$Br$_4$Cl$_2$N$_7$O$_4$Zn	C$_{25}$H$_{19}$Br$_2$Cl$_2$N$_6$NiO$_{2.5}$	C$_{24}$H$_{17}$Br$_2$Cl$_2$N$_6$O$_{2.5}$Zn	C$_{24}$H$_{16.5}$Br$_4$N$_6$NiO$_{2.25}$	C$_{24}$H$_{16}$Br$_4$N$_6$O$_2$Zn
Mr	629.93	636.63	718.83	721.02	965.43	732.85	725.53	803.22	805.44
Crystal system	Triclinic	Triclinic	Triclinic	Triclinic	Triclinic	Triclinic	Triclinic	Triclinic	Monoclinic
Space group	P-1	P-1	P-1	P-1	P-1	P-1	P-1	P-1	C2/c
a (Å)	9.991(9)	10.041(8)	10.036(8)	10.086(1)	9.717(9)	11.549(1)	10.133(1)	10.083(1)	20.620(2)
b (Å)	12.177(1)	12.248(1)	12.177(1)	12.241(1)	12.657(1)	12.221(1)	12.207(8)	12.158(1)	10.369(7)
c (Å)	13.367(1)	13.490(1)	13.657(9)	13.713(2)	14.592(1)	12.292(1)	13.554(2)	13.750(1)	12.405(7)
α (°)	64.032(9)	63.171(9)	64.071(7)	116.119(1)	107.224(9)	103.363(7)	63.610(9)	64.703(9)	90
β (°)	72.843(8)	71.655(7)	72.653(6)	97.971(1)	98.582(8)	114.799(9)	72.041(9)	72.992(9)	92.500(6)
γ (°)	79.131(8)	78.268(7)	78.726(7)	101.776(8)	98.639(9)	102.242(7)	79.837(7)	80.167(8)	90
V (Å^3)	1393.6(3)	1401.6(2)	1428.5(2)	1436.9(3)	1658.8(3)	1435.3(2)	1427.0(3)	1455.1(3)	2649.8(3)
F (000)	638	642	710	709	940	726	714	777	1552
Z	2	2	2	2	2	2	2	2	4
D$_c$ (g cm^{-3})	1.501	1.508	1.671	1.666	1.933	1.696	1.689	1.823	2.019
μ (mm^{-1})	1.115	1.292	3.698	3.854	5.764	3.682	3.882	6.192	6.993
θ range (°)	3.41,25.10	3.30,25.10	3.42,25.10	3.40,25.10	3.44,25.10	3.41,25.10	3.40,25.10	3.41,25.10	3.29,25.10
Ref. meas./ indep.	9470,4952	9385,4967	9613,5073	8586,4941	10833,5900	10472,5102	9633,5055	9887,5073	7791,2363
Obs. ref.[I > 2σ(I)]	3083	3648	3444	2978	3287	2704	3253	2735	1345
R$_{int}$	0.0498	0.0349	0.0347	0.0700	0.0474	0.0698	0.0376	0.0593	0.0954
R$_1$ [I ≥ 2σ(I)] ^{a}	0.0724	0.0631	0.0720	0.1308	0.0621	0.0701	0.0674	0.0936	0.0582
ωR$_2$(all data)^b	0.2424	0.2001	0.2062	0.3176	0.1233	0.1932	0.1947	0.2839	0.0931
Goof	1.041	1.053	1.034	1.090	1.022	1.063	1.042	1.028	0.986

IR spectroscopy

The infrared spectra of ligands H_2L^n (n=i-v) and complexes **chapt1-1–chapt1-9** exhibited comparable characteristics. This paper exclusively focuses on the characterization of the infrared spectra of H_2L^i and complexes **chapt1-1** and **chapt1-2**. The repetition of infrared spectroscopy analysis for different ligands and complexes will be avoided. The infrared (IR) spectrum of H_2L^i has distinctive bands at 1578 cm^{-1} and 1527 cm^{-1}, which can be attributed to the stretching vibrations of –CH=N–.[55] Additionally, a peak at 3288 cm^{-1} may be ascribed to the stretching vibrations of hydroxyl. The spectral band observed at a wavenumber of 3052 cm^{-1} is assigned to the C–H stretching vibration mode occurring on the benzene ring. Additionally[55], the spectral band observed at a wavenumber of 1257 cm^{-1} corresponds to the C–O stretching vibration mode associated with the phenolic hydroxyl group.[56] The infrared spectra of complexes **chapt1-1** and **chapt1-2** exhibit comparable distinctive peaks. The stretching vibration peaks observed in complexes **chapt1-1** and **chapt1-2** can be identified as follows: the band at 1528 cm^{-1} corresponds to the stretching of the –CH=N– vibration. The C–O stretching vibration exhibits peaks at approximately 1289 cm^{-1}, while the stretching vibration peaks of M-N and M–O are observed at roughly 413 and 449 cm^{-1}, respectively.[57,58] The involvement of metal ions in coordination is observed to have an impact on the location of the vibration peak.

PXRD

The confirmation of metal complex formation and crystallinity was achieved through the utilization of powder X-ray diffraction (PXRD) technique. The X-ray diffraction patterns of samples **chapt1-1–chapt1-9** were experimentally obtained throughout the angular range of 2θ = 5-50°. The simulated data for these complexes were obtained using the Mercury software, represented as black data, whereas the experimental test values were represented as red. The experimental X-ray diffraction (PXRD) patterns of compounds **chapt1-1–chapt1-9** exhibited a strong agreement with the simulated patterns, suggesting that compounds **chapt1-1–chapt1-9** possess high phase purities.

Anticancer Activity

The Key Laboratory of Pharmaceutical Sciences at Guangxi Normal University conducted a study to investigate the tumor cell inhibition rate and toxicity of complexes **chapt1-1–chapt1-9** and their respective ligands. The reference substance used was DMSO, while cisplatin served as the control agent. The MTT method was employed to measure the inhibitory rate of the complexes on various cell lines, including HepG2 cancer cell line, NCI-H460 cancer cell line, MGC80-3 cancer cell line, BEL-7404 cancer cell line, HL-7702 normal liver cell line, and others. The resulting IC$_{50}$ values are presented in Table 1-3.

Table 1-2 The Inhibition rate on different cells of chapt1-1-chapt1-9 and H₂Lⁱ-H₂Lᵛ (%).

Complexes	HepG2	NCI-H460	MGC80-3	BEL-7404	HL-7702
H₂Lⁱ	38.06±1.06	25.03±0.43	32.12±1.14	37.14±1.74	28.06±1.26
chapt1-1	40.22±0.33	58.18±0.63	40.99±1.32	55.54±1.49	31.02±0.51
chapt1-2	60.13±1.42	42.13±1.76	57.14±0.55	40.21±1.02	30.99±1.77
H₂Lⁱⁱ	32.85±0.75	20.16±0.67	30.24±1.23	36.09±0.65	25.09±1.65
chapt1-3	38.55±1.12	56.11±0.71	35.06±1.42	50.13±0.67	34.06±1.03
chapt1-4	57.02±0.77	40.16±1.17	54.03±1.69	38.25±0.41	29.01±1.85
H₂Lⁱⁱⁱ	32.12±1.01	30.11±0.43	28.36±1.25	28.79±1.47	26.36±1.17
chapt1-5	38.96±1.17	40.12±0.91	39.36±0.31	41.26±1.45	33.02±0.46
H₂Lⁱᵛ	30.18±1.54	18.64±1.09	27.09±0.78	34.84±1.16	24.88±0.95
chapt1-6	37.56±1.07	54.02±1.25	32.42±1.76	41.02±1.06	37.88±0.54
chapt1-7	55.02±0.75	35.02±1.94	50.99±0.56	35.09±0.49	30.12±0.46
H₂Lᵛ	29.04±1.65	15.36±0.69	25.36±1.24	30.15±0.39	24.56±2.05
chapt1-8	32.91±1.47	50.14±1.09	29.14±1.78	40.32±2.02	33.06±2.06
chapt1-9	48.02±1.04	30.12±0.79	50.34±1.11	32.53±1.88	25.03±0.46
cisplatin	55.15±1.18	60.63±0.99	50.88±3.69	47.58±2.65	60.63±0.99

Table 1-3 The IC₅₀ on different cells of complexes chapt1-1-chapt1-9 and H₂Lⁱ-H₂Lᵛ (μM)

Complexes	HepG2	NCI-H460	MGC80-3	BEL-7404	HL-7702
H₂Lⁱ	86.09±1.08	115.06±0.65	91.04±1.11	70.33±1.66	116.06±1.33
chapt1-1	43.09±0.49	**10.11±0.68**	39.66±1.40	**12.13±1.52**	87.25±0.57
chapt1-2	**9.52±1.39**	29.63±1.81	**10.75±0.59**	42.06±1.06	87.99±1.79
H₂Lⁱⁱ	94.18±0.69	153.84±0.78	104.32±1.26	75.06±0.61	130.26±1.78
chapt1-3	57.86±1.15	**10.89±0.83**	54.12±1.47	20.14±0.62	81.09±1.09
chapt1-4	**10.58±0.79**	36.09±1.21	**15.64±1.72**	62.03±0.39	99.56±1.93
H₂Lⁱⁱⁱ	120.12±1.06	>150	>150	>150	>150
chapt1-5	60.12±1.19	35.03±0.94	50.21±0.35	29.56±1.33	83.29±0.58
H₂Lⁱᵛ	105.48±1.51	186.03±1.13	112.06±0.95	83.06±1.20	140.16±1.04
chapt1-6	53.06±1.10	**11.42±1.22**	89.03±1.79	39.69±1.11	72.03±0.61
chapt1-7	15.06±0.76	57.14±1.91	19.86±0.63	86.06±0.54	89.03±0.57
H₂Lᵛ	108.25±1.72	195.06±0.77	135.64±1.31	92.32±0.44	141.09±2.01
chapt1-8	88.45±1.24	20.15±1.16	104.12±1.89	44.03±2.05	82.06±2.01
chapt1-9	25.18±1.06	73.13±0.82	20.12±1.04	23.06±1.47	131.02±0.51
cisplatin	14.06±0.33	15.03±0.73	15.59±1.09	17.02±0.46	16.01±1.23

The investigation involved assessing the inhibitory rate of complexes **chapt1-1–chapt1-9** and H₂Lⁱ-H₂Lᵛ on cancer cell lines. This assessment was conducted following a 48-hour treatment with a dose of 20 μM. The observed effects of the nine complexes on the aforementioned cancer cell lines are evident in Table 1-2 and Table 1-3. The complexes **chapt1-1–chapt1-9** exhibited a higher inhibition rate on cancer cells compared to the respective ligands' inhibition rate on cancer cells. Among the several cancer cells tested, complex **chapt1-1** exhibited a higher inhibition rate on NCI-H460 and BEL-7404 cells compared to the other three cell lines. The inhibition rates observed were 58.18 ± 0.63% and 55.54 ± 1.49% respectively. The inhibitory effect of complex **chapt1-1** on NCIH460 was found to be comparable to that of cisplatin, with an inhibition rate of 60.63 ± 0.99%. On the other hand, complex **chapt1-1** exhibited a superior inhibitory effect on BEL-7404 compared to cisplatin, with an inhibition rate of 47.58 ± 2.65%. The corresponding IC₅₀ values for complex **chapt1-1** on NCIH460 and BEL-7404 were determined to be 10.11 ± 0.68 μM and 12.13 ± 1.52 μM, respectively. Notably, both IC$_{50}$ values were lower than the IC$_{50}$ values of cisplatin on these two cancer cell lines. Complex **chapt1-2** exhibited a higher inhibition rate on HepG2 and MGC80-3 cancer cells compared to the other three cell lines. The inhibition rates were measured at 60.13 ± 1.42% and 57.14 ± 0.55% respectively, surpassing the inhibitory effect of cisplatin. Additionally, the corresponding IC50 values for complex **chapt1-2** were 9.52 ± 1.39 μM and 10.75 ± 0.59 μM, which were lower than the IC$_{50}$ value of cisplatin. Several other complexes exhibited inhibitory effects on the aforementioned cancer cell lines, as indicated in Table 1-2 and Table 1-3 for further information.

The sensitivity of HepG2 cells to the synthesized complexes and ligands decreased in the following order: **chapt1-2** > **chapt1-4** > cisplatin > **chapt1-7** > **chapt1-9** > **chapt1-1** > **chapt1-3** > **chapt1-5** > **chapt1-6** > **chapt1-8** > H$_2$L^{i-v}, For NCI-H460, the sensitivity is as follows: **chapt1-1** > **chapt1-3** > **chapt1-6** > cisplatin > **chapt1-8** > **chapt1-2** > **chapt1-5** > **chapt1-4** > **chapt1-7** > **chapt1-9** > H$_2$L^{i-v}, For MGC80-3, the sensitivity is as follows: **chapt1-2** > cisplatin > **chapt1-4** > **chapt1-7** > **chapt1-9** > **chapt1-1** > **chapt1-5** > **chapt1-3** > **chapt1-6** > **chapt1-8** > H$_2$L^{i-v}, For BEL-7404, the sensitivity is as follows: **chapt1-1** > cisplatin > **chapt1-3** > **chapt1-9** > **chapt1-5** > **chapt1-6** > **chapt1-8** > **chapt1-2** > **chapt1-4** > **chapt1-7** > H$_2$L^{i-v}.

The results of the MTT test indicated that the complexes **chapt1-1**–**chapt1-9** exhibited a reduced inhibition rate on the HL-7702 human normal liver cell line compared to cisplatin. The IC$_{50}$ value of the HL-7702 human normal liver cell line was found to be greater than that of cisplatin. A larger IC$_{50}$ value is indicative of a lower inhibition rate in normal human cells, suggesting a reduced toxicity in normal human hepatocytes. In the context of tumor cells, a higher inhibition rate corresponds to a lower IC$_{50}$ value, which signifies a more favorable treatment outcome in terms of its impact on tumor cells.[59] The data presented in Table 1-2 and Table 1-3 demonstrates that complexes **chapt1-1**–**chapt1-9** exhibited inhibitory effects on cancer cell lines. Notably, certain complexes shown superior inhibitory effects on tumor cells compared to cisplatin, while also demonstrating reduced toxicity on HL-7702 human normal hepatocytes. This observation implies that there is potential for conducting comprehensive studies on these compounds as potential therapeutic agents against tumors.

Through a comparative analysis of compounds **chapt1-1**–**chapt1-2** and **chapt1-8**–**chapt1-9**, it has been observed that the electronegativity of halogen atoms present on the ligands exerts a notable influence on the anticancer efficacy of the complexes. The enhancement of the anticancer activity of the complexes is observed with the increase in electronegativity of the halogen atoms present on the ligands. Upon comparing the compounds **chapt1-3–chapt1-4 and chapt1-6–chapt1-7'**, it was seen that the compound including halogen atoms with a greater electronegativity on the pyridine ring exhibited a higher level of anti-cancer activity compared to the compound containing halogen atoms with a greater electronegativity on the benzene ring.

Hirshfeld surface analysis
The generation of Hirshfeld surfaces and 2D fingerprint plots from crystal data of compound **chapt1-1** was facilitated by employing the Crystal Explorer software,[60] as depicted in Figure

1-3. The fingerprint plots possess the capability to undergo decomposition, hence emphasizing the presence of proximate interactions among the constituent parts[61]. The Hirshfeld surfaces of compound **chapt1-1**, when seen using color mapping techniques for dnorm, shape index, and three-dimensional curved shape, provide insights into the distinct intermolecular interactions that exist within the crystal lattice. The stable molecular packing observed in complex **chapt1-1** can be attributed to the presence of close contact contacts, as indicated by the red spots depicted on the dnorm surfaces (Figure 1-2a). The red regions observed in the image mostly consist of N–H···O hydrogen bonds. Conversely, the white area on the surface is characterized by H···H bonds, while the blue area exhibits minimal contact between atoms due to their significant distance from each other. The lack of a red and blue triangle bow pattern observed in the Shape index indicates the absence of π···π interactions in the complex or C–H···π bonds (Figure 1-2b). The aforementioned outcome was validated by Curvedness and corresponded to its three-dimensional molecular representation (Figure 1-2c).

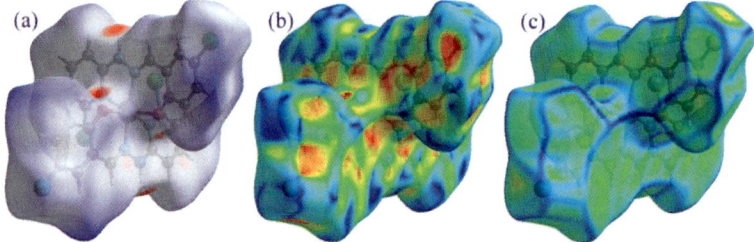

*Figure 1-2. Hirshfeld surfaces of **chapt1-1** mapped with a. d_{norm}, b. shape index and c. curvedness*

In order to conduct a quantitative analysis of the impact of intermolecular interactions on the molecular surface, a two-dimensional fingerprint was examined.[62,63] The respective values of the complex **chapt1-1** interactions, H···H, Cl···H/H···Cl, and C···H/H···C account for 24.7%, 22.2%, and 17.6% of the total, collectively over half of the entire value (Figure 1-3). The complex exhibits hydrogen bonding, with the O···H/H···O bond contributing 7.0% of the overall interactions. Additionally, the N···H/H···N bonds account for 2.1% of the complex's interactions, while the van der Waals forces between Cl and Cl atoms contribute 4.8% of the overall interactions. The carbon atom serves as the primary structural element in the complex, with carbon-hydrogen (C···H) bonds being prevalent on nearly all surfaces. This facilitates the interaction of other forces, enabling the formation of complexes by molecular stacking.

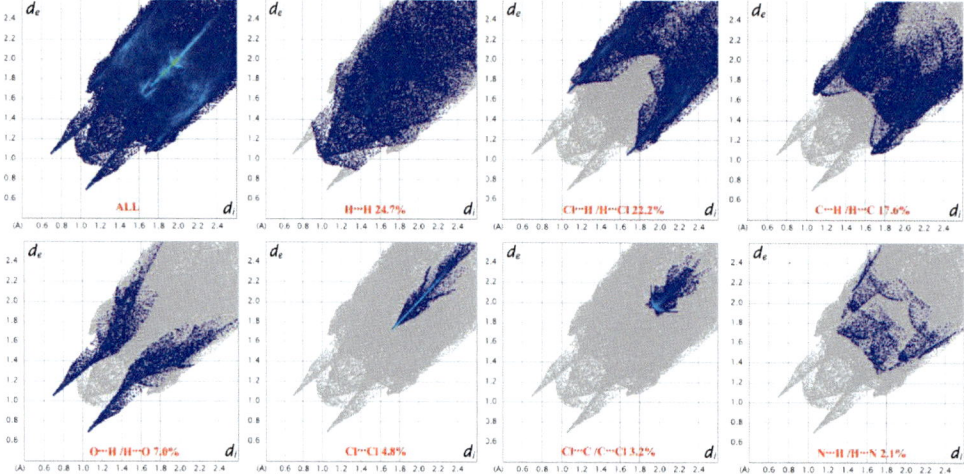

Figure 1-3. 2D Fingerprint plots of chapt1-1, with all element interactions and resolved element interactions between H···H, Cl···H/H···Cl, C···H/H···C, O···H/H···O, Cl···Cl, Cl···C/C···Cl, N···H/H···N contacts in percentages

In this study, a collection of H_2L^i-H_2L^v ligands derived from salicylaldehyde Schiff-base were synthesized, along with their corresponding nickel and zinc complexes. Similar framework compositions have been identified by the investigation of single-crystal diffraction using X-ray techniques. The MTT method was employed to assess the inhibition rates and IC_{50} values of six cell lines, namely HepG2, NCI-H460, MGC80-3, BEL-7404, and HL-7702. The testing period spanned from day 1 to day 9. According to the results obtained, '**complex chapt1-2**' shown higher levels of antitumor activity against HepG2 (60.13 ± 1.42) and MGC80-3 (57.14 ± 0.55) compared to other complexes. Furthermore, Complex **chapt1-2** exhibited superior antitumor activity compared to cisplatin (55.13 ± 1.18) and (50.88 ± 3.69). Complex **chapt1-1** demonstrated enhanced anticancer efficacy against BEL-7404 cells (55.54 ± 1.49), surpassing that of cisplatin (47.58 ± 2.65). Complexes **chapt1-1-chapt1-9** have demonstrated a specific inhibitory action on cancer cells, with a lower rate of inhibition on normal cells and less toxicity compared to cisplatin. The findings demonstrate the involvement of metal complexes in the inhibition of cancer cell proliferation, suggesting their potential therapeutic significance. Furthermore, the Hirshfeld surface analyses conducted on '**complex chapt1-1**' revealed that the interaction between hydrogen atoms (H···H) plays a crucial role in stabilizing the process of self-assembly.

References

1. Deng, Z.; Fang, C.; Ma, X.; Li, X.; Zeng, Y. J.; Peng, X. S. One Stone Two Birds: Zr-Fc Metal-Organic Framework Nanosheet for Synergistic Photothermal and Chemodynamic Cancer Therapy. *ACS. Appl. Mater. Inter.*, 2020, *12(18)*, 20321-20330.
2. Chen, Z. N.; Zhang, S. P.; Shao, J. P.; Su, F. Synthesis, Structure, and in Vitro Antigastric Cancer Activity Evaluation of Two New Zn(II) and Cd(II)-Organic Frameworks. *J. Coord. Chem.*, 2019, *72(11)*, 1833-1844.
3. Ke, C. L.; Dong, F.; Wang, P. R. Research on the Enhancement Mechanism of Dihydromyricetin on the Inhibitory Role of Cisplatin Towards Breast Cancer Cell Activity. *J. Biomater. Tiss. Eng.*, 2022, *12(5)*, 989-995.
4. Sui, X.; Tang, X. L.; Wu, X.; Liu, Y. S. Identification of ERCC8 as a Novel Cisplatin-Resistant Gene in Esophageal Cancer Based on Genome-Scale CRISPR/Cas9 Screening. *Biochem. Biophys. Res. Commun.*, 2022, *593*, 84-92.
5. Shi, Z. D.; Hao, L.; Han, X. X.; Wu, Z. X.; Pang, K.; Dong, Y.; Qin, J. X.; Wang, G. Y. Targeting HNRNPU to Overcome Cisplatin Resistance in Bladder Cancer. *Mol. Cancer.*, 2022, *21(1)*, 21-37.
6. Corte-Real, L.; Teixeira, R. G.; Girio, P.; Comsa, E.; Moreno, A.; Nasr, R.; Baubichon-Cortay, H.; Avecilla, F.; Marques, F. Methyl-Cyclopentadienyl Ruthenium Compounds with 2,2'-Bipyridine Derivatives Display Strong Anticancer Activity and Multidrug Resistance Potential. *Inorg. Chem.*, 2018, *57(8)*, 4629-4639.
7. Zheng, X. H.; Xia, L. X.; Mao, Z. W. The New Anticancer Platinum Complex Designed Based on Nucleic Acid. *Prog. Chem.*, 2016, *28(7)*, 1029-1038.
8. Ma, Y. Y.; Su, Z.; Zhou, L. M.; He, L. C.; Hou, Z. Y.; Zou, J. H.; Cai, Y.; Chang, D.; Xie, J. B.; Zhu, C. Biodegradable Metal-Organic-Framework-Gated Organosilica for

Tumor-Microenvironment-Unlocked Glutathione-Depletion-Enhanced Synergistic Therapy. *Adv. Mater.*, 2022, *34(12)*, 2107560.

9. Sun, R. W. Y.; Zhang, M.; Li, D.; Li, M. A.; Wong, A. S. T. Enhanced Anti-Cancer Activities of a Gold(III) Pyrrolidinedithiocarbamato Complex Incorporated in a Biodegradable Metal-Organic Framework. *J. Inorg. Biochem.*, 2016, *163*, 1-7.

10. Chen, Y. T.; Zhang, S. N.; Wang, Z. F.; Wei, Q. M.; Zhang, S. H. Discovery of Thirteen Cobalt(II) and Copper(II) Salicylaldehyde Schiff-Base Complexes that Induce Apoptosis and Autophagy in Human Lung Adenocarcinoma A549/DDP Cells and that can Overcome Cisplatin Resistance in Vitro and in Vivo. *Dalton. Trans.*, 2022, *51(10)*, 4068-4078.

11. Ceramella, J.; Iacopetta, D.; Catalano, A.; Cirillo, F.; Lappano, R.; Sinicropi, M. S. A Review on the Antimicrobial Activity of Schiff-Bases: Data Collection and Recent Studies. *Antbiotics-Basel.*, 2022, *11(2)*, 191.

12. More, M. S.; Joshi, P. G.; Mishra, Y. K.; Khanna, P. K. Metal Complexes Driven from Schiff-Bases and Semicarbazones for Biomedical and Allied Applications: A Review. *Mater. Today Chem.*, 2019, *14*, 100195.

13. Przybylski, P.; Huczynski, A.; Pyta, K.; Brzezinski, B.; Bartl, F. Biological Properties of Schiff-Bases and Azo Derivatives of Phenols. *Curr. Org. Chem.*, 2009, *13*, 124-148.

14. Chandra, A.; Das, D.; Castro, J. O.; Naskar, K.; Jana, S.; Frontera, A.; Ray, P. P.; Sinha, C. Cd(II) Coordination Polymer of Fumaric Acid and Pyridyl-Hydrazide Schiff-Base: Structure, Photoconductivity, and Theoretical Interpretation. *Inorg. Chim. Acta*, 2021, *518*, 120253.

15. Zhang, Q. K.; Yue, C. P.; Zhang, Y.; Lu, Y. L.; Hao, Y. P.; Miao, Y. L.; Li, J. P.; Liu, Z. Y. Six Metal-Organic Frameworks Assembled from Asymmetric Triazole Carboxylate Ligands: Synthesis, Crystal Structures, Photoluminescence Properties, and Antibacterial Activities. *Inorg. Chim. Acta*, 2018, *473*, 112-120.

16. Iacopetta, D.; Ceramella, J.; Catalano, A.; Saturnino, C.; Bonomo, M. G.; Franchini, C.; Sinicropi, M. S. Schiff-Bases: Interesting Scaffolds with Promising Antitumoral Properties. *Appl. SCI. Basel.*, 2021, *11(4)*, 1877.

17. Matela, G.; Schiff-Bases, and Complexes: A Review on Anti-Cancer Activity. *Anti-Cancer Agent. Me*, 2020, *20(16)*, 1908-1917.

18. Obeid, A.; El-Shekeil, A.; Al-Aghbari, S.; Al-Shabi, J. Anticancer, DNA cleavage, and Antimicrobial Activity Studies of Some New Schiff-Base Titanium(IV) Vomplexes. *J. Coord. Chem.*, 2012, *65 (15)*, 2762-2770.

19. Gerz, I.; Jannuzzi, S. A. V.; Hylland, K. T.; Negri, C.; Wragg, D. S.; Oien-Odegaard, S.; Tilset, M.; Olsbye, U.; DeBeer, S.; Amedjkouh, M. Structural Elucidation, Aggregation, and Dynamic Behaviour of N,N,N,N-Copper(I) Schiff-Base Complexes in Solid and in Solution: A Combined NMR, X-Ray Spectroscopic and Crystallographic Investigation. *Eur. J. Inorg. Chem.*, 2021, *2021(46)*, 4762-4775.

20. Malik, M. A.; Dar, O. A.; Gull, P.; Wani, M. Y.; Hashmi, A. A. Heterocyclic Schiff-Base Transition Metal Complexes in Antimicrobial and Anticancer Chemotherapy. *Medchemcomm.*, 2018, *9(3)*, 409-436.

21. Szymanska, M.; Pospieszna-Markiewicz, I.; Manka, M.; Insinska-Rak, M.; Dutkiewicz, G.; Patroniak, V.; Fik-Jaskolka, M. A. Synthesis and Spectroscopic

Investigations of Schiff-Base Ligand and Its Bimetallic Ag(I) Complex as DNA and BSA Binders. *Biomolecules*, 2021, *11(10)*, 1449.

22. Li, L. J.; Yan, Q. Q.; Liu, G. J.; Yuan, Z.; Lv, Z. H.; Fu, B.; Han, Y. J.; Du, J. L. Synthesis Characterization and Cytotoxicity Studies of Platinum (II) Complexes with Reduced Amino Pyridine Schiff-Base and Its Derivatives as Ligands. *Biosci. Biotechnol. Biochem.*, 2017, *81(6)*, 1086-1089.

23. Damercheli, M.; Dayyani, D.; Behzad, M.; Mehravi, B.; Ardestani, M. S. New Salen-Type Manganese (III) Schiff-Base Complexes Derived from Meso-1,2-Diphenyl-1,2-Ethylenediamine: In Vitro Anticancer Activity, Mechanism of Action, and Molecular Docking Studies. *J. Coord. Chem.*, 2015, *68(9)*, 1500-1513.

24. Karthiyayini, B.; Kadalmani, B.; Akbarsha, M. A. Cytotoxic Cobalt (III) Schiff-Base Complexes: in Vitro Anti-Proliferative, Oxidative Stress and Gene Expression studies in Human Breast and Lung Cancer Cells. *Biometals*, 2021, *35*, 67-85.

25. Yan, L.; Liu, F. W.; Liu, H. M. Synthesis, Structure and Biological Activities of Novel Furanosyl Schiff-Base Derivatives. *Chin. J. Chem.*, 2011, *31(10)*, 1639-1642.

26. Adhikari, A.; Kumari, N.; Adhikari, M.; Kumar, N.; Tiwari, A. K.; Shukla, A.; Mishra, A. K.; Datta, A. Zinc Complex of Tryptophan Appended 1,4,7,10-Tetraazacyclododecane as Potential Anticancer Agent: Synthesis and Evaluation. *Bioorg. Med. Chem.*, 2017, *25(13)*, 3483-3490.

27. Wang, Z.; Zhou, X.; Wei, Q.; Qin, Q.; Li, J.; Tan, M.; Zhang, S. Novel Bifluorescent Zn(II)–Cryptolepine–Cyclen Complexes Erigger Apoptosis Induced by Nuclear and Mitochondrial DNA Damage in Cisplatin-Resistant Lung Tumor Cells. *Eur. J. Med. Chem.*, 2022, *238*, 114418.

28. Mendiguchia, B. S.; Pucci, D.; Mastropietro, T. F.; Ghedini, M.; Crispini, A. Non-Classical Anticancer Agents: On The Way to Water Soluble Zinc(II) Heteroleptic Complexes. *Dalton Trans.*; 2013, *42(19)*, 6768-6774.

29. Darawsheh, M.; Ali, H. A.; Abuhijleh, A. L.; Rappocciolo, E.; Akkawi, M.; Jaber, S.; Maloul, S.; Hussein, Y. New Mixed Ligand Zinc(II) Complexes Based on the Antiepileptic Drug Sodium Valproate and Bioactive Nitrogen-Donor Ligands. Synthesis, Structure and Biological Properties. *Eur. J. Med. Chem.*, 2014, *82*, 152-163.

30. Icsel, C.; Yilmaz, V. T.; Aydinlik, S.; Aygun, M. Zn(II), Cd(II) and Hg(II) Saccharinate Complexes with 2,6-Bis(2-Benzimidazolyl)Pyridine as Promising Anticancer Agents in Breast and Lung Cancer Cell Lines Via ROS-Induced Apoptosis. *Dalton Trans.*, 2020, *49(23)*, 7842–7851.

31. Cao, Q.; Yang, J.; Zhang, H.; Hao, L.; Yang, G. G.; Ji, L. N.; Mao, Z. W. Traceable In-Cell Synthesis and Cytoplasm-to-Nucleus Translocation of a Zinc Schiff-Base Complex as a Simple and Economical Anticancer Strategy. *Chem. Commun.*, 2019, *55(54)*, 7852-785.

32. S Siters, K. E.; Sander, S. A.; Devlin, J. R.; Morrow, J. R. Bifunctional Zn (II) Complexes for Recognition of Non-Canonical Thymines in DNA Bulges and G-Quadruplexes. *Dalton Trans.*, 2015, *44(8)*, 3708-3716.

33. Abdel-Rahman, L. H.; Al-Farhan, B. S.; Al Zamil, N. O.; Noamaan, M. A.; El-Sayed H.; Ahmed, M. S. Synthesis, Spectral Characterization, DFT Calculations, Pharmacological Studies, CT-DNA Binding and Molecular Docking of Potential N, O-

Multidentate Chelating Ligand and Its VO(II), Zn(II) and ZrO(II) Chelates. *Bioorg. Chem.*, 2021, *114*, 105106.

34. Qin, L. Q.; Liang, C. J.; Zhou, Z.; Qin, Q. P.; Wei, Z. Z.; Tan, M. X.; Liang, H. Mitochondria-Localizing Curcumin-Cryptolepine Zn(II) Complexes and Their Antitumor Activity. *Bioorg. Med. Chem.*, 2021, *30*, 115948.

35. Gao, E.; Sun, N.; Zhang, S.; Ding, Y.; Qiu, X.; Zhan, Y.; Zhu, M. Synthesis, Structures, Molecular Docking, Cytotoxicity and Bioimaging Studies of Two Novel Zn(II) Complexes. *Eur. J. Med. Chem.*, 2016, *121*, 1-11.

36. Lin, W.; Buccella, D.; Lippard, S. J. Visualization of Peroxynitrite-Induced Changes of Labile Zn^{2+} in the Endoplasmic Reticulum with Benzoresorufin-Based Fluorescent Probes. *J. Am. Chem. Soc.*, 2013, *135(36)*, 13512-13520.

37. Zhang, S.; Wang, Z.; Tan, H. Novel Zinc(II)-Curcumin Molecular Probes Bearing Berberine and Jatrorrhizine Derivatives as Potential Mitochondria-Targeting Antineoplastic Drugs. *Eur. J. Med. Chem.*, 2022, *243*, 114736.

38. Wang, Z.; Nong, Q.; Yu, H.; Qin, Q.; Pan, F.; Tan, M.; Liang H.; Zhang, S. Complexes of Zn(II) with Mixed Tryptanthrin Derivative and Curcumin Chelating Ligands as a New Promising Anticancer Agents. *Dalton Trans.*, 2022, *51(13)*, 5024-5033.

39. Gao, E.; Qi, Z.; Qu, Y.; Ding, Y.; Zhan, Y.; Sun, N.; Zhang, S.; Qiu, X.; Zhu, M. Two Novel Dinuclear Ellipsoid Ni(II) and Co(II) Complexes Bridged by 4,5-Bis([Pyrazol-1-yl)phthalic Acid: Synthesis, Structural Characterization and Biological Evaluation. *Eur. J. Med. Chem.*, 2017, *136*, 235-245.

40. Flamme, M.; Cressey, P. B.; Lu, C.; Bruno, P. M.; Eskandari, A.; Hemann, M. T.; Hogarth, G.; Suntharalingam, K. Induction of Necroptosis in Cancer Stem Cells Using a Nickel(II)-Dithiocarbamate Phenanthroline Complex. *Chem. Eur. J.*, 2017, *23(40)*, 9674-9682.

41. Heng, M. P.; Sim, K. S.; Tan, K. W. Nickel and Zinc Complexes of Testosterone N4-Substituted Thiosemicarbazone: Selective Cytotoxicity Towards Human Colorectal Carcinoma Cell Line HCT 116 and Their Cell Death Mechanisms. *J. Inorg. Biochem.*, 2020, *208*, 111097.

42. Banaspati, A.; Raza M. K.; Goswami, T. K. Ni(II) Curcumin Complexes for Cellular Imaging and Photo-Triggered in Vitro Anticancer Activity. *Eur. J. Med. Chem.*, 2020, *204*, 112632.

43. Balachandran, C.; Haribabu, J.; Jeyalakshmi, K.; Bhuvanesh, N. S. P.; Karvembu, R.; Emi, N.; Awale, S. Nickel(II) Bis(Isatin Thiosemicarbazone) Complexes Induced Apoptosis Through Mitochondrial Signaling Pathway and G0/G1 Cell cycle Arrest in IM-9 Cells. *J. Inorg. Biochem.*, 2018, *182*, 208-221.

44. Masaryk, L.; Tesarova, B.; Choquesillo-Lazarte, D.; Milosavljevic, V.; Heger, Z.; Kopel, P. Structural and Biological Characterization of Anticancer Nickel(II) Bis(benzimidazole) Complex. *J. Inorg. Biochem.*, 2021, *217*, 111395.

45. Icsel, C.; Yilmaz, V. T.; Aydinlik, S.; Aygun, M. New Manganese(II), Iron(II), Cobalt(II), Nickel(II) and Copper(II) Saccharinate Complexes of 2,6-Bis(2-Benzimidazolyl)pyridine as Potential Anticancer Agents. *Eur. J. Med. Chem.*, 2020, *202*, 112535.

46. Liao, L. S.; Chen, Y.; Mo, Z. Y.; Hou, C.; Su, G. F.; Liang, H.; Chen, Z. F. Ni(II), Cu(II) and Zn(II) Complexes with the 1-Trifluoroethoxyl-2,9,10-trimethoxy-7-oxoaporphine Ligand Simultaneously Target Microtubules and Mitochondria for Cancer Therapy. *Inorg. Chem. Front.*, 2021, *8(9)*, 2225-2247.

47. Elsayed, S. A.; Badr, H. E.; di Biase, A.; El-Hendawy, A. M. Synthesis, Characterization of Ruthenium(II), Nickel(II), Palladium(II), and Platinum(II) Triphenylphosphine-based Complexes Bearing an ONS-Donor Chelating Agent: Interaction with Biomolecules, Antioxidant, in Vitro Cytotoxic, Apoptotic Activity and Cell Cycle Analysis. *J. Inorg. Biochem.*, 2021, *223*, 111549.

48. Bisceglie, F.; Orsoni, N.; Pioli, M.; Bonati, B.; Tarasconi, P.; Rivetti, C.; Amidani, D.; Montalbano, S.; Buschini, A. Cytotoxic Activity of Copper(II), Nickel(II) and Platinum(II) Thiosemicarbazone Derivatives: Interaction with DNA and the H2A Histone Peptide. *Metallomics*, 2017, *11(10)*, 1729-1742.

49. Bera, P.; Aher, A.; Brandao, P.; Manna, S. K.; Bhattacharyya, I.; Mondal, G.; Jana, A.; Santra, A.; Bera, P. Anticancer Activity, DNA Binding and Docking Study of M(II)-Complexes (M = Zn, Cu and Ni) Derived from a New Pyrazine-Thiazole Ligand: Synthesis, Structure and DFT. *New J. Chem.*, 2021, *45(27)*, 11999–12015.

50. Terenzi, A.; Lötsch, D.; van Schoonhoven, S.; Roller, A.; Kowol, C. R.; Berger, W.; Keppler, B. K.; Barone, G. Another Step Toward DNA Selective Targeting: Ni(II) and Cu(II) Complexes of a Schiff-Base Ligand Able to Bind Gene Promoter G-quadruplexes. *Dalton Trans.*, 2016, *45(18)*, 7758-7767.

51. Hosseini-Kharat, M.; Zargarian, D.; Alizadeh, A. M.; Karami, K.; Saeidifar, M.; Khalighfard, S.; Dubrulle, L.; Zakariazadeh, M.; Cloutier, J. P.; Sohrabijame, Z. In Vitro and in Vivo Antiproliferative Activity of Organo-Nickel SCS-pincer Complexes on Estrogen Responsive MCF7 and MC4L2 Breast Cancer Cells. Effects of amine fragment substitutions on BSA binding and cytotoxicity. *Dalton Trans.*, 2018, *47(47)*, 16944-16957.

52. Illán-Cabeza, N. A.; Jiménez-Pulido, S. B.; Hueso-Ureña, F.; Ramírez-Expósito, M. J.; Sánchez-Sánchez, P.; Martínez-Martos, J. M.; Moreno-Carretero, M. N. Effects on Estrogen-Dependent and Triple Negative Breast Cancer Cells Growth of Ni(II), Zn(II) and Cd(II) Complexes with the Schiff-Base Derived from Pyridine-2-carboxaldehyde and 5,6-diamino-1,3-dimethyluracil Explored Through the Renin-angiotensin System (RAS)-regulating Aminopeptidases. *J. Inorg. Biochem.*, 2018, *185*, 52-62.

53. Sheldrick, G. M. Crystal Structure Refinement with SHELXL. *Acta Crystallogr. Sect. C: Struct. Chem.*, 2015, *71(1)*, 3-8.

54. Dolomanov, O. V.; Bourhis, L. J.; Gildea, R. J.; Howard, J. A. K.; Puschmann, H. OLEX2: A Complete Structure Solution, Refinement and Analysis Program. *J. Appl. Cryst.*, 2009, *42(2)*, 339-341.

55. Kasare, M. S.; Dhavan, P. P.; Shaikh, A. H. I.; Jadhav, B. L.; Pawar, S. D. Novel Schiff-Base Scaffolds Derived from 4-aminoantipyrine and 2-Hydroxy-3-methoxy-5-(phenyldiazenyl)benzaldehyde: Synthesis, Antibacterial, Antioxidant and Anti-Inflammatory. *J. Mol. Recognit.*, 2022, *35(9)*, e2976.

56. Habibi, M.; Beyramabadi, S. A.; Allameh, S.; Khashi, M.; Morsali, A.; Pordel, M.; Khorsandi-Chenarboo, M. Synthesis, Experimental and Theoretical Characterizations

of a New Schiff-Base Derived from 2-Pyridincarboxaldehyde and Its Ni (II) Complex. *J. Mol. Struct.*, 2017, *1143*, 424-430.

57. Hassan, A. M.; Nassar, A. M.; Hussien, Y. Z.; Elkmash, A. N. Synthesis, Characterization and Niological Evaluation of Fe(III), Co(II), Ni(II), Cu(II), and Zn(II) Complexes with Tetradentate Schiff-Base Ligand Derived from Protocatechualdehyde with 2-Aminophenol. *Appl. Biochem. Biotech.*, 2012, *167*, 581-594.

58. Zhang, S.; Jiang, Y.; Zhong, X. Synthesis, Crystal Structure, Peoperties and Thermoanalysis of [Cu(TSSB)(Phen)]·1.5H$_2$O. *Chin. J. Inorg. Chem.*, 2004, *20(8)*, 959-963.

59. Hussain, I.; Ullah, A.; Khan, A. U.; Khan, W. U.; Ullah, R.; Naser, A. A. S. A. A.; Mahmood, H. M. Synthesis, Characterization and Biological Activities of Hydrazone Schiff-Base and Its Novel Metals Complexes. *Sains. Malays.*, 2019, *48(7)*, 1439-1446.

60. Hajibabaei, M.; Zendehdel, R.; Panjali, Z. Imidazole-Functionalized Ag/MOFs as Promising Scaffolds for Proper Antibacterial Activity and Toxicity Reduction of Ag Nanoparticles. *J. Inorg. Organomet. P.*, 2020, *30*, 4622-4626.

61. Chinthamreddy, A.; Karreddula, R.; Pitchika, G. K.; SurendraBabu, M. S. Synthesis, Characterization of [Co(BDC)(Phen)H$_2$O] and [Co(BDC)(DABCO)] MOFs, π..π Interactions, Hirshfeld Surface Analysis and Biological Activity. *J. Inorg. Organomet. P.*, 2021, *31*, 1381-1394.

62. Xu, T. Y.; Li, J. M.; Han, Y. H.; Wang, A. R.; He, K. H.; Shi, Z. F. A New 3D Four-Fold Interpenetrated Dia-Like Luminescent Zn(II)-Based Metal-Organic Framework: The Sensitive Detection of Fe^{3+}, Cr$_2$O$_7^{2-}$, and CrO$_4^{2-}$ in Water, and Nitrobenzene in Ethanol. *New J. Chem.*, 2020, *44(10)*, 4011-4022.

63. Chen, Z. H.; Fan, Y. P.; Wang, J. M.; Yang, L.; Zhang, S. H. Penta-Nuclear Fe(III) Cluster: Synthesis, Structure, Magnetic Properties and Hirshfeld Surface Analysis. *Chemistryselect*, 20187, *3(34)*, 9841-9844.

Chapter 2

4-amino-1,2,4-Triazole Schiff Base Two-Dimensional Zn/Cd Coordination Polymers and their Electrochemiluminescent Efficiency

Introduction

The design and synthesis of novel coordination polymers (CPs) have gained attention due to their potential applications in fields like photoluminescence, magnetism, catalysis, gas storage, and nonlinear optics.[1-13] However, controlling CP synthesis is challenging due to sensitivity to reaction conditions and intermolecular interactions.[14-17] The selection of appropriate organic ligands, such as 1,2,4-triazole ligands, can control versatile structures, resulting in unique polynuclear compounds. The investigation of 4-amino-1,2,4-triazole Schiff base metal complexes is of interest.[18,19]

Hirshfeld surface analysis describes molecule surface characteristics, while the dnorm surface describes close intermolecular interactions in crystals using a red-white-blue color scheme. The 2-D fingerprint plot quantitatively analyzes the nature and type of intermolecular interactions within a crystal, making these techniques popular in studying crystal interactions.[20-23]

Electrochemical luminescence (ECL) is a process where reactants generate light through co-reactants and annihilation. It has potential applications in chemical/biochemical sensors, molecular logic gates, molecular memories, and display devices. ECL can study the binding of luminescent metal complexes to DNA and interact with surfactants.[25-27] Coreactant ECL is used in environmental assays, clinical diagnostics, biowarfare agent detection, and molecular diagnostics. Transition metal complexes, which are "green" and exhibit good ECL activity, may be an alternative for sensing applications.[28-30]

Experimental

Materials and physical measurements

The study used commercially available chemicals without purification. FT-IR spectra were recorded using KBr pellets, while elemental analyses were performed using a Perkin-Elmer 240 elemental analyzer. TGA measurements were made by heating the crystalline sample. PXRDs of '**chapt2-1–chapt2-4**' were determined using a PANalytical X'Pert3 powder diffractometer, and X-ray crystal structures were determined using an Agilent G8910A CCD diffractometer using SHELXL crystallographic software. Photoluminescence was tested using a Hitachi F-4600 fluorescence spectrophotometer, and electrochemical luminescence tests were performed using an MPI-A Electrochemical workstation.

Syntheses

The study synthesized HL1 by refluxing a mixture of 3,5-dibromo-2-hydroxybenzaldehyde, 4-amino-1,2,4-triazole, and ethanol in a flask. A beige precipitate appeared, which was rinsed three times with fresh ethanol and dried at 40°C for 12 hours. The anal. calc. for HL1 was $C_9H_6Br_2N_4O$, with a calculated calc. of C, 31.24, H, 1.75, and N, 16.19%. The IR data for HL1 showed a range of values from 3454 to 570 w.

HL2 was prepared similarly to HL1, replacing 3,5-dibromo-2-hydroxybenzaldehyde with 3,5-dichloro-2-hydroxybenzaldehyde. It was obtained in a 97% yield, with anal. calc. of $C_9H_6Cl_2N_4O$ (Mr = 257.08) and IR data of 3145 w, 1591 w, 1521 s, 1463 s, 1377 m, 1318 s, 1230 s, 1071 s, 870 m, 737 w, 634 w.

The study synthesized $[Zn(L1)_2]_n$ (**chapt2-1**) by combining $Zn(Ac)_2·2H_2O$, HL1, DMF, and deionized water in a vial at 90°C for 72 hours. Yellow block crystals of **chapt2-1** were collected, washed with fresh ethanol, and dried in air. The anal. calc. for **chapt2-1** was $C_{18}H_{10}Br_4N_8O_2Zn$ (Mr = 755.33), with a calculated value of C, 28.62; H, 1.33; N, 14.83. The IR data for **chapt2-1** showed a range of values from 3410 s to 473 w.

The study synthesized $[Cd(L1)_2]_n$ (**chapt2-2**), replacing $Zn(Ac)_2·2H_2O$ with $Cd(Ac)_2·2H_2O$. Yellow block crystals of **chapt2-2** were collected, washed with fresh ethanol, and dried in air. The anal. calc. for **chapt2-2** was $C_{18}H_{10}Br_4N_8O_2Cd$ (Mr = 802.38), with a calculated C, 26.94, H, 1.26, and N, 13.96%. The IR data for **chapt2-2** showed various values, including 3444, 3120, 1593, 1517, 1455, 1405, 1211, 1152, 1061, 864, 700, 622, and 415 w.

The study synthesized $[Zn(L2)_2]_n$ (**chapt2-3**), replacing HL1 with HL2. Yellow block crystals of **chapt2-3** were collected, washed with fresh ethanol, and dried in air. The anal calc. for **chapt2-3** was $C_{18}H_{10}Cl_4N_8O_2Zn$ (Mr = 577.51), with a calculated value of C, 37.43; H, 1.75; N, 19.40%. The IR data for 3 showed a range of values from 3117 m to 461 w.

The study synthesized $[Cd(L2)_2]_n$ (**chapt2-4**), replacing $Zn(Ac)_2·2H_2O$ with $Cd(Ac)_2·2H_2O$. Yellow block crystals of 4 were collected, washed with fresh ethanol, and dried in air. The anal calc. for **chapt2-4** was $C_{18}H_{10}Cl_4N_8O_2Cd$, with a calculated value of 34.62; H, 1.61; N, 17.94%. The IR data for **chapt2-4** showed various values, including 3130 m, 1602 s, 1516 m, 1457 s, 1347 w, 1214 m, 1057 s, 859 w, 761 w, 627 w, and 466 w.

Crystal structure determination

The diffraction data of complexes **chapt2-1-chapt2-4** were collected using an Agilent G8910A CCD diffractometer with graphite monochromated Mo-Kα radiation. The data were integrated with the SAINT program, solved using direct methods using SHELXS-97,[31-34] and refined using full-matrix least-squares on F^2. An empirical absorption correction was applied with the program SADABS.[34] Non-hydrogen atoms were refined anisotropically, while hydrogen atoms were positioned geometrically and refined as riding. Calculations and graphics were performed with SHELXTL. For **chapt2-4** the highest peaks in residual electron density were located 1.30 Å from atom Br2, 1.25 Å from atom Cl2, and 1.08 Å from atom Cd1, respectively. The deepest residual electron density hole was located 1.13 Å from atom Br2 and 0.91 Å from atom Cl2. The crystallographic details are provided in Table 2-1, and selected bond lengths and angles for **chapt2-1**-**chapt2-4** are listed in Table 2-2.

Table 2-1 Crystallographic data for complexes chapt2-1-chapt2-4

Complexes	chapt2-1	chapt2-2	chapt2-3	chapt2-4
formula	$C_{18}H_{10}Br_4N_8O_2Zn$	$C_{18}H_{10}Br_4N_8O_2Cd$	$C_{18}H_{10}Cl_4N_8O_2Zn$	$C_{36}H_{20}Cl_8N_{16}O_4Cd_2$
formula weight	755.33	802.38	577.51	1236.08
temperature	298	298	298	298
crystal system	Monoclinic	Tetragonal	Monoclinic	Tetragonal
space group	$P2_1/c$	$P4_32_12$	$P2_1/c$	$P4_12_12$
a (Å)	12.6370 (6)	7.8274 (3)	12.1364 (8)	7.7613 (4)
b (Å)	8.9158 (3)	7.8274 (3)	8.6903 (4)	7.7613 (4)
c (Å)	10.3960 (4)	36.8134 (15)	10.3966 (4)	35.852 (3)
β (°)	100.151 (4)	90	100.145 (5)	90
V (Å^3)	1152.97 (8)	2255.5 (2)	1079.37 (10)	2159.6 (3)
$F(000)$	720	1512	576	1224
Z	2	4	2	4
D_c (g·cm^{-3})	2.176	2.363	1.777	1.921
μ (mm^{-1})	8.031	8.090	1.669	1.542
θ range (°)	3.03, 25.01	3.09, 26.36	3.08, 25.10	2.86, 25.09
Obs. reflns	1598	2014	1640	1679
R_{int}	0.0348	0.0328	0.0218	0.0453
R_1 [$I \geq 2\sigma(I)$]^a	0.0708	0.0399	0.0415	0.0787
wR_2(all data)^a	0.1987	0.0674	0.1098	0.2216
GOOF	1.020	1.059	1.007	1.002
$\Delta\rho$(max, min) (e Å^{-3})	2.845, −2.404	0.568, -0.515	1.181, -1.066	1.374, -0.911

$^a R_1 = \Sigma ||F_o| - |F_c||/\Sigma |F_o|$. $^b wR_2 = [\Sigma w(|F_o^2|-|F_c^2|)^2/\Sigma w(|F_o^2|)^2]^{1/2}$

Table 2-2 Selected bond lengths (Å) and angles (°) for complexes chapt2-1-chapt2-4.

Complexes	chapt2-1	chapt2-2	chapt2-3	chapt2-4
M1-O1	2.013(6)	2.195(4)	2.013(2)	2.187(3)
M1-N2^i	2.194(7)	2.317(5)	2.191(3)	2.290(11)
M1-N4	2.202(8)	2.459(5)	2.187(3)	2.445(12)
O1-M1-O1^{iii}	180.000(1)	162.6(2)	180.0	162.7(6)
O1-M1-N2^i	92.1(3)	85.50(15)	92.50(10)	83.6(4)
O1-M1-N2^{ii}	87.9(3)	107.73(15)	87.50(10)	109.5(4)
N2^i-M1-N2^{ii}	180.0(3)	83.2(2)	180.00(9)	84.7(6)
O1-M1-N4	84.2(3)	76.79(15)	84.38(10)	76.1(4)

O1ⁱⁱⁱ-M1-N4	95.8(3)	92.25(15)	95.62(10)	93.0(4)
N2ⁱ-M1-N4	95.1(3)	158.38(16)	94.35(11)	156.1(4)
N2ⁱⁱ-M1-N4	84.9(3)	90.40(18)	85.65(11)	90.2(4)
N4-M1-N4ⁱⁱⁱ	180.000(1)	102.5(3)	180.0	103.2(6)
Symmetry codes	(i) −x, −y−1, −z; (ii) x, 1.5−y, z+0.5; (iii)−x, 1.5+y, 1.5−z	(i) x, y−1, z; (ii) y, x−1, 1−z; (iii)1+y, x−1, 1−z	(i) −x, −y−1, −z; (ii) x, 1.5−y, z+0.5; (iii)−x, 1.5+y, 1.5−z	(i) 1+x, y, z; (ii) y, 1+x, 1−z; (iii) y, x, 1−z

Photoluminescence

The photoluminescence properties of compounds **chapt2-1-chapt2-4** were studied in the solid state at room temperature using an F-4600 fluorescence spectrophotometer.

Electrochemical luminescence

Electrochemical luminescence tests were conducted using an MPI-A Electrochemical workstation, utilizing a standard three-electrode cell with a reference electrode of Ag/AgCl, an auxiliary electrode of platinum wire, and a working electrode of glassy carbon with a diameter of 1 mm, supported by 0.1 mol L⁻¹ potassium peroxydisulfate in DMF.

Results and discussion

Description of the crystal structure

The single-crystal X-ray diffraction analysis of $[Zn(L^i)_2]_n$ reveals that **chapt2-1** and **chapt2-3** are homogeneous complexes, so only complex **chapt2-1** is analyzed.

The $[Zn(L1)_2]$ monomer of **chapt2-1** crystallizes in the monoclinic space group $P2_1/c$, with the metal zinc atom at the inversion center and six-coordinate. The Zn(II) center is bonded to two (L1)⁻¹ ions at an equatorial position through the chelating phenolic hydroxyl oxygen O1 and its adjacent Schiff base group nitrogen N4, with bond lengths of 2.013(6) and 2.202(8) Å, respectively(Figure 2-1). The Zn atom forms a distorted octahedral geometry, with the L1 ligand displaying the $\mu_2:\eta^1:\eta^1:\eta^1$ coordination mode (Scheme 2-1).

The L1 ligand forms a staircase-shaped chain connecting two Zn(II) ions, forming a 2-D network with a length of 11.246 Å (Figure 2-2). The network includes Zn ions and triazol inside the plane, while the benzene ring and bromine atoms lie outside. All 2D layers are stacked in parallel in **chapt2-1** and **chapt2-3**, with larger distances in **chapt2-1** due to repulsion between adjacent halogen atoms.

The $[Cd(L1)_2]$ monomer of **chapt2-2** crystallizes in the tetragonal space group $P4_32_12$ (Figure 2-3). It consists of one Cd(II) ion and two HL1 ligands, each six-coordinated by two oxygen atoms and four nitrogen atoms of four HL1 ligands. This results in a distorted octahedral geometry. The L1 ligand acts as a bridge to link adjacent Cd(II) atoms through its atz ring, forming a 1D chain. The 1D chains of **chapt2-2** and **chapt2-4** are different from those of **chapt2-1** and **chapt2-3**, with the 1D chain being perpendicular to each other. The 1-D chain further constructs two-dimensional (2D) grid-like layers(Figure 2-4), each composed of 20-membered metallocycles. The 2-D network structure has all Cd ions in one plane, and the distance between neighboring layers in **chapt2-2** is slightly larger than that in **chapt2-4**, possibly due to the repulsion between halogen atoms. The C–X⋯π and C–H⋯X interactions create a three-dimensional supramolecular network (Figure 2-5), as shown in the Hirshfeld surface and fingerprint plot analysis.

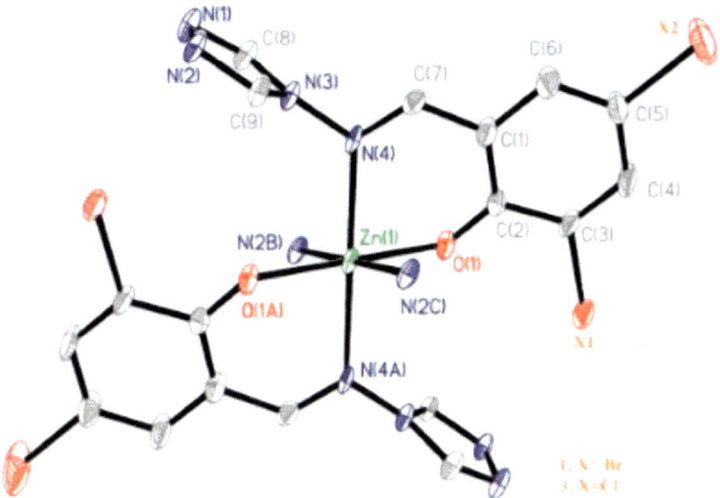

Figure 2-1. Structures of chapt2-1 and chapt2-3 crystals

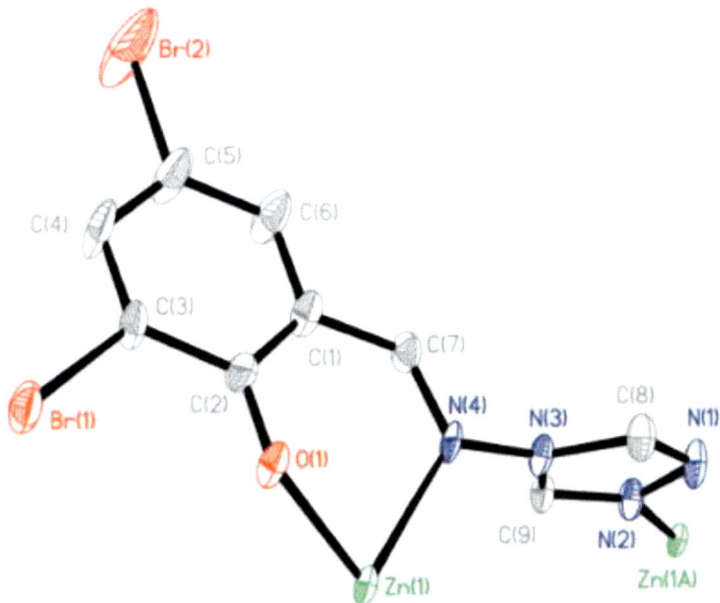

Scheme 2-1. Mode of coordination of the HL1 ligand.

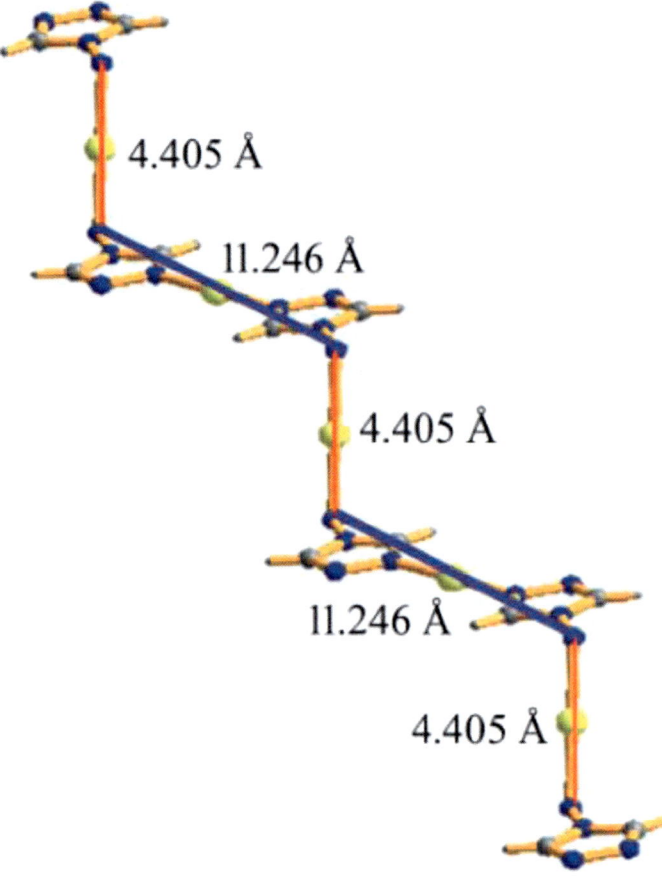

Figure 2-2. Staircase-shaped [Cd(Li)₂]ₙ (i = 1 or 2) chain. The X-ray diffraction analysis of a single crystal reveals that elements chapt2-2 and chapt2-4 have the same crystal structure and crystallize in the tetragonal crystal system. Consequently, only complex chapt2-2 is examined here.

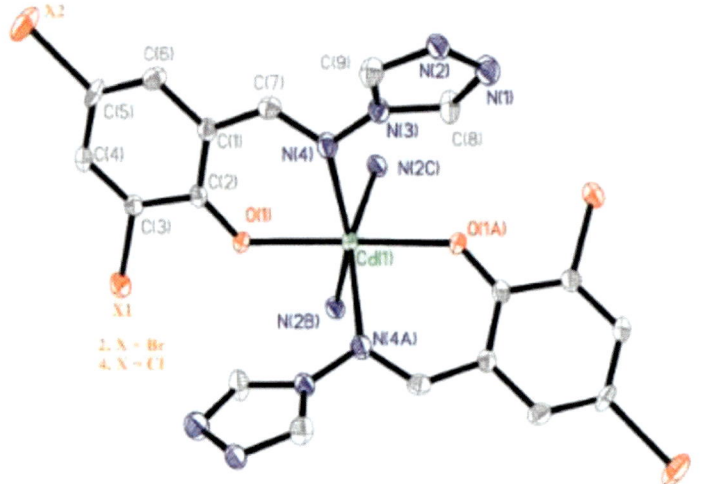

Figure 2-3. The crystal structures of chapt2-2 and chapt2-4, respectively.

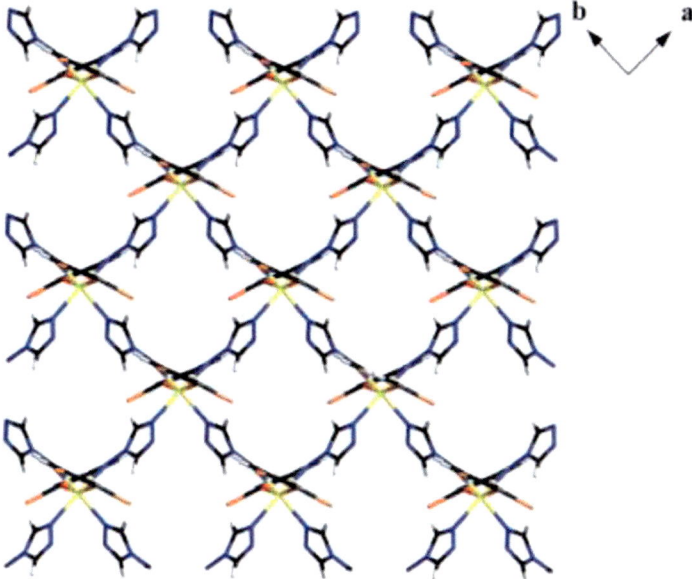

Figure 2-4. The 2D configuration of chapt2-2

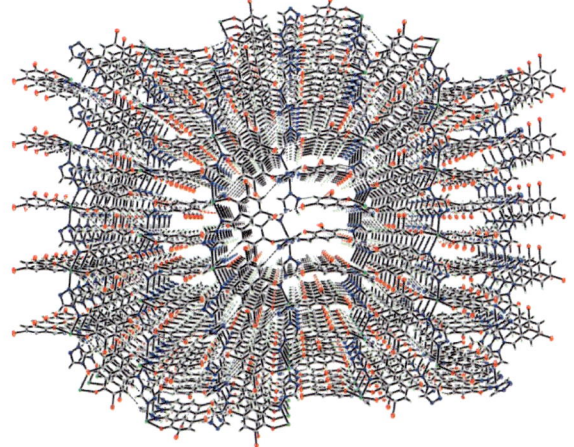

Figure 2-5. 3D structure of chapt2-2.

Hirshfeld surface and fingerprint plot analysis

The Hirshfeld surface analysis is a method used to visualize intermolecular interactions in crystal structures using 3D molecular surface contours. It is based on the electron distribution calculated as the sum of spherical atom electron densities. The pro-molecule's electron distribution dominates the pro-crystal's distribution, and the Hirshfeld surface is defined as the ratio of pro-molecule to pro-crystal electron densities equal to 0.5.

The 2-D fingerprint plot is a crucial tool for Hirshfeld surface analysis, allowing quantitative analysis of intermolecular interactions within crystals (Figure 2-6). It highlights close contacts between elements, separating contributions from different interaction types. The X-H interaction is significant, with a spike in donor and acceptor regions, indicating C-H-X interactions. H-H contacts are also significant, with C-X contacts playing a significant role in the total 2-D fingerprint plot. Other contacts are also observed(Table 2-3).

Thermogravimetric analysis

Considering the fact that pyrazole based MOFs are well-known for their high thermal stability, we investigated the thermal analysis of all the compounds in this work. All the samples were heated in a platinum crucible at a rate of 10 °C min^{-1} under a nitrogen atmosphere within the temperature range of 25–1200 °C (Figure 2-7). Complexes **chapt2-1–chapt2-4** exhibit higher thermal stability. Complexes **chapt2-1–chapt2-4** began to decompose at a temperature of 260 °C, 272 °C, 251 °C and 280 °C, respectively. On comparison with the decomposition temperature of **chapt2-1–chapt2-4**, we found that the thermal stability of **chapt2-2** and **chapt2-4** is higher than that of **chapt2-1** and **chapt2-3**.

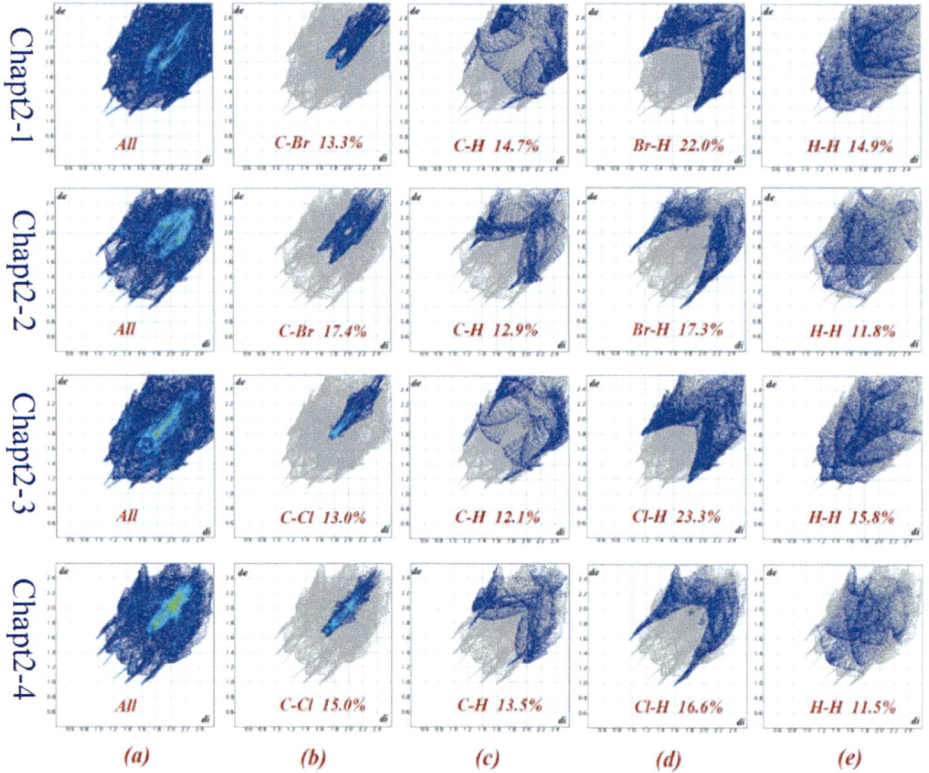

Figure 2-6. Fingerprint plots of chapt2-1-chapt2-4: full (a) and resolved into CX (b) and CH (c), XH (d), and HH (e) contacts displaying the proportions of contacts contributing to the total Hirshfeld surface area of chapt2-1-chapt2-4.

Table 2-3. Surface force summary sheet of chapt2-1-chapt2-4

Complexes	X···H	H···H	C···X	C···H	N···X	N···H	Other
chapt2-1	22.0%	14.9%	13.3%	14.7%	1.9%	8.8%	24.4%
chapt2-2	17.3%	11.8%	17.4%	12.9%	10.2%	10.3%	20.1%
chapt2-3	23.3%	15.8%	13.0%	12.1%	2.3%	8.7%	24.8%
chapt2-4	16.6%	11.5%	15.0%	13.5%	9.8%	11.5%	22.1%

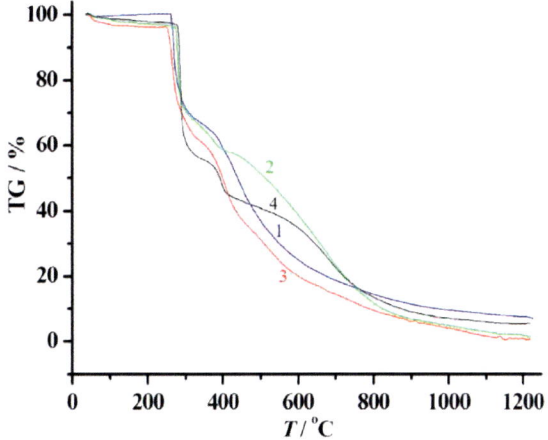

Figure 2-7 Thermogravimetric analysis of compounds chapt2-1–chapt2-4

Solid state luminescence properties

Previous studies have shown that coordination compounds containing d^{10} metal centers such as Zn(II) and Cd(II) may exhibit excellent luminescence properties and have potential applications as photo-active materials and chemical sensors.[28,35-37]

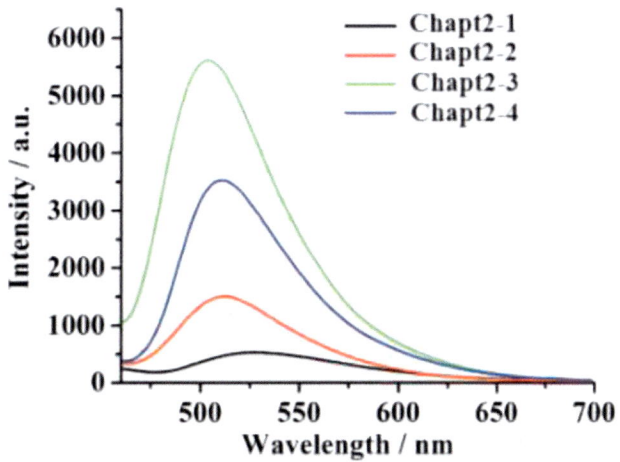

Figure 2-8. Solid-state photoluminescence emission spectra of chapt2-1-chapt2-4 at ambient temperature.

The study examines the solid-state photoluminescence properties of compounds **chapt2-1–chapt2-4** at room temperature (Figure 2-8). It found that compounds exhibit green fluorescence emission bands at 513 nm, 512 nm, 520 nm, and 513 nm, possibly due to ligand-to-metal charge-transfer[38-40]. HL1-based complexes have stronger fluorescence intensity than HL2-based complexes, possibly due to different halogen substituents. Fluorescence efficiency decreases with halogen substituent atomic number.

The study presents two photos of complexes **chapt2-1–chapt2-4**, HL1 and HL2 exposed to 365 nm UV-light and visible light at a concentration of 10^{-4} mol L^{-1}. In visible light, the solutions show a slight light color, while HL2 appears colorless. However, under 365 nm UV light, the color becomes deeper, with HL2 complexes **chapt2-3** and **chapt2-4** exhibiting an obvious glow. This indicates that these complexes emit stronger light under UV-light irradiation.

ECL properties of chapt2-1–chapt2-4 and the ligands HL1 and HL2

The study examines the redox properties of pure complexes **chapt2-1–chapt2-4** and ligands HL1 and HL2 using cyclic voltammetry (CV, Figure 2-9). The results show that when $K_2S_2O_8$ is added to the solution, an oxidation peak in the cathodic current at -1.6 V and a reduction peak at -0.90 V are observed. The CV curves for the other three complexes are similar to that of **chapt2-1**. The phase purities of **chapt2-1–chapt2-4** were checked by PXRD.

The maximum luminous intensity of HL1, HL2, and complexes **chapt2-1–chapt2-4** is around 2000, 3125, 2880, 2500, 2800, and 3250 a.u., respectively(Figure 2-10). These intensities maintain stability after six or seven circulations. HL2 has a larger maximum luminous intensity than HL1, possibly due to differences in electronegativity of the halogen atom. Luminous intensities of **chapt2-1** and **chapt2-2** are larger than HL1, while **chapt2-1** is larger than **chapt2-2**. Cd, a highly toxic heavy metal, may cause health and environmental concerns. The maximum luminous intensity of **chapt2-4** is larger than HL2, but the maximum luminous intensity of **chapt2-3** is smaller than HL2.

The study uses $Ru(bpy)_3^{3+}$ as a standard[41] for ECL yield(Figure 2-11), resulting in ECL yields of 0.44, 0.69, 0.64, 0.56, 0.62, and 0.72 for HL1, HL2, and complexes **chapt2-1–chapt2-4**. The introduction of the Zn ion may strengthen the spin-orbit coupling effect and enhance ECL emission. The six complexes exhibit stronger ECL emission and higher stability, potentially guiding the design of novel polymers ECL materials.

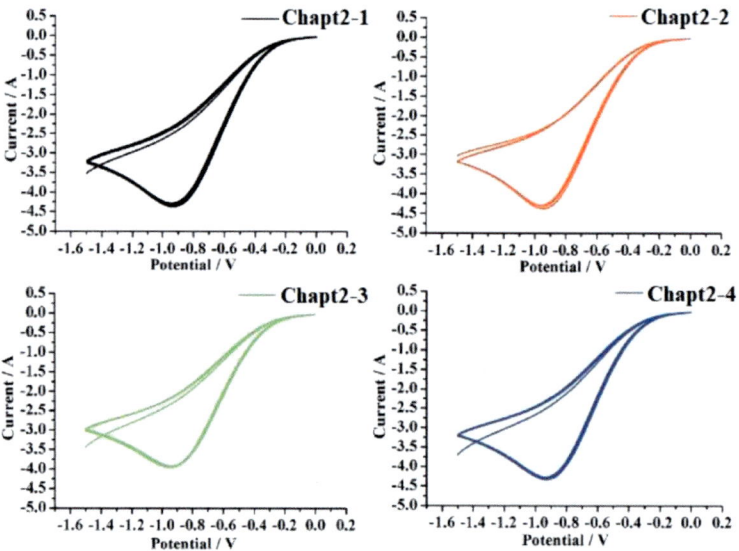

Figure 2-9. chapt2-1–chapt2-4 (1×10^{-6} mol L^{-1}) cyclic voltammogram in DMF with 0.1 mol L^{-1} $K_2S_2O_8$

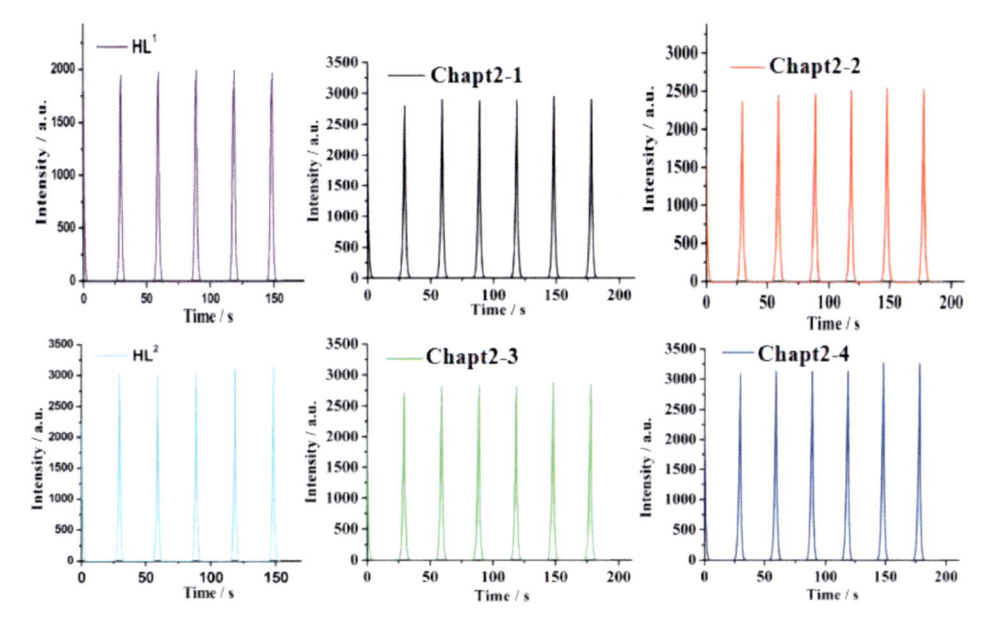

Figure 2-10. Electrochemical luminescence for chapt2-1–chapt2-4, HL1 and HL2.

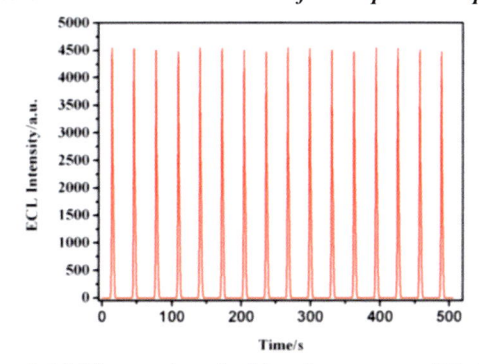

Figure 2-11 Electrochemical luminescence of Ru(bpy)$_3^{3+}$[52].

Conclusion

We have successfully synthesized four coordination complexes having mononuclear 2D structures with HL1 and HL2, together with different acetate salts, Zn^{2+} for **chapt2-1** and **chapt2-3**, and Cd^{2+} for **chapt2-2** and **chapt2-4**, respectively. The Hirshfeld surface analysis results indicate that C–H⋯X (X = Br, Cl) interactions play a considerable role in stabilizing the self-assembly process. Besides, these four transition metal complexes manifest high stability and stronger ECL emissions, and can be a useful guide for the design of novel polymers ECL materials.

References

1. Yu, C. X.; Wang, K. Z.; Li, X. J.; Liu, D.; Ma, L. F.; Liu, L. L. Highly Efficient and Facile Removal of Pb^{2+} from Water by Using a Negatively Charged Azoxy-Functionalized Metal-Organic Framework. Cryst. Growth Des., 2020, 20(8), 5251-5260.

2. Yu, C. X.; Hu, F. L.; Song, J. G.; Zhang, J. L.; Liu, S. S.; Wang, B. X.; Meng, H.; Liu, L. L.; Ma, L. F. Ultrathin Two-Dimensional Metal-Organic Framework Nanosheets Decorated with Tetra-Pyridyl Calix[4]Arene: Design, Synthesis and Application in Pesticide Detection. Sensor. Actuat. B-Chem., 2020, 310, 127819.

3. Zhao, Y.; Wang, L.; Fan, N. N.; Han, M. L.; Yang, G. P.; Ma, L. F. Porous Zn(II)-Based Metal–Organic Frameworks Decorated with Carboxylate Groups Exhibiting High Gas Adsorption and Separation of Organic Dyes. Cryst. Growth Des., 2018, 18(11), 7114-7121.
4. Wu, Y. P.; Tian, J. W.; Liu, S.; Li, B.; Zhao, J.; Ma, L. F.; Li, D. S.; Lan, Y. Q.; Bu, X. Bi-Microporous Metal-Organic-Frameworks with Cubane [M$_4$(OH)$_4$] (M= Ni, Co) Clusters and Pore Space Partition for Electrocatalytic Methanol Oxidation Reaction. Angew. Chem. Int. Ed., 2019, 58(35), 12185-12189.
5. Pang, J. Y.; Jiang, T. L.; Ke, Z. L.; Xiao, Y.; Li, W. Z.; Zhang, S. H.; Guo, P. H. Wood Cellulose Nanofibers Grafted with Poly(ε-caprolactone) Catalyzed by ZnEu-MOF for Functionalization and Surface Modification of PCL Films, Nanomaterials, 2023, 13(13), 1904.
6. Dutta, A.; Pan, Y.; Liu, J. Q.; Kumar, A. Multicomponent Isoreticular Metal-Organic Frameworks: Principles, Current Status and Challenges, Coord. Chem. Rev., 2021, 445, 214074.
7. Chen, Y. T.; Chen, Z.; Yuan, L. Y.; Xiao, Y.; Zhang, S. H.; Li, N. Adsorption of PO$_4^{3-}$, Cd(II), Pb(II), Cu(II), AsO$_3^{3-}$, and AsO$_4^{3-}$ Using a Carbonised Mn-Based Metal–Organic Framework, Arab. J. Chem., 2023, 16(8), 104950.
8. Singh, A.; Singh, A. K.; Liu, J.; Kumar, A. Syntheses, Design Strategies, and Photocatalytic Charge Dynamics of Metal–Organic Frameworks (MOFs): a Catalyzed Photo-Degradation Approach towards Organic Dyes, Catal. Sci. Technol., 2021, 11(12), 3946–3989.
9. Zhao, Y.; Yang, X. G.; Lu, X. M.; Yang, C. D.; Fan, N. N.; Yang, Z. T.; Wang, L. Y.; Ma, L. F. {Zn6} Cluster Based Metal-Organic Framework with Enhanced Room-Temperature Phosphorescence and Optoelectronic Performances. Inorg. Chem., 2019, 58(9), 6215-6221.
10. Liu, J. Q.; Luo, Z. D.; Pan, Y.; Singh, A. K.; Trivedi, M.; Kumar, A. Recent Developments in Luminescent Coordination Polymers: Designing Strategies, Sensing Application and Theoretical Evidences, Coord. Chem. Rev., 2020, 406, 213145.
11. Gao, Q. F.; Jiang, T. L.; Li, W. Z.; Tan, D. F.; Zhang, X. H.; Pang, J. Y.; Zhang, S. H. Porous and Stable Zn-Series Metal–Organic Frameworks as Efficient Catalysts for Grafting Wood Nanofibers with Polycaprolactone via a Copolymerization Approach. Inorg. Chem., 2023, 62(8), 3464-3473.
12. Wang, J.; Zhou, L.; Rao, C.; Wang, G. L.; Jiang, F.; Singh, A.; Kumar, A.; Liu, J. Q. Two 3D Supramolecular Isomeric Zn(II)-MOFs as Photocatalysts for Photodegradation of Methyl Violet Dye, Dyes Pigments, 2021, 190, 109285.
13. Zhang, C.; Qin, Y.; Ke, Z. L.; Yin, L. L.; Xiao, Y.; Zhang, S. H. Highly Efficient and Facile Removal of As(V) from Water by Using Pb-MOF with Higher Stable and Fluorescence, Appl. Organomet. Chem., 2023; 37(5), e7066.
14. Braga, D.; Grepioni, F.; Tedesco, E.; Wadepohl, H.; Gebert, S. C–H...O Hydrogen Bonding in Crystalline Complexes Carrying Methylidyne (μ_3-CH$_2$) and Methylene (μ_2-CH$_2$) Ligands: Adatabase Study. J. Chem. Soc., Dalton Trans., 1997, (10), 1727-1732.

15. Davies, P. J.; Veldman, N.; Grove, D. M.; Spek, A. L.; Lutz, B. T. G.; vanKoten, G. Organoplatinum Building Blocks for One-Dimensionalhydrogen-Bonded Polymeric Structures. Angew. Chem. Int. Ed. Engl., 1996, 35, 1959–1961.
16. James, S. L.; Verspui, G.; Spekb, A. L.; Koten, G. Organometallic Polymers: an Infinite Organoplatinum Chain in the Solid State Formed by (C≡CH...ClPt) Hydrogen Bonds. J. Chem. Soc. Chem. Commun., 1996, 11, 1309–1310.
17. Copp, S. B.; Subramanian, S.; Zaworotko, M. J. Supramolecular Chemistry of Manganese Complex [Mn(CO)$_3$(μ$_3$-OH)]$_4$: Assembly of a Cubic Hydrogen-Bonded Diamondoid Network with 1,2-Diaminoethane. J. Am. Chem. Soc., 1992, 114(22), 8719-8720.
18. Zeng, Y. M.; Zhang, H. Y.; Zhang, Y. J.; Ji, F. H.; Liang, J. L.; Zhang, S. H. Synthesis, Crystal Structures, Fluorescence, Electrochemiluminescent Properties, and Hirshfeld Surface Analysis of Four Cu/Mn Schiff-Basecomplexes. Appl. Organomet. Chem., 2020, 34(8), e5712.
19. Chen, Q.; Ma, X. D.; Li, G. Z.; Zhang, S. H.; Hu, Z. G.; Xiao, Y. Highly Sensitive Detection Trace Moisture, Atrazinem 3-Hydroxytyramine Hydrochloride Based on 4-Amino-1,2,4Triazole Schiff Based Coordination Polymers ; Advances in Materials Science Research, 2021, 45(2), 69-112.
20. Spackman,. M. A.; Jayatilaka, D. Hirshfeld Surface Analysis. CrystEngComm., 2009, 11(1), 19-32.
21. Zhang, J. L.; Zhang, C. L.; Xiao, Y.; Qin, Y.; Zhang, S. H. Two Novel Trinuclear Cluster-Based Coordination Polymers with 2, 6-Di-imidazol-1-yl-pyridine: Solvothermal Syntheses, Crystal Structures, Properties and Hirshfeld Surface Analysis. Supramol. Chem., 2016, 28(3-4), 231-238.
22. Mahmoudi, G.; Castiñeiras, A.; Garczarek, P.; Bauzá, A.; Rheingold, A. L.; Kinzhybalo, V.; Frontera, A. Synthesis, X-ray Characterization, DFT Calculations and Hirshfeld Surface Analysis of Thiosemicarbazone Complexes of Mn+ Ions (n= 2, 3; M= Ni, Cd, Mn, Co and Cu). CrystEngComm., 2016, 18(6), 1009-1023.
23. Nakagawa, T.; Hasegawa, Y.; Kawai, T. Nondestructive Luminescence Intensity Readout of a Photochromic Lanthanide(III) Complex. Chem. Commun., 2009, (37), 5630-5632.
24. Li, S.; Tao, H.; Li, J. Molecularly Imprinted Electrochemical Luminescence Sensor Based on Enzymatic Amplification for Ultratrace Isoproturon Determination. Electroanalysis, 2012, 24(7), 1664-1670.
25. Wang, Q. L.; Chen, M. M.; Zhang, H. Q.; Wen, W.; Zhang, X. H.; Wang, S. F. Selective and Sensitive Determination of Ochratoxin A Based on a Molecularly Imprinted Electrochemical Luminescence Sensor. Anal. Methods, 2015, 7(24), 10224-10228.
26. Feng, C.; Ma, Y. H.; Zhang, D.; Li, X. J.; Zhao, H. Highly Efficient Electrochemiluminescence Based on Pyrazolecarboxylic Metal Organic Framework. Dalton Trans., 2016, 45(12), 5081-5091.

27. Zheng, L.; Chi, Y.; Dong, Y.; Lin, J.; Wang, B. Electrochemiluminescence of Water-Soluble Carbon Nanocrystals Released Electrochemically from Graphite. J. Am. Chem. Soc., 2009, 131(13), 4564-4565.
28. Fan, F. R. F.; Park, S.; Zhu, Y.; Ruoff, R. S.; Bard, A. J. Electrogenerated Chemiluminescence of Partially Oxidized Highly Oriented Pyrolytic Graphite Surfaces and of Graphene Oxide Nanoparticles. J. Am. Chem. Soc., 2009, 131(3), 937-939.
29. Sheldrick, G. M. SHELXS-97, Program for the Solution of Crystal Structures." Göttingen University, Germany, 1997.
30. Sheldrick, G. M. SHELXL–97, Program for Crystal Structure Refinement, Göttingen University, Germany, 1997.
31. Sheldrick, G. M. Crystal Structure Refinement with SHELXL. Acta. Crystallogr. C., 2015, 71(1), 3-8.
32. Sheldrick, G. M. A Short History of SHELX. Acta Crystallogr., Sect. A: Found. Crystallogr, 2008, 64(1), 112-122.
33. Wei, G. H.; Yang, J.; Ma, J. F.; Liu, Y. Y.; Li, S. L.; Zhang, L. P. Syntheses, Structures and Luminescent Properties of Zinc(II) and Cadmium(II) Coordination Complexes Based on New Bis(imidazolyl)ether and Different Carboxylate Ligands. Dalton Trans., 2008, (23), 3080-3092.
34. Chen, W.; Wang, J. Y.; Chen, C.; Yue, Q.; Yuan, H. M.; Chen, J. S.; Wang, S. N. Photoluminescent Metal−Organic Polymer Constructed from Trimetallic Clusters and Mixed Carboxylates. Inorg. Chem., 2003, 42(4), 944-946.
35. Zhang, S. H.; Zhao, R. X.; Li, G. Z.; Zhang, H. Y.; Huang, Q. P.; Liang, F. P. Room Temperature Syntheses, Crystal Structures and Properties of Two New Heterometallic Polymers Based on 3-Ethoxy-2-Hydroxybenzaldehyde Ligand. J. Solid. State. Chem., 2014, 220, 206-212.
36. Huo, P.; Chen, T.; Hou, J. L.; Yu, L.; Zhu, Q. Y.; Dai, J. Ligand-to-Ligand Charge Transfer within Metal–Organic Frameworks Based on Manganese Coordination Polymers with Tetrathiafulvalene-Bicarboxylate and Bipyridine Ligands. Inorg. Chem., 2016, 55(13), 6496-6503.
37. Tsai, C. N.; Mazumder, S.; Zhang, X. Z.; Schlegel, H. B.; Chen, Y. J.; Endicott, J. F. Are Very Small Emission Quantum Yields Characteristic of Pure Metal-to-Ligand Charge-Transfer Excited States of Ruthenium(II)-(Acceptor Ligand) Chromophores?. Inorg. Chem., 2016, 55(15), 7341-7355.
38. Chen, Z. H.; Zhang, S. H.;, Zhang, S. M.; Sun, Q. C.; Xiao, Y.; Wang, K. Cadmium-Based Coordination Polymers from 1D to 3D: Synthesis, Structures, and Photoluminescent and Electrochemiluminescent Properties. ChemPlusChem, 2019, 84(2), 190-202.
39. Richter, M. M. Electrochemiluminescence (ecl). Chem. Rev., 2004, 104(6), 3003-3036.

Chapter 3

Five novel dinuclear copper (II) complexes: Crystal structures, properties, Hirshfeld surface analysis, and vitro antitumor activity study

Introduction

Schiff bases are versatile organic compounds. They demonstrate multifaceted bonding modes that associate with metal ions and form intermediate and basic components to synthesize chemicals and new products in industry. Schiff bases exhibit pharmacological properties that have broad applications in medicine,[1-4] optical,[5,6] electrochemical,[7,8] magnetic,[9-15] luminescence,[16-18] and catalytic materials[19-21]. The synthesis of Schiff bases has been studied extensively based on intermolecular interactions, especially to describe molecular crystal formations.[22-23]

Rosenberg and colleagues revolutionized chemotherapy with platinum drugs such as cisplantin,[24] but the side-effects of the platinum-based anticancer drugs prompted the synthesis of non-platinum metal-based drugs[25-27]. Inclusion of copper complexes in medical applications is based on extensive research on its biological chemistry, resulting in the use of many Schiff bases in medicine, and it has encouraged further studies on copper(II) complexes derived from Schiff base ligands[28-34]. This article describes the synthesis of five copper (II) complexes made from the reaction of $Cu(NO_3)_2$ and three Schiff base ligands (H_2bdhc, H_2bchc and H_2bbhc) in the test tube. The MTT method assessed the antiproliferative capabilities of complexes **chapt3-1–chapt3-5** against a panel of human tumor cells, including BEL-7404, Hep-G2, NCI-H460, T-24, MGC-803, A549, SK-OV-3 and normal human liver HL-7702 cells.

Methodology

Materials and physical measurements: The study procured the unpurified chemicals commercially. They conducted the elemental analyses (CHN) using an PE 2400 series II elemental analyzer. They recorded the FT–IR spectra using KBr pellets in the ranges 4000–400 cm^{-1} on a BioRad FTS-7 spectrophotometer. The authors recorded the UV–vis spectra ranging between 200-800 nm on a UV-2450 spectrophotometer. A Hitachi F-4600 fluorescence spectrophotometer conducted the luminescence spectra at room temperature. A Quantum

Design PPMS model 600 magnetometer performed the magnetic measurements to 5 T for **chapt3-1**.

Syntheses of complexes **chapt3-1**–**chapt3-5** comprising of [Cu$_2$(bdhc)(CH$_3$OH)(NO$_3$)(dmf)$_2$] **chapt3-1**, [Cu$_2$(bdhc)(CH$_3$CH$_2$OH)(NO$_3$)(dmf)$_2$] **chapt3-2**, [Cu$_2$(bchc)(CH$_3$CH$_2$OH)(NO$_3$)(dmf)$_2$] **chapt3-3**, [Cu$_2$(bchc)(CH$_3$OH)(NO$_3$)(dmf)$_2$] **chapt3-4**, and [Cu$_2$(bbhc)(H$_2$O)(dmf)$_2$]·NO$_3$H$_2$O **chapt3-5**: A mixture was prepared with H$_3$bdhc (0.5 mmol, 0.313 g), DMF (3 mL), CH$_2$Cl$_2$ (2 mL) and placed in a test tube. The authors added 5 mL of methanol solution with Cu(NO$_3$)$_2$·H$_2$O in the tube and sealed it. Dark crystals were collected after 8 days and washed with methanol and air-dried. For the next two complexes, most steps were same except that the methanol was replaced by ethanol. Complex **chapt3-3** was prepared in a similar way to **chapt3-2**, except that the H$_3$bdhc was replaced by H$_3$bchc. Dark Green crystals of **chapt3-2** and **chapt3-3** were collected by filtration, washed with ethanol and air dried. Complex **chapt3-4** preparation was similar to **chapt3-3**, except that the ethanol was replaced by methanol. Complex **chapt3-5** was prepared in a similar way to **chapt3-1**, except that the H$_3$bdhc was replaced by H$_3$bbhc. Dark Green crystals of **chapt3-4** and **chapt3-5** were collected by filtration, washed with ethanol and air dried.

Crystal structure determination: An Agilent G8910A CCD diffractometer with graphite monochromated Mo-Ka radiation collected the diffraction data. The study integrated the raw frame data with the SAINT program. The SHELXS-97 solved the structures by direct methods, refined by full matrix least-squares on F^2. The program SADABS was used for an empirical absorption correction[35]. All non-hydrogen atoms were refined aniso-tropically. All hydrogen atoms were positioned geometrically and refined as riding. SHELXTL was used for calculations and graphics[35]. Table 3-1 lists the crystallographic data and structure refinement parameters. Selected bond lengths and angles for complexes **chapt3-1**-**chapt3-5** is given in Table 3-2.

Table 3-1. Crystal data and structure refinement for complexes chapt3-1–chapt3-5

Compound	**chapt3-1**	**chapt3-2**	**chapt3-3**	**chapt3-4**	**chapt3-5**
Formule.	C$_{22}$H$_{25}$Br$_4$Cu$_2$N$_7$O$_9$	C$_{23}$H$_{27}$Br$_4$Cu$_2$N$_7$O$_9$	C$_{23}$H$_{27}$Cl$_4$Cu$_2$N$_7$O$_9$	C$_{22}$H$_{25}$Cl$_4$Cu$_2$N$_7$O$_9$	C$_{21}$H$_{27}$Br$_2$Cu$_2$N$_7$O$_{10}$
Form. weight	977.19	992.24	814.42	800.37	824.40
Crystal system	Monoclinic	Monoclinic	Monoclinic	Monoclinic	Monoclinic
Space group	$P2_1/c$	$P2_1/c$	$P2_1/c$	$P2_1/n$	$P2_1/c$
a/Å	17.913 (1)	17.915 (1)	17.494 (1)	19.171 (1)	6.410 (1)
b/Å	9.178 (1)	9.179 (2)	9.144 (1)	9.311 (1)	24.053 (1)
c/Å	20.920 (1)	20.930 (1)	20.752 (1)	19.288 (1)	18.815 (1)
a/°	90.00	90.00	90.00	90.00	90.00
b/°	107.72 (1)	107.71 (3)	107.28(1)	116.11 (1)	93.39 (1)
c/°	90.00	90.00	90.00	90.00	90.00
V/Å^3	3276.0 (2)	3278.8 (1)	3169.9 (1)	3091.5 (2)	2895.7 (2)
Z	4	4	4	4	4
$F(000)$	1904	1936	1644	1616	1640
$Dcal$./g cm^{-3}	1.983	2.010	1.706	1.720	1.891
μ/mm^{-1}	6.234	6.231	1.739	1.782	4.287
θ range/°	3.01–25.01	3.44–25.01	2.87–25.10	2.96–25.00	3.18–25.00
Ref. coll./unique	5714/4119	5744/4402	5622/4632	5444/4508	5104/3687
R_{int}	0.0296	0.0246	0.0212	0.0190	0.0303
Completeness	99.2	99.6	99.7	99.8	99.6
Parameters	378	411	412	405	386
GOOF	1.020	1.002	1.009	1.007	1.006

R_1 [$I > 2r(I)$][a,b]	0.0430	0.0347	0.0351	0.0298	0.0422
wR_2 (all data)[a,b]	0.1074	0.0781	0.0865	0.0719	0.0894
Residues/e Å^{-3}	—1.135, 1.714	—0.595, 1.282	—0.334, 0.729	—0.292, 0.273	—0.632, 0.586

$^a R_1 = \Sigma||F_o| - |F_c||/\Sigma|F_o|$. $^b wR_2 = [\Sigma w(|F_o^2|-|F_c^2|)^2/\Sigma w(|F_o^2|)^2]^{1/2}$

Table 3-2 Matal-ligand Bond lengths(Å) and Angles (deg) in Chapt3-1–Chapt3-5

Compound	chapt3-1	chapt3-2	chapt3-3	chapt3-4	chapt3-5
Cu1–O1	1.889(4)	1.887(2)	1.887(2)	1.886(2)	1.881(3)
Cu1–N1	1.950(4)	1.951(2)	1.953(2)	1.951(2)	1.937(4)
Cu1–O5	1.958(3)	1.957(2)	1.964(2)	1.961(2)	1.960(3)
Cu1–N3	1.995(4)	1.990(2)	1.985(2)	1.986(2)	1.979(3)
Cu1–O9	2.530(4)	2.537(2)	2.539(2)	2.551(2)	/
Cu2–O3	1.878(4)	1.875(2)	1.883(2)	1.870(2)	1.895(3)
Cu2–N4	1.942(4)	1.942(2)	1.940(2)	1.943(2)	1.949(4)
Cu2–O4	1.953(3)	1.947(2)	1.946(2)	1.951(2)	1.973(3)
Cu2–O2	1.958(4)	1.956(2)	1.957(2)	1.947(2)	1.936(3)
Cu2–O6	2.435(4)	2.436(2)	2.435(2)	2.386(2)	2.283(4)
Cu1···Cu2	4.791(1)	4.972(1)	4.791(1)	4.784(1)	4.792(1)
O1–Cu1–N1	91.4(2)	91.4(1)	91.3(1)	91.2(1)	91.5(1)
O1–Cu1–O5	87.8(2)	88.0(1)	87.9(1)	88.4(1)	88.9(1)
N1–Cu1–O5	176.8(2)	176.8(1)	176.7(1)	176.2(1)	173.7(1)
O1–Cu1–N3	171.4(2)	171.4(1)	171.5(1)	171.2(1)	171.9(1)
N1–Cu1–N3	81.0(2)	81.1(1)	81.3(1)	81.1(1)	81.3(1)
O5–Cu1–N3	99.5(2)	99.3(1)	99.2(1)	99.0(1)	98.7(1)
O3–Cu2–N4	94.4(2)	94.0(1)	94.2(1)	94.2(1)	93.6(1)
O3–Cu2–O4	93.3(2)	93.3(1)	93.6(1)	92.6(1)	90.0(1)
N4–Cu2–O4	166.7(2)	167.0(1)	166.1(1)	166.7(1)	169.5(1)
O3–Cu2–O2	171.2(2)	171.5(1)	172.1(1)	171.5(1)	169.3(1)
N4–Cu2–O2	81.2(2)	81.7(1)	81.5(1)	81.7(1)	81.8(1)
O4–Cu2–O2	89.7(2)	89.5(1)	89.4(1)	90.0(1)	93.0(1)
O3–Cu2–O6	92.9(2)	92.6(1)	92.2(1)	91.4(1)	92.5(1)
N4–Cu2–O6	92.6(2)	92.4(1)	93.4(1)	93.0(1)	99.0(1)
O4–Cu2–O6	97.8(2)	97.9(1)	97.9(1)	98.3(1)	90.7(1)
O2–Cu2–O6	94.9(2)	95.0(1)	94.6(1)	96.3(1)	97.7(1)

Hirshfeld surface calculations of **Chapt3-1–Chapt3-5**: The CrystalExplorer program was used to calculate the Molecular Hirshfeld surface calculations.[36] When the CIF file of **Chapt3-1–Chapt3-5** were read into the CrystalExplorer program, all bond lengths to hydrogen were automatically modified to typical standard neutron values (C-H = 1.083 Å, N-H = 1.009 Å and O-H = 0.983 Å)[37]. Here, all the Hirshfeld surfaces were generated using a high(standard) surface resolution. The 3D dnorm surfaces were mapped by using a fixed color scale of 0.76 (red) to 2.4 (blue). The 2D fingerprint plots were displayed by using the standard 0.4–2.6 Å view with the de and di distance scales displayed on the graph axes.

Results and discussion

Structural description: Figure 3-1 shows the similarity in the structures of complexes **Chapt3-1–Chapt3-5**, except for the terminal ligands and the halogen substituents of the Schiff base ligands. Thus, the authors analyzed only complex **Chapt3-1**. Single-crystal X-ray diffraction analysis shows complex **Chapt3-1** belonged to the monoclinic with space group of $P2_1/c$, with

2₁ axial and a dinuclear copper complex. Two Cu (II) ions, one bdhc ligand, one methanol terminal ligand, one nitrate and two DMF terminal ligands contributed to the dinuclear copper complex.

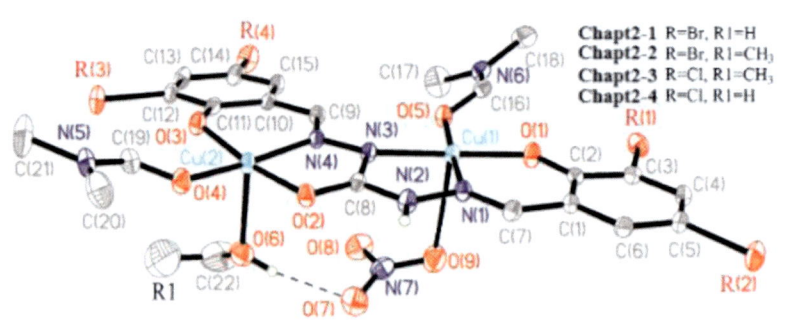

Figure 3-1. Chapt3-1-Chapt3-4 crystal structures

A single terminal DMF molecule, one oxygen atom from nitrate, and one oxygen and two nitrogen atoms from bdhc ligand with O9 atom in the apical position coordinated the distorted tetragonal pyramid geometry containing the Cu1 ion. Similarly, Cu2 appeared to be in a distorted tetragonal pyramid geometry coordinated by one terminal DMF molecule, one oxygen atom from methanol molecule, and two oxygen and one nitrogen atoms from bdhc ligand with O6 atom in the apical position. The authors attribute the existence of Cu1 and Cu2 from the John-teller effect.[38,39] Scheme 3-1 depicts the unique bdhc ligand as a tri-anion in a $\mu_2:\eta^1:\eta^1:\eta^1:\eta^1:\eta^1:\eta^1$ coordination mode. Intramolecular distance between the Cu1···Cu2 of **Chapt3-1–Chapt3-4** are 4.791(1) Å, 4.972(1) Å, 4.791(1) Å, 4.784(1) Å, respectively.

It should be noted that the dimer of **Chapt3-1** was constructed through double weak Cu···N interaction(Cu1-N3^i, 3.359 Å, symmetry code: (i) 2 - x, - y, 1 - z). The dimer also created a 1D supramolecular chain via N-H···O hydrogen bonds (N2-H2···O8^{vii}, 2.877(1) Å, symmetry code: (vii) 2 - x, 1 - y, 1 - z, Figure 3-2). The 1D supramolecular chain was formed by 3D network through Br···Br interaction (Br2···Br2^{ii}, 3.538 Å; Br2···Br2^{iii}, 3.880 Å; Br3···Br4^{iv}, 3.880 Å; symmetry code: (ii) 3- x, 1- y, 1- z; (iii) 1 + x, y, z; (iv) 1- x, 0.5 + y, 0.5- z.)[40] and weak C-H···Br hydrogen bonds (C20-H20A···Br2^v, 3.720 Å; C22-H22C···Br4^{vi}, 3.843 Å, symmetry code: (v) 1 + x, y, z; (vi) x, 1 + y, z.) and C-H···O hydrogen bond (C6-H6···O6^{vii}, 3.431 Å, symmetry code: (vii) 2- x, 1- y, 1- z.)

Scheme 3-1. Mode of coordination of Schiff base ligands

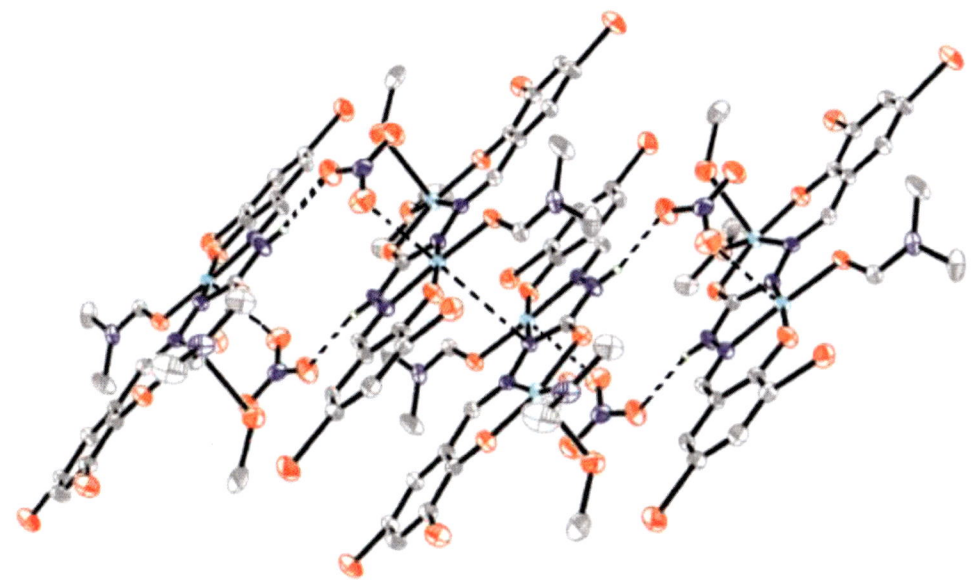

Figure 3-2. 1D chain of Chapt3-1

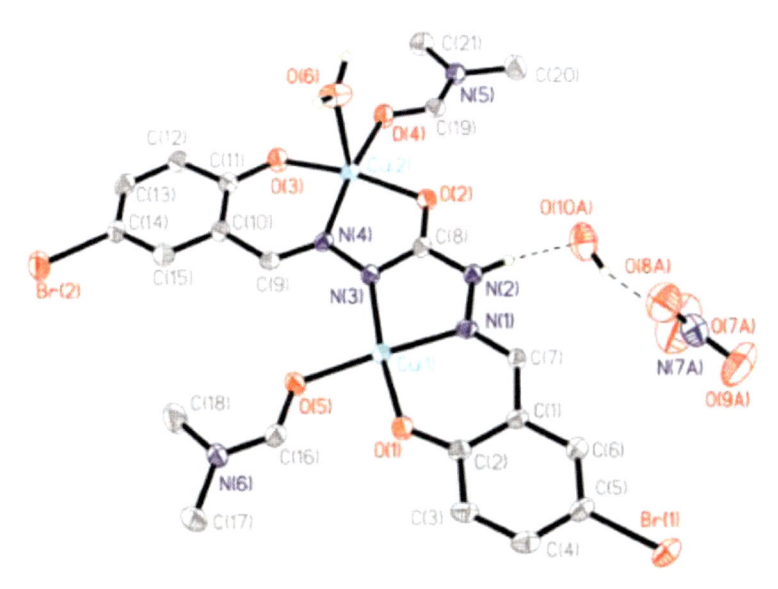

Figure 3-3. The crystal structure of Chapt3-5.

The structure of complex **Chapt3-5** was different from **Chapt3-1–Chapt3-4**, with NO$_3$ ion being free in **Chapt3-5** but was coordinated with Cu1 ion in the rest (Figure 3-3). The dinuclear copper complex developed from two Cu (II) ions, one bbhc ligand, two DMF terminal ligands, one coordination water molecule, one counter anion nitrate and one lattice water molecule. The Cu1 ion appeared coordinated in a slightly distorted square–planar geometry by two nitrogen atoms and one oxygen atom from a bbhc ligand and one oxygen atom form DMF molecule. However, the coordination geometry of the Cu2 ion and intramolecular between Cu1⋯Cu2 of all complexes were similar. The 1-D chain was constructed by weak Cu⋯O interaction and the 1-D chain further formed double chain through strong O-H⋯O hydrogen bonds.

Hirshfeld surface analysis: Figure 3-4 presents the molecular Hirshfeld surface of the five compounds to describe the surface features. The close intermolecular interactions were identified by the dnorm surface and their values were mapped onto the Hirshfeld surface with a three-color scheme: where red regions were associated with the closer intermolecular contacts than r^{vdW} (van der Waals (vdW) radii); the blue regions corresponded to longer intermolecular contacts than r^{vdW}; and the white regions corresponded to the distance of intermolecular contacts as exactly the r^{vdW}. The short contacts of NH and OH interactions associated with the N-HO and O-HO hydrogen bonds are depicted by the red regions (Figure 3-4, Table 3-3). The primary intermolecular interactions of the five complexes are HH contacts which are reflected in the middle of the scattered point of the 2D fingerprint plots (the percentage of HH contacts of **Chapt3-1–Chapt3-5** are 22.7%, 25.5%, 26.4%, 23.3%, and 29.5%, respectively). Figure 3-5 shows the XH interactions of complex **Chapt3-1** as depicted by a spike in the bottom left (donor) area of the fingerprint plot, and the HX interactions are represented by a spike in the bottom right (acceptor) region of the fingerprint plot. Table 3-4 summarizes the percentage of contacts of complexes **Chapt3-1–Chapt3-5**.

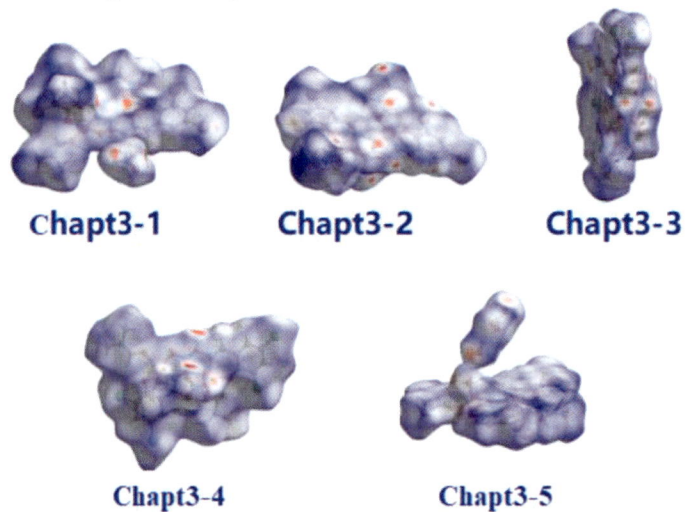

Figure 3-4. Complexes Chapt3-1-Chapt3-5 Hirshfeld surface mapped with dnorm.

Table 3-3 The percentages of contacts between different element pairs contributed to the total Hirshfeld Surface area of molecules (X = Cl, Br).

Complex	H–H	C–H	O–H	X–H	C–C	C–O	Br–Br	Other
Chapt3-1	22.7	8.1	21.0	20.4	3.0	3.3	3.8	17.7
Chapt3-2	25.5	8.2	19.2	24.0	3.2	2.5	3.7	13.7
Chapt3-3	26.4	8.7	19.2	23.9	3.2	2.6	2.9	13.1
Chapt3-4	23.3	7.7	23.0	22.0	3.4	3.1	2.5	15.0
Chapt3-5	29.5	10.4	25.5	13.0	1.6	1.3	2.9	15.8

UV–vis spectrum: Fig 3-6 depicts the spectra of complexes **Chapt3-1–Chapt3-5**. Usually, no absorption bands have been reported above 400 nm in polar and nonpolar solvents[41]. However, a considerable broad band was observed at 407, 414, 424, 415, and 415 nm for **Chapt3-1–Chapt3-5**, respectively. It suggested that the five molecules existed from ligand-to-metal-charge-transfer (LMCT)[42,43]. Also, the UV–vis spectra of **Chapt3-1–Chapt3-5** showed another peak at 273 nm, 270 nm, 268 nm, 269 nm, and 270 nm, respectively and the complexes **Chapt3-1–Chapt3-5** showed two same peaks at 415 nm and 270 nm.

Fluorescence properties: Figure 3-7 shows the fluorescence properties of complexes **Chapt3-1–Chapt3-5**. After photoexcitation at 380 nm, H₃bchc, H₃bbhc, and H₃bdhc ligands showed a green luminescent emission band with the maximum at 561, 566, and 563 nm, respectively. Excitation at 416 nm the complexes **Chapt3-1–Chapt3-5** showed a green luminescent emission band with the maximum at 632, 632, 632, 632, and 630 nm, respectively. Fig 3-8,3-9, 3-10 shows the luminescent properties of **Chapt3-1–Chapt3-3** in DMF solvent. The fluorescence intensity of complexes **Chapt3-1–Chapt3-3** increased when the concentration of the solution was reduced and indicated the fluorescence concentration self-quenching effect in the solution of **Chapt3-1–Chapt3-3**.

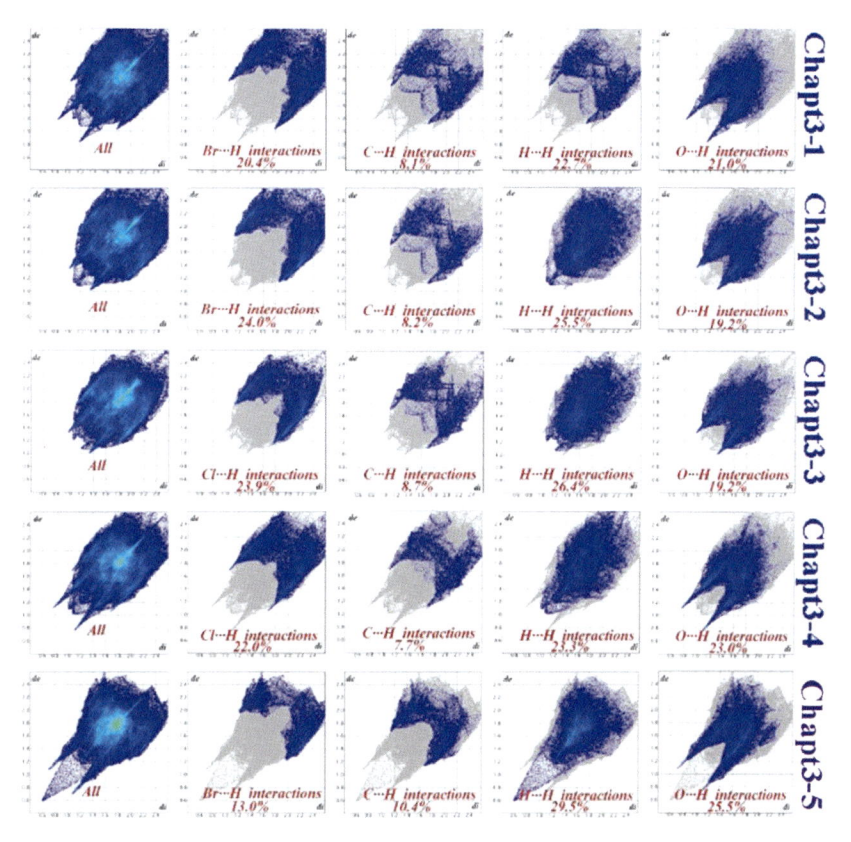

Figure 3-5. Fingerprint plots of Chapt3-1–Chapt3-5: Full (1) and resolved into X⋯H (2), C⋯H (3), H⋯H (4) and O⋯H (5) contacts displaying the proportions of contacts contributing to the total Hirshfeld Surface area of molecules

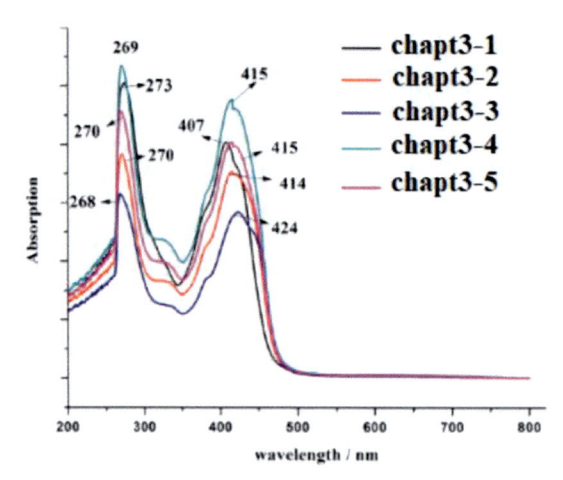

Figure 3-6. The UV–vis spectra of complexes Chapt3-1–Chapt3-5 in DMF medium [3 × 10⁻⁵ (M)] are shown

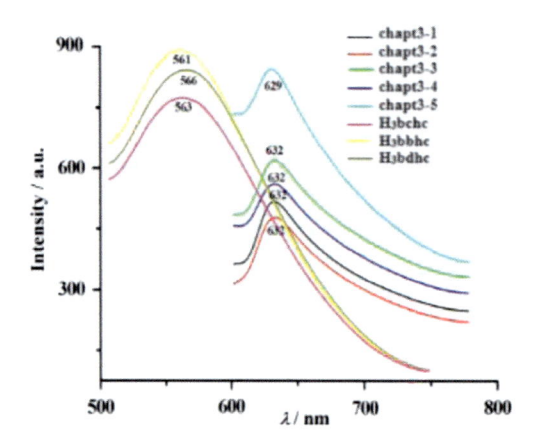

Figure 3-7. Solid-state emission spectra of the Chapt3-1–Chapt3-5 and H₃bchc, H₃bbhc, and H₃bdhc ligands at room temperature.

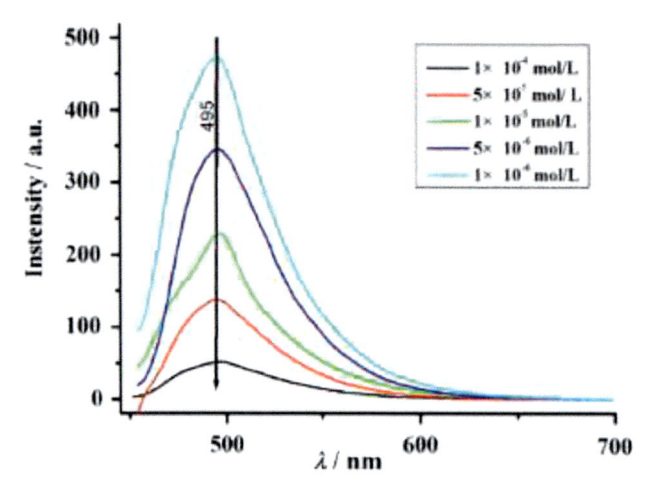

Figure 3-8. Spectral luminescence in a solvent of the complex Chapt3-1

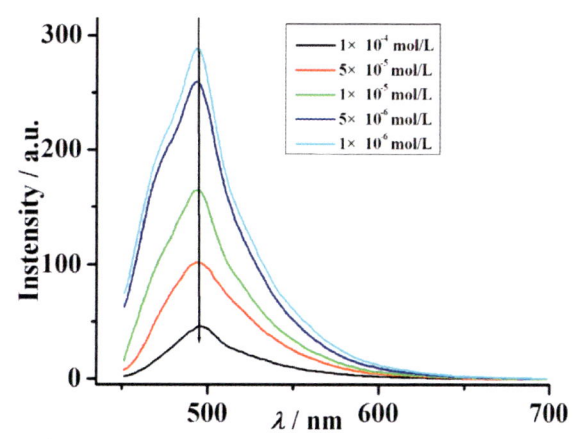

Figure 3-9. Solvent luminescence spectrum of the complex Chapt3-2.

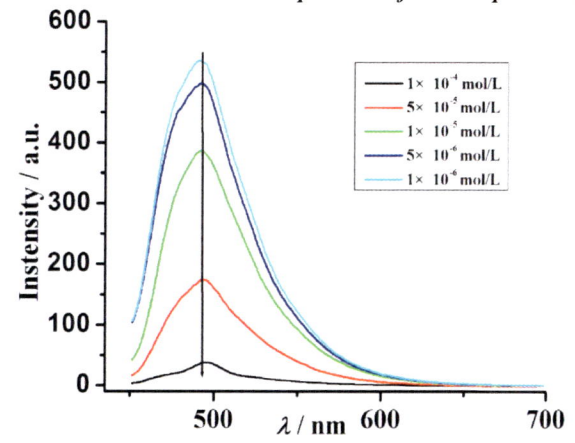

Figure 3-10. Solvent luminescence spectrum of the complex Chapt3-3.

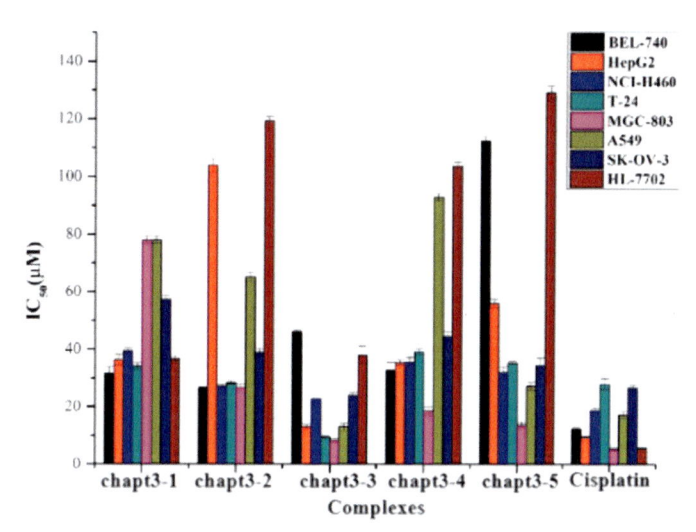

Figure 3-11. The IC50 (μM) values of complex Chapt3-1–Chapt3-5 and cisplatin against eight different cell lines for 48 hours.

In-vitro antitumor: Table 3-4 shows the cytotoxicity outcomes of complexes **Chapt3-1 and Chapt3-5** against BEL-7404, Hep-G2, NCI-H460, T-24, MGC-803, A549, and SKOV-3. Complex 3 induced higher inhibitory rates against Hep-G2, NCI-H460, T-24, MGC-803, A549, and SK-OV-3 cells than other complexes. The inhibitory rates of complexes **Chapt3-1** and -**Chapt3-5** against BEL-740 and HepG2 were higher than 30%. All complexes fared better than cisplatin against HL-7702. Next, the IC$_{50}$ levels were determined, as shown in Figure 3-11 and Table 3-5. All complexes showed high IC$_{50}$ values against BEL-7404, HepG2, NCI-H460, MGC-803 cells. Complexes **Chapt3-2** and **Chapt3-4** showed selective toxicity on BEL-7404. IC$_{50}$ values for Complex **Chapt3-3** of 9.41 μM, 12.96 μM, and 24.09 μM had higher cytotoxicity against T-24, A549, SK-OV-3 cells, respectively. Further, T-24 cells showed the highest sensitivity to complex **Chapt3-3** with an IC$_{50}$ value of 9.41 ± 0.49 μM, which increased approximately 3-fold compared with the cisplatin. The results indicated the potential of complex **Chapt3-3** as an anti-cancer drug compared to others. Also, the apical position of ethanol in complex **Chapt3-2** and **Chapt3-3** had easy release than methanol in others, supporting the candidature of complex **Chapt3-3** against cancer.

Table 3-4 The inhibitory effect on different cells of complexes **chapt3-1–chapt3-5** and cisplatin(%)

Complex	BEL-740	HepG2	NCI-H460	T24	MGC-830	A549	SK-OV-3	HL-7702
Chapt3-1	33.45±1.54	37.66±1.41	24.75±1.79	30.71±1.38	25.67±1.76	39.29±1.52	28.24±1.78	45.59±1.74
Chapt3-2	45.71±1.42	20.38±2.58	34.88±1.96	30.72±2.39	41.87±2.94	35.17±2.13	36.06±0.66	15.38±1.34
Chapt3-2	19.85±0.16	53.82±1.93	44.15±2.73	56.45±1.20	59.35±3.12	53.39±4.37	41.91±2.02	32.93±1.59
Chapt3-4	35.47±0.15	38.96±2.39	35.79±1.43	28.45±1.50	47.38±1.54	13.94±1.25	26.94±2.63	17.97±3.91
Chapt3-5	22.90±3.62	22.78±1.42	30.08±2.46	30.83±3.39	50.38±3.87	34.96±3.19	34.65±1.01	11.53±0.81
Cisplatin	55.15±1.18	60.63±0.99	50.88±3.69	37.38±3.39	71.35±1.46	21.14±3.4	46.56±0.92	73.58±2.30

Table 3-5 'The IC50^a on different cells of complexes **chapt3-1–chapt3-5** and cisplatin (μM)

Complex	BEL-740	HepG2	NCI-H460	T24	MGC-830	A549	SK-OV-3	HL-7702
Chapt3-1	31.68±2.37	36.41±1.81	39.42±1.02	34.22±1.18	78.07±1.38	78.07±1.38	57.35±1.33	36.77±0.91
Chapt3-2	26.67±0.39	103.96±2.25	27.31±0.51	28.44±0.60	26.78±1.02	65.09±1.65	38.89±1.49	119.44±1.42
Chapt3-2	46.04±0.65	13.04±0.75	22.86±0.14	9.41±0.49	8.29±0.60	12.96±1.30	24.09±1.01	37.99±3.02
Chapt3-4	32.85±2.79	35.48±0.88	35.67±1.52	39.19±1.16	18.43±1.53	92.96±1.29	44.53±1.58	103.71±1.50
Chapt3-5	112.47±1.53	56.04±1.48	32.22±1.78	35.41±0.49	13.76±1.01	29.35±1.32	34.53±2.59	128.30±2.31
Cisplatin	12.41±0.38	9.48±0.35	18.89±1.02	28.07±1.88	5.43±0.45	17.35±1.24	26.77±0.89	5.63±0.32

^{a} IC$_{50}$ values are presented as the mean ± SD (standard error of the mean) from five independent experiments.

Magnetic property of complex **Chapt3-1**: Figure 3-12 depicts the magnetic susceptibility of **Chapt3-1**. The spin–orbit coupling of the two Cu (II) ions induced a $\chi_M T$ product of 0.53 cm^{3}Kmol^{-1} at room temperature. Under 50 K, $\chi_M T$ of **Chapt3-1** remained constant till 2 K. To fit and interpret magnetic susceptibility data of 1, all possible magnetic pathways were assessed. The intramolecular antiferromagnetic interaction in **Chapt3-1** was as expected based on the exchange pathway contributed by one dinitrogen bridge between two Cu(II) ions of the dinuclear unit. Subsequently, the dimeric nature of the **Chapt3-1** can be easily simplified to a Cu(II) dimer skeleton as schematized. Keeping the above considerations in mind, to calculate the magnetic exchange interaction (*J*)

$$\chi_M = \frac{2Ng^2\beta^2}{kT} \times \frac{1}{3 + e^{-2J/kT}} \quad (1)$$

$$R = \sum \left[\frac{(\chi_m T)_{exp} - (\chi_m T)_{cal}}{(\chi_m T)_{cal}}\right]^2 \quad (2)$$

between the copper centers in **Chapt3-1**, the magnetic data was fitted to be modified Bleaney-Bowers equation expression for two interacting Cu(II) ions (S = 1/2)[44] with isotropic spin Hamiltonian in the form $\hat{H} = -J_1\hat{S}_1\hat{S}_2$ and it is given by Eq. (1). The best curve fitting gave *g* = 1.99, J_1 = -85.1 cm1, and R = 2.86 x 10^{-4}. The R represents the agreement factor and it is defined in Eq. (2). The negative *J* value represents the obvious antiferromagnetic coupling between two Cu(II) centers in **Chapt3-1**.

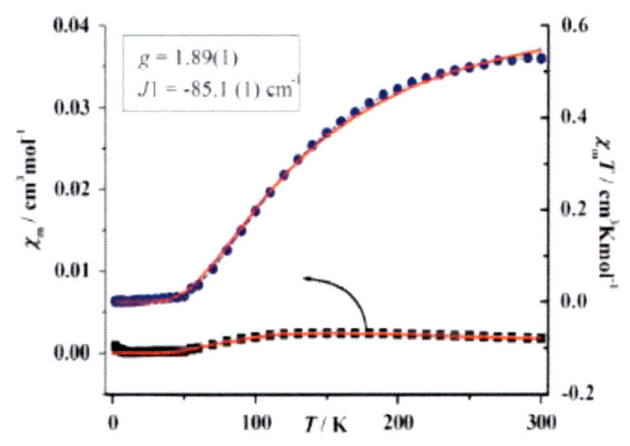

Figure 3-12. Plot of $\chi_M T$ and χ_M versus T for chapt3-1 in a 1000 Oe field. The solid lines indicate the optimal data fits as described in the text'.

Conclusion

To conclude, in-vitro antitumor activity showed chapt3-3 with a high apoptosis-inducing ability against T-24, A549, SK-OV-3. Hirshfeld surface and fingerprint plot analysis of **chapt3-1–chapt3-5** revealed that the close contacts of these five complexes were dominated by H···H, X···H (X = Cl, Br), O···H, and C···H interactions. There are significant N-H···O, O-H···O, and C-H···X (X = Cl, Br) interactions noted in all five compounds. The fluorescence concentration self-quenching effect was observed in the solution of **chapt3-1–chapt3-5**. On the other hand, magnetic studies revealed that there were antiferromagnetic interactions between two Cu(II) ions.

References

1. Jia, Y.; Li, J. B. Molecular Assembly of Schiff Base Interactions: Construction and Application. Chem. Rev., 2015, 115(3), 1597-1621.
2. Zhang, S. M.; Zhang, H. Y.; Qin, Q. P.; Fei, J. W.; Zhang, S. H. Syntheses, Crystal Structures and Biological Evaluation of Two New Cu(II) and Co(II) Complexes Based on (E)-2-(((4H-1,2,4-Triazol-4-Yl)Imino)Methyl)-6-Methoxyphenol. J. Inorg. Biochem., 2019, 193, 52-59.
3. Peterson, M. D.; Holbrook, R. J.; Meade, T. J.; Weiss, E. A. Photoinduced Electron Transfer from PbS Quantum Dots to Cobalt(III) Schiff Base Complexes: Light Activation of a Protein Inhibitor. J. Chem. Soc., 2013, 135(35), 13162-13167.
4. Chen, Y. T.; Ke, Z. L.; Yuan, L. Y.; Liang, M. X.; Zhang, S. H. Hydrazylpyridine Salicylaldehyde-Copper(II)-1,10-Phenanthroline Complexes as Potential Anticancer Agents: Synthesis, Characterization and Anticancer Evaluation. Dalton Trans., 2023, 52, 12318-12331.
5. Li, L. J.; Hua, X. X.; Huang, Y. Y.; Yang, X. Y.; Wang, C.; Du, J. L. Synthesis and Characterize of Multifunctional Schiff Base and Cu(II) Complex: An Optical Property Investigation. Inorg. Nano-Met. Chem., 2014, 44(2), 291-294.
6. Kumar, R. A.; Arivanandhan, M.; Hayakawa, Y. Recent Advances in Rare Earth-Based Borate Single Crystals: Potential Materials for Nonlinear Optical and Laser Applications. Prog. Cryst. Growth Ch., 2013, 59(3), 113-132.

7. Pelayo-Vázquez, J. B.; González, F. J.; Leyva, M. A.; Campos, M.; Torres, L. A.; Rosales-Hoz, M. J. A Ruthenium Carbonyl Cluster Containing a Hydroquinone Ligand: A Layered Structure with a Polymetallic Species. Structure and Electrochemical Characterization. J. Organomet. Chem., 2012, 716, 289-293.
8. Balić, T.; Marković, B.; Medvidović-Kosanović, M. Electrochemical and Structural Analysis of a Novel Symmetrical Bis-Schiff Base with Herringbone Packing Motif. J. Mol. Struct., 2015, 1084, 82-88.
9. Xiao, Y.; Qin, Y.; Yi, M.; Zhu, Y. A Disc-Like Heptanuclear Nickel Cluster Based on Schiff Base: Synthesis, Structure, Magnetic Properties and Hirshfeld Surface Analysis. J. Clust. Sci., 2016, 27(6), 2013-2023.
10. Vigato, P. A.; Peruzzo, V.; Tamburini, S. Acyclic and Cyclic Compartmental Ligands: Recent Results and Perspectives. Coordin. Chem. Rev., 2012, 256, 953-1114.
11. Sessoli, R.; Gatteschi, D. Quantum Tunneling of Magnetization and Related Phenomena in Molecular Materials. Angew. Chem. Int. Edit., 2003, 42(3), 268-297.
12. Yang, L.; Zhang, S. H.; Wang, W.; Guo, J. J.; Huang, Q. P.; Zhao, R. X.; Zhang, C. L.; Muller, G. Ligand Induced Diversification from Tetranuclear to Mononuclear Compounds: Syntheses, Structures and Magnetic Properties. Polyhedron, 2014, 74, 49-56.
13. Alborés, P.; Rentschler, E. A Co36 Cluster Assembled from the Reaction of Cobalt Pivalate with 2,3-Dicarboxypyrazine. Angew. Chem. Int. Edit., 2009, 48(49), 9366-9370.
14. Zhao, B.; Gao, H. L.; Chen, X. Y.; Cheng, P.; Shi, W.; Liao, D. Z.; Yan, S. P.; Jiang, Z. H. A Promising MgII-Ion-Selective Luminescent Probe: Structures and Properties of Dy-Mn Polymers with High Symmetry. Chem. Eur. J., 2005, 12(1), 149-158.
15. Xiao, Y.; Liu, Y. Q.; Li, G.; Huang, P. Microwave-Assisted Synthesis, Structure and Properties of a Co-Crystal Compound with 2-Ethoxy-6-Methyliminomethyl-Phenol. Supramol. Chem., 2015, 27, 161-166.
16. Bozoklu, G.; Gteau, C.; Imbert, D.; Pécaut, J.; Robeyns, K.; Filinchuk, Y.; Memon, F.; Muller. G.; Mazzanti, M. Metal-Controlled Diastereoselective Self-Assembly and Circularly Polarized Luminescence of a Chiral Heptanuclear Europium Wheel. J. Am. Chem. Soc., 2012, 134(20), 8372-8375.
17. Hu, S.; Yu, F. Y.; Zhang, P.; Lin D. R. In Situamination and Side Group Effect of Multifunctional Heterocyclic Thione Ligand toward Discrete and Polymeric Cluster Constructions. Dalton Trans., 2013, 42, 7731-7740.
18. Xiao, Y.; Huang, P.; Wang, W. Ligand Structure Induced Diversification from Dinuclear to 1D Chain Compounds: Syntheses, Structures and Fluorescence Properties. J. Clust. Sci., 2015, 26(4), 1091-1102.
19. Fu, H.; Lu, Y.; Wang, Z.; Liang, C.; Zhang, Z. M.; Wang, E. Three Hybrid Networks Based on Octamolybdate: Ionothermal Synthesis, Structure and Photocatalytic Properties. Dalton Trans., 2012, 41(14), 4084-4090.
20. Zhao, Y.; Chen, K.; Fan, J.; Okamura, T. A.; Lu, Y.; Luo, L.; Sun, W. Y. Structural Modulation of Silver Complexes and Their Distinctive Catalytic Properties. Dalton Trans., 2014, 43(5), 2252-2258.

21. Zhao, Y.; Zhai, L. L.; Fan, J.; Chen, K.; Sun, W. Y. Silver(I) Complexes of 4-(2-Oxazolinyl)Pyridine: Counteranion Dependent Structural Diversity. Polyhedron, 2012, 46, 16-24.
22. Luo, Y. H.; Zhang, C. G.; Xu, B.; Sun, B. W. A Cocrystal Strategy for the Precipitation of Liquid 2,3-Dimethyl Pyrazine with Hydroxyl Substituted Benzoic Acid and a Hirshfeld Surfaces Analysis of Them. Crystengcomm, 2012, 14(20), 6860-6868.
23. Loots, L.; Barbour, L. J. A Simple and Robust Method for the Identification of π–π Packing Motifs of Aromatic Compounds. Crystengcomm, 2012, 14(1), 300-304.
24. Rosenberg, B.; Vancamp, L.; Trosko, J. E.; Mansour, V. H. Platinum Compounds: a New Class of Potent Antitumour Agents. Nature, 1969, 222, 385-386.
25. Jung, Y. W.; Lippard, S. J. Direct Cellular Responses to Platinum-Induced DNA Damage. Chem. Rev., 2007, 107, 1387-1407.
26. Hartinger, C. G.; Dyson, P. J. Bioorganometallic Chemistry—from Teaching Paradigms to Medicinal Applications. Chem. Soc. Rev., 2009, 38(2), 391-401.
27. Chen, Z. F.; Shi, Y. F.; Liu, Y. C.; Hong, X.; Geng, B.; Peng, Y.; Liang, H. TCM Active Ingredient Oxoglaucine Metal Complexes: Crystal Structure, Cytotoxicity, and Interaction with DNA. Inorg. Chem., 2012, 51, 1998-2009.
28. Zhang, Q. Q.; Zhang, F.; Wang, W. G.; Wang, X. L. Synthesis, Crystal Structure and DNA Binding Studies of a Binuclear Copper(II) Complex with Phenanthroline. J. Inorg. Biochem., 2006, 100(8), 1344-1352.
29. Mazur, L.; Modzelewska-Banachiewicz, B.; Paprocka, R.; Zimecki, M.; Wawrzyniak, U. E.; Kutkowska, J.; Ziółkowska, G. Synthesis, Crystal Structure and Biological Activities of a Novel Amidrazone Derivative and Its Copper(II) Complex — A Potential Antitumor Drug. J. Inorg. Biochem., 2012, 114, 55-64.
30. Lovejoy, D. B.; Jansson, P. J.; Brunk, U. T.; Wong, J.; Ponka, P.; Richardson, D. R. Antitumor Activity of Metal-Chelating Compound Dp44mT Is Mediated by Formation of a Redox-Active Copper Complex That Accumulates in Lysosomes. Cancer Res., 2011, 71(17), 5871-5880.
31. Qiao, X.; Ma, Z. Y.; Xie, C. Z.; Xue, F.; Zhang, Y. W.; Xu, J. Y.; Yan, S. P. Study on Potential Antitumor Mechanism of a Novel Schiff Base Copper(II) Complex: Synthesis, Crystal Structure, DNA Binding, Cytotoxicity and Apoptosis Induction Activity. J. Inorg. Biochem., 2011, 105, 728-737.
32. Da Silveira, V. C.; Luz, J. S.; Oliveira, C. C.; Graziani, I.; Ciriolo, M. R.; Da Costa Ferreira. A. M. Double-Strand DNA Cleavage Induced by Oxindole-Schiff Base Copper(II) Complexes with Potential Antitumor Activity. J. Inorg. Biochem., 2008, 102, 1090-1103.
33. Li, X.; Fang, C.; Zong, Z.; Cui, L. S.; Bi, C. F.; Fan, Y. H. Synthesis, Characterization and Anticancer Activity of Two Ternary Copper(II) Schiff Base Complexes. Inorg. Chim. Acta, 2015, 432, 198-207.
34. Konarikova, K.; Andrezalova, L.; Rapta, P.; Slovakova, M.; Durackova, Z.; Laubertova, L.; Zitnanova, I. Effect of the Schiff Base Complex Diaqua-(N-Salicylidene-L-Glutamato)Copper(II) Monohydrate on Human Tumor Cells. Eur. J. Pharm., 2013, 721, 178-184.
35. Sheldrick, G. M. A Short History of SHELX. Acta. Cryst. A., 2008, 64, 112-122.

36. McKinnon, J. J.; Spackman, M. A.; Mitchell, A. S. Novel Tools for Visualizing and Exploring Intermolecular Interactions in Molecular Crystals. Acta Cryst. B., 2004, 60, 627-668.
37. Allen, F. H.; Kennard, O.; Watson, D. G.; Brammer, L.; Orpen, A. G.; Taylor, R. Tables of Bond Lengths Determined by X-ray and Neutron Diffraction. Part 1. Bond Lengths in Organic Compounds. J. Chem. Soc. Perkin Trans. II., 1987, S1-S19.
38. Bersuker, I. B. Modern Aspects of the Jahn-Teller Effect Theory and Applications to Molecular Problems. Chem. Rev., 2001, 101, 1067-1114.
39. Cutsail III, G. E.; Stein, B. W.; Subedi, D.; Smith, J. M.; Kirk, M. L.; Hoffman, B. M. EPR, ENDOR, and Electronic Structure Studies of the Jahn-Teller Distortion in an FeV Nitride. J. Am. Chem. Soc., 2014, 136, 12323-12336.
40. Zordan, F.; Brammer, L.; Sherwood, P. Supramolecular Chemistry of Halogens: Complementary Features of Inorganic (M-X) and Organic (C-X`) Halogens Applied to M-X···X`-C Halogen Bond Formation. J. Am. Chem. Soc., 2005, 127, 5979-5989.
41. Bilge, S.; Kiliç, Z.; Hayvali, Z.; Hökelek, T.; Safran, S. Intramolecular Hydrogen Bonding and Tautomerism in Schiff Bases: Part VI. Syntheses and Structural Investigation of Salicylaldimine and Naphthaldimine Derivatives. J. Chem. Sci., 2009, 127, 989-1001.
42. Zhang, S. H.; Zhao, R. X.; Li, G.; Zhang, H. Y.; Huang, Q. P.; Liang, F. P. Room Temperature Syntheses, Crystal Structures and Properties of Two New Heterometallic Polymers Based on 3-Ethoxy-2-Hydroxybenzaldehyde Ligand. J. Solid. State Chem., 2014, 220, 206-212.
43. Wei, Y. Q.; Yu, Y. F.; Wu, K. C. Highly Stable Five-Coordinated Mn(II) Polymer [Mn(Hbidc)]n (Hbidc=1H-Benzimidazole-5,6-Dicarboxylate): Crystal Structure, Antiferromegnetic Property, and Strong Long-Lived Luminescence. Cryst. Growth Des., 2008, 8, 2087-2089.
44. Liu, X. Y.; Liu, H. X.; Cen, P. P.; Zhou, H. L.; Song, W. M.; Hu, Q. L. Auxiliary Ligand-Triggered Assembly of Two Dinuclear Cu(II) Compounds with a Pyridylhydrazone Derivative: Synthesis, Crystal Structure and Magnetic Property. Inorg. Chim. Acta., 2016, 447, 12-17.

Chapter 4

Syntheses, Crystal structures, and Magnetic Properties of a Novel Decanuclear Copper Cluster Based on 3- amino-1,2,4 triazole Schiff Base at Room Temperature

Significant advancements have been achieved over the last ten years in the field of ferromagnetic and antiferromagnetic polynuclear metal clusters or cluster-based coordination polymers. These developments have led to the emergence of intriguing structural and functional applications, including optical, adsorbent, magnetic, catalytic, electronic, and fluorescent materials. Initially, single-molecule magnets (SMMs) were found, and these compounds have since been extensively studied for their ability to store information, making them promising candidates for the synthesis of innovative clusters.

In recent times, there has been a notable surge in research interest surrounding copper coordination compounds due to their diverse range of biological activities. These activities encompass antibacterial, antiviral, antileukemic, anticancer, anti-inflammatory, and anti-neurodegenerative properties. In recent times, there has been a growing interest in the utilization of copper compounds as viable alternatives to platinum-based compounds for their potential efficacy as anticancer agents. The primary area of interest for our research group pertains to the examination of the magnetic properties exhibited by copper coordination complexes. The utilization of Schiff bases in the synthesis of polynuclear clusters has been extensively employed. Mark Murrie documented the existence of two pentanuclear Mn(III) complexes, namely (HNEt$_3$)The chemical compound [Mn^{III}$_5$(μ_3-O)$_2$(CH$_3$COO)$_4$(L1)$_4$] is a subject of interest in academic research.The chemical formula 4CH$_3$-CN.4H$_2$O can be represented as (HNEt$_3$)[Mn^{III}$_5$(μ_3-O)$_2$(CH$_3$COO)$_4$(L2)$_4$]. The chemical reaction involves the conversion of N-(2-hydroxy-3-methoxybenzylene) (referred to as H$_2$L1) to CH$_3$CN and 2CH$_3$OH. In our study, we have documented the synthesis and characterization of two tetranuclear manganese(II) complexes. The first complex is denoted as [Mn$_4$(L3)$_2$(-MeCOO)$_{5.168}$(CHO$_2$)$_{0.832}$], where L3 represents N-salycilene-3,5-diamino-1,2,4-triazole. The second combination is labeled as [Mn$_4$(L4)$_2$(MeCOO)$_6$], with L4 also being N-salycilene-3,5-diamino-1,2,4-triazole. HL3 refers to a chemical compound with the systematic name 2-[(6-chloro-pyridin-2-yl)-hydrazonomethyl].The compound -6-methoxy-phenol is referred to as HL4, which is the chemical name for 2-[(6-bromo-pyridin-2-yl)- hydrazonomethyl].The compound referred to as 6-methoxyphenol is of interest in this study. Based on the aforementioned considerations, we suggest the utilization of the 3-amino-1,2,4-triazole derivative, namely (E)-2-(((4H-1,2,4-triazol-3-yl)imino)methyl)-6-methoxy phenol (referred to as H$_2$L), as a directing agent for the production of a decanuclear copper cluster. This cluster is denoted as [Cu$_{10}$(L)$_8$(CH$_3$COO)$_2$(μ$_3$-OH)$_2$]·(DMF)$_2$·(H$_2$O)$_5$ (referred to as **chapt4-1**). The core of {Cu$_{10}$O$_4$(N$_{2triazol}$)$_8$} exhibits prevalent antiferromagnetic interactions mostly due to the presence of μ$_3$-OH and μ$_2$-O$_{phenoxo}$ bridged binding modes.

Experimental Section

The Materials and Equipment

All chemicals and solvents utilized in the study were obtained commercially and employed without undergoing any purifying procedures. The PXRD spectra were acquired utilizing a PANalytical X'Pert 3 powder diffractometer. The elemental studies, specifically carbon, hydrogen, and nitrogen (CHN), were conducted with a Perkin-Elmer 2400 elemental analyzer. The Fourier-transform infrared (FT-IR) spectra were obtained by measuring KBr pellets using a Bio-Rad FTS-7 spectrophotometer over the wavenumber range of 4000 to 400 cm^{-1}. The X-ray single crystal structures were found using a SuperNova diffractometer, namely the Single source at offset, Eos configuration. Magnetic measurements were conducted using a Quantum Design PPMS model 600 magnetometer to assess the effects under an applied field of 1000 Oe at temperatures ranging from 2 to 300 K.

Synthesis

Construction of H$_2$L

A solution containing 2-Hydroxy-3-methoxy-benzaldehyde (10 mmol, 1.522 g), 3-amino-1,2,4-triazole (Hataz, 10 mmol, 0.8404 g), and ethanol (20 mL) was prepared in a 100 mL three-necked flask. The combination was subjected to reflux at a temperature of 353 K for a duration of 2 hours. The solution underwent a color transformation to a brown hue and was subjected to enrichment at a temperature of 353 K for a duration of 2 hours. A brown powder was obtained through the process of filtration, followed by washing with ethanol (3 x 9.5 mL), and subsequent air drying. The resulting yield was determined to be 2.095 g, approximately 96% of the expected yield based on Hataz. The percentage composition of H$_2$L, C$_{10}$H$_{10}$N$_4$O$_2$ (Mr = 218.21) was determined as follows: C, 55.04%; H, 4.62%; N, 25.68%. The experimentally obtained values were found to be: C, 54.95%; H, 4.69%; N, 25.73%. The infrared (IR) data for H$_2$L (KBr, cm^{-1}) are as follows: 3090 (strong), 2985 (medium), 1665 (weak), 1581 (weak), 1519 (medium), 1479 (strong), 1438 (strong), 1359 (weak), 1286 (medium), 1255 (strong), 1156 (strong), 1074 (strong), 976 (weak), 728 (medium), 627 (weak), and 472 (weak). The proton nuclear magnetic resonance (^{1}H NMR) spectrum was recorded at a frequency of 500 MHz in dimethyl sulfoxide (DMSO). The chemical shifts (δ) and coupling constants (J) for the observed peaks are as follows: a broad peak at δ 9.87 (^{1}H), a doublet at δ 9.165 (J = 5 Hz, 3H), a doublet at δ 7.375 (J = 5 Hz, 1H), a doublet at δ 7.145 (J = 5 Hz, 1H), a triplet at δ 6.90 (J = 10 Hz, 1H), and a singlet at δ 3.85 (3H).

Construction of chapt4-1

A solution containing Cu(CH$_3$COO)$_2$·H$_2$O (0.5 mmol, 0.099 g), H$_2$L (0.5 mmol, 0.1091 g), DMF (5 mL), and acetonitrile (5 mL) was subjected to stirring for a duration of 10 minutes at ambient temperature. The combination was introduced into a microbottle reactor and allowed to react at ambient temperature for a duration of one week. Rhombohedral blue crystals of chapt4-1 were successfully synthesized, with a yield of 0.085 g, about 61.75% depending on the amount of Cu^{II} used. The analysis of compound **chapt4-1**, $C_{90}H_{96}Cu_{10}N_{34}O_{29}$ (molecular weight = 2753.51 g/mol), yielded the following percentages: carbon (C) 39.26%, hydrogen (H) 3.51%, and nitrogen (N) 17.29%. The elemental composition of the sample was determined to be as follows: carbon (C) at a mass fraction of 39.14%, hydrogen (H) at a mass fraction of 3.59%, and nitrogen (N) at a mass fraction of 17.37%. The infrared (IR) spectrum for compound **chapt4-1** (KBr, cm^{-1}) exhibits the following characteristic peaks: a broad peak at 3294 cm^{-1}, a sharp peak at 1662 cm^{-1}, a medium peak at 1513 cm^{-1}, a sharp peak at 1413 cm^{-1}, a weak peak at 1236 cm^{-1}, a sharp peak at 1154 cm^{-1}, a sharp peak at 1032 cm^{-1}, a weak peak at 833 cm^{-1}, weak peaks at 819 cm^{-1}, 673 cm^{-1}, and 558 cm^{-1}.

The measurement of magnetic properties

To prevent any loss of solvent, the magnetic properties measurements were conducted on crushed crystals obtained from recently isolated samples. The granules were combined with a lubricating substance and encapsulated within gelatin shells. The magnetic susceptibilities were determined by conducting measurements in an applied field of 1000 Oe. The molar susceptibility (χ_m) was adjusted for the presence of the sample holder and the diamagnetic effect of all atoms using Pascal's tables.

Structure of Crystal Determination

The diffraction data for compound **chapt4-1** was obtained using a SuperNova Single source with an offset Eos, employing graphite monochromated Mo–Kα radiation ($\lambda = 0.71073$ Å). The θ scan mode was utilized within the angular range of 2.82° to 25.01° (**chapt4-1**). The raw frame data were processed using the CrysAlisPro software. The structure of compound 1 was determined through the application of direct methods using SHELXT. Subsequently, a refinement process was conducted using full-matrix least-squares on F^2, employing the SHELXL-2018 software within the OLEX-2 graphical user interface. The application of an empirical absorption correction was conducted using spherical harmonics, which was performed within the SCALE3 ABSPACK scaling method. Anisotropic refinement was performed on all atoms except for hydrogen. The positions of all hydrogen atoms were determined geometrically and improved using the riding model. Several computer applications commonly used in scientific research include CrysAlis PRO, developed by Agilent Technologies and available in Version 1.171.37.35, SHELXL, and Olex2. The summary of crystal data, data collecting, and structural refinement details may be found in Table 4-1. The bond lengths and angles for compound **chapt4-1** have been documented in Table 4-2.

Table 4-1. The refining of crystal data and structures for chapt4-1 is being discussed.

Formula	$C_{90}H_{96}Cu_{10}N_{34}O_{29}$
Fw	2753.51
Crystal system	Monoclinic
Space group	*I2/c*
a (Å)	14.736(1)
b (Å)	28.713(1)
c (Å)	28.898(1)
α (°)	90
β (°)	97.944(3)
γ (°)	90

V (Å^3)	12109.9(6)		
F(000)	5584		
Z	4		
D_c (g cm^{-3})	1.510		
μ (mm^{-1})	1.800		
θ range (°)	2.82–25.01		
Ref. meas. / indep.	26517/ 10643		
Obs. ref.[$I > 2\sigma(I)$]	8027		
R_{int}	0.0311		
R_1 [$I \geq 2\sigma(I)$] [a]	0.0590		
ωR_2(all data)[b]	0.2004		
Goof	1.065		
$\Delta\rho$(max, min) (e Å^{-3})	1.090, -0.625		
CCDC	2017049		

[a] $R_1 = \Sigma||F_o| - |F_c||/\Sigma|F_o|$. [b] $wR_2 = [\Sigma w(|F_o^2|-|F_c^2|)^2/\Sigma w(|F_o^2|)^2]^{1/2}$.

Table 4-2. The bond lengths (Å) and angles (in degrees) for chapt4-1 are presented below.

Cu1–O5	1.867(5)	Cu3–N6	1.984(5)
Cu1–O7	1.938(4)	Cu3–N3	1.988(5)
Cu1–N9	1.978(6)	Cu3–N11	2.013(5)
Cu1–O10	1.992(6)	Cu3–O11	2.039(4)
Cu1–O8	2.322(5)	Cu3–N14	2.216(5)
Cu2–N7	1.959(5)	Cu4–O1	1.927(4)
Cu2–O7	1.970(4)	Cu4–N15	1.954(5)
Cu2–O9	1.994(5)	Cu4–N1	1.972(5)
Cu2–N10	2.007(5)	Cu4–O11	2.130(4)
Cu2–N13	2.190(5)	Cu4–N2	2.229(5)
Cu5–O3	1.889(4)	Cu5–N4^i	1.988(5)
Cu5–O11	1.937(4)	Cu5–N5	1.995(5)
Cu1···Cu2	2.924(1)	Cu2···Cu3	3.560(5)
Cu5···Cu3	3.154(1)	Cu4···Cu5	3.696(5)
Cu4···Cu3	3.323(4)		
O5–Cu1–O7	169.1(2)	N6–Cu3–N3	159.5(2)
O5–Cu1–N9	93.0(2)	N6–Cu3–N11	92.7(2)
O7–Cu1–N9	89.3(2)	N3–Cu3–N11	93.6(2)
O5–Cu1–O10	91.1(3)	N6–Cu3–O11	84.8(2)
O7–Cu1–O10	91.3(2)	N3–Cu3–O11	86.7(2)
N9–Cu1–O10	154.8(2)	N11–Cu3–O11	173.2(2)
O5–Cu1–O8	94.1(2)	N6–Cu3–N14	97.1(2)
O7–Cu1–O8	75.4(2)	N3–Cu3–N14	100.5(2)
N9–Cu1–O8	116.4(2)	N11–Cu3–N14	102.8(2)
O10–Cu1–O8	88.0(2)	O11–Cu3–N14	83.9(2)
N7–Cu2–O7	164.6(2)	O1–Cu4–N15	87.6(2)
N7–Cu2–O9	88.6(2)	O1–Cu4–N1	91.3(2)
O7–Cu2–O9	88.7(2)	N15–Cu4–N1	178.5(2)
N7–Cu2–N10	90.6(2)	O1–Cu4–O11	150.3(2)
O7–Cu2–N10	85.7(2)	N15–Cu4–O11	85.6(2)
O9–Cu2–N10	155.5(2)	N1–Cu4–O11	94.8(2)
N7–Cu2–N13	110.6(2)	O1–Cu4–N2	125.5(2)
O7–Cu2–N13	84.8(2)	N15–Cu4–N2	91.5(2)
O9–Cu2–N13	97.3(2)	N1–Cu4–N2	90.0(2)
N10–Cu2–N13	105.9(2)	O11–Cu4–N2	83.6(2)
O3–Cu5–O11	164.2(2)	O3–Cu5–N5	93.1(2)

O3−Cu5−N4ⁱ	84.4(2)	O11−Cu5−N5	95.3(2)
O11−Cu5−N4ⁱ	89.2(2)	N4ⁱ−Cu5−N5	171.0(2)
Cu1−O7−Cu2	96.9(2)	Cu5−O11−Cu3	104.9(2)
Cu3−O11−Cu4	105.7(2)	Cu5−O11−Cu4	130.6(2)

Symmetry code: (i) 1.5 + x, 0.5 + y, 0.5 + z.

Outcomes and Analysis

The Detailed Description of the Crystal Structure

The utilization of single-crystal X-ray diffraction techniques has provided evidence that compound **chapt4-1** is a decanuclear cluster containing copper. This cluster has a crystalline structure that belongs to the monoclinic crystal system, with the *I2/c* space group (as depicted in Figure 4-1 and Scheme 4-1). The researchers discovered that the asymmetric unit of compound **chapt4-1** is composed of a unit consisting of [Cu$_5$(L)$_4$(-CH$_3$COO)(μ$_3$-OH)]. In this study, it is seen that five copper atoms exhibit distinct coordination environments. The Cu1 atom is coordinated with three O and one N atoms from two distinct L ligands [Cu1-O5 = 1.867(5) Å; Cu1-O7 = 1.938(4) Å; Cu1-O8 = 2.322(5) Å; Cu1-N9 = 1.978(6) Å], as well as one O atom from an acetate group [Cu1-O10 = 1.992(6) Å]. This coordination arrangement results in the formation of a distorted tetragonal pyramid. It is important to acknowledge that the τ_5 value exhibits a numerical approximation of 0.24, indicating its proximity to zero. The Cu2 atom exhibits a coordination geometry characterized by a distorted tetragonal pyramid. This coordination is achieved through the bonding of one oxygen (O) atom and three nitrogen (N) atoms from three distinct L ligands. The bond lengths for these interactions are as follows: Cu2-N7 = 1.959(5) Å, Cu2-O7 = 1.970(4) Å, Cu2-N10 = 2.007(5) Å, and Cu2-N13 = 2.190(5) Å. Additionally, one oxygen atom from an acetate group forms a bond with the Cu2 atom, with a bond length of Cu2-O9 = 1.994(5) Å. In this context, the value of τ_5 is determined to be 0.15, which might be considered as approaching zero. The Cu3 atom exhibits coordination with four N atoms from four distinct L ligands, resulting in the formation of a tetragonal pyramid shape. The bond lengths between Cu3 and the N atoms are as follows: Cu3-N6 = 1.984(5) Å, Cu3-N3 = 1.988(5) Å, Cu3-N11 = 2.013(5) Å, and Cu3-N14 = 2.216(5) Å. Additionally, Cu3 is coordinated with one μ$_3$-OH, with a bond length of Cu3-O11 = 2.039(4) Å. The coordination number, denoted as τ_5, is calculated to be 0.23. The Continuous Shape Measure (CShM) computations revealed that the coordination environment of the Cu4 atom is positioned at an intermediate point between a square pyramid and a trigonal bipyramid, with a value of τ_5 equal to 0.47. This value is in close proximity to the median value of 0.5. In this context, Cu4 is coordinated by three nitrogen (N) atoms and one oxygen (O) atom from three distinct ligands, denoted as L. The bond lengths are as follows: Cu4-O1 = 1.927(4) Å, Cu4-N15 = 1.954(5) Å, Cu4-N1 = 1.972(5) Å, Cu4-N2 = 2.229(5) Å. Additionally, there is one hydroxide ion (OH-) coordinated to Cu4, denoted as μ_3-OH, with a bond length of Cu4-O11 = 2.130(4) Å. It is intriguing to note that the coordination number of Cu1, Cu2, Cu3, and Cu4 is five, whereas the coordination number of Cu5 is four. In this case, the Cu5 atom exhibits a distorted parallelogram geometry coordination, wherein it is coordinated by one O atom and two N atoms from two separate L ligands. The distances between Cu5 and the coordinating atoms are as follows: Cu5-N5 = 1.995(5) Å, Cu5-O3 = 1.889(4) Å, Cu5-N4ⁱ = 1.988(5) Å (symmetry code: (i) 1.5 + x, 0.5 + y, 0.5 + z). Additionally, Cu5 is also coordinated by one μ_3-OH ligand, with a Cu5-O11 distance of 1.937(4) Å.

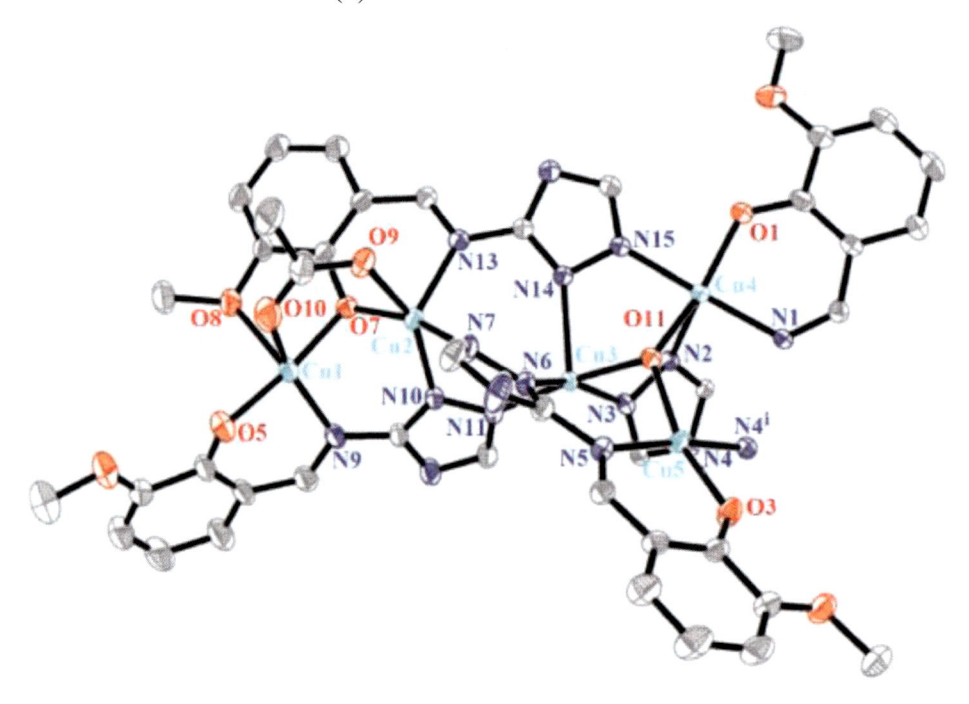

Figure 4-1. The asymmetric unit of chapt4-1, excluding hydrogen atoms and solvent molecules.

Scheme 4-1. The asymmetric unit of chapt4-1, excluding hydrogen atoms and solvent molecules.

Furthermore, the bond valence model can be utilized to ascertain the atomic valences of five copper ions. Based on the proposed model, the aggregate of bond valences encompassing an ion is equivalent to its ionic charge or valence. In this study, the bond valences (s) were determined using the formula $s = \exp[r_0 - r]/B$, where B is equal to 0.37. The values of r_0 were obtained from the reference, with $r_0 = 1.679$ for Cu(II)-O pairs and $r_0 = 1.61$ for Cu(II)-N pairs. It is apparent that the computed bond valence sums exhibit a high level of concordance with the anticipated atomic valence values. Consequently, it can be inferred that the five Cu cations possess a valence state of undetermined magnitude. The user's text does not contain any information to be rewritten. The decanuclear copper cluster was created by linking and assembling the asymmetric unit $[Cu_5(L)_4(CH_3COO)(\mu_3\text{-}OH)]$ of compound **chapt4-1**, utilizing two triazol of the L ligand as bridging units. There is a weak interaction between the $[Cu_5(L)_4(CH_3COO)(\mu_3\text{-}OH)]$ complex and the solvent water (Cu5-O12, 2.828(5) Å). The decanuclear copper cluster forms 3D supramolecular networks through extensive O–H···O hydrogen bonding interactions (O11-H11···O15, 2.802(9) Å; O12-H12A···O14[ii], 2.993(10) Å; O12-H12B···O14[iv], 2.926(10) Å; symmetry codes: (ii) x + 1/2,-y + 3/2, z; (iv)-x + 1/2,-y + 3/2,-z + 1/2). Additionally, weak C-H···O hydrogen bonds are observed (C1-H1B···O16[i], 3.564(19) Å; C10- H10A···O14[ii], 3.422(9) Å; C48-H48C···O15[iii], 3.19(2) Å; symmetry codes: (i) -x + 1, y, -z + 1/2; (iii) -x, y, -z + 1/2), as well as weak C-H···N hydrogen bonds (C46-H46···N14, 3.251(16) Å; C46-H46···N15, 3.300(17) Å). It is important to acknowledge that the ligand L exhibits three distinct coordination modes: the first mode is μ_4-L-$\kappa^6O^1,O^2:O^2,N^1,N^2,N^3$ (Scheme 4-2a), the second mode is μ_3-L-κ^4O^1,N^1,N^2,N^3 (Scheme 4-2b), and the third mode is μ_4-L-$\kappa^5O^1,N^1,N^2,N^3,N^4$ (Scheme 4-2c).

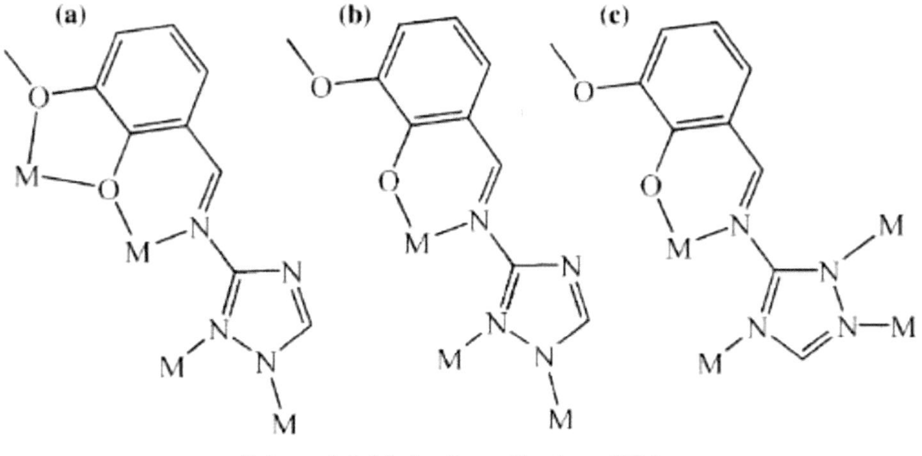

Scheme 4-2. Mode of coordination of H₂L

Magnetic Qualities

The magnetic susceptibilities (χ_M) of **chapt4-1** were determined through the measurement of crushed single crystalline samples. The phase purity of **chapt4-1** was confirmed by examining the PXRD patterns. The direct current (DC) magnetic susceptibilities of a sample were measured under an applied magnetic field of 1 kilo-Oersted (kOe) over a temperature range of 2 to 300 Kelvin (K).

Figure 4-2 presents plots depicting the relationship between the molar magnetic susceptibility (xM) and the product of the molar magnetic susceptibility and temperature ($\chi_M T$) for ten Cu^{II} ions. At room temperature, the observed $\chi_M T$ value is significantly more than the predicted spin-only value for the ten non-interacting Cu^{II} ions. The spin-only value is calculated using the equation $\chi_M T = 10(N\beta^2 g^2/3k)S(S+1)$, where N, β, g, k, S, and T represent their conventional definitions. Assuming g = 2.1 and S = 1/2, the spin-only value is 3.75 cm³ Kmol⁻¹. However, the observed $\chi_M T$ value at normal temperature is 10.04 cm³Kmol⁻¹. As the temperature falls, the value of $\chi_M T$ exhibits a progressive reduction, ultimately reaching its minimum value of 4.01 cm³ Kmol⁻¹ at a temperature of 2 K. The observed magnetic behavior in **chapt4-1** suggests the presence of an anti-ferromagnetic coupling among the ten Cu^{II} ions or a zero-field splitting effect in the ground state.

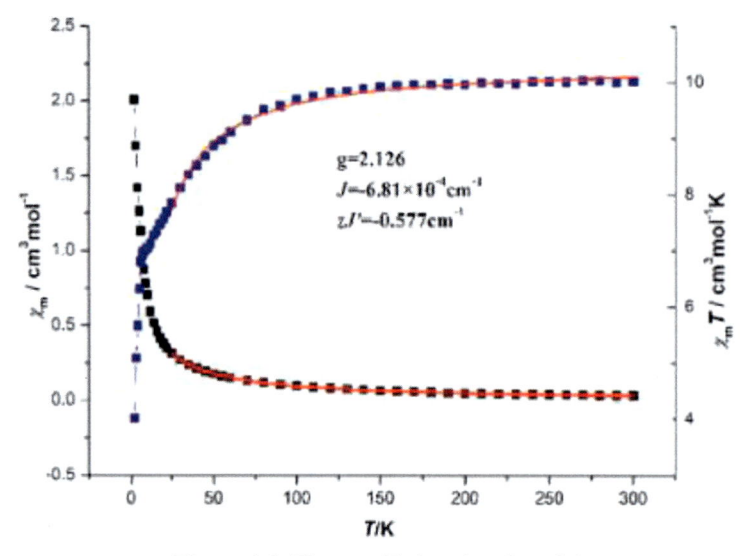

Figure 4-2. The xm -T plots for chapt4-1

The reciprocal susceptibility (χ_M^{-1}) above 50 K can be described by the Curie-Weiss equation ($\chi_M = C/(T - \theta)$), where the Weiss constant (θ) is -5.52 K and the Curie constant (C) is 10.22 cm³Kmol⁻¹. The presence of intramolecular antiferromagnetic interactions among the ten Cu^{II} ions is further corroborated by the negative Weiss constant.

The two samples were fitted to the exchange Hamiltonian (Eq. 1) and the equation for vM (Eq. 2) to determine their respective dates.

$$\hat{H} = -2J_1(\hat{S}_1\hat{S}_5 + \hat{S}_2\hat{S}_5 + \hat{S}_3\hat{S}_5 + \hat{S}_4\hat{S}_5 + \hat{S}_1\hat{S}_2 + \hat{S}_2\hat{S}_3 + \hat{S}_3\hat{S}_4 + \hat{S}_4\hat{S}_1)$$

(1)

$$\chi_M = \frac{2N g^2 \beta^2}{kT} \times \frac{9e^{2J/kT} + 55e^{6J/kT} + 140e^{12J/kT} + 180e^{20J/kT} + 165e^{30J/kT} + 91e^{42J/kT}}{4 + 27e^{2J/kT} + 55e^{6J/kT} + 70e^{12J/kT} + 54e^{20J/kT} + 33e^{30J/kT} + 13e^{42J/kT}}$$

(2)

The coupling constant between the Cu^{II} ions is denoted by J. In the temperature range of 300–30 K, the most suitable fit resulted in the following values: g = 2.126, J = -6.81 × 10⁻⁴ cm⁻¹, and zJ = -0.577 cm^{-1}, as depicted in Figure 4-2. The findings suggest that there exists a somewhat feeble antiferromagnetic interaction among ten Cu^{II} ions. The findings from previous research on hydroxo- and phenoxo-bridged copper(II) compounds suggest that the total coupling in these systems can be affected by the lengths between copper atoms (Cu-Cu distances) and the angles formed by copper-oxygen-copper bonds (Cu-O-Cu angles). In general, it can be observed that there exists an inverse relationship between the distance separating copper (Cu) atoms, denoted as Cu-Cu distance, and the strength of the exchange interaction. When the Cu–O–Cu angle is 97.51°, it is anticipated that ferromagnetic interactions would occur. Conversely, if the angle exceeds 97.51°, the interaction through the Cu–O–Cu pathway is mostly anti-ferromagnetic, with the amplitude of this interaction increasing as the angle increases. In the first case, there are three magnetic exchange angles greater than 97.51°, specifically measuring 104.9(2), 105.7(2), and 130.6(2)°, respectively (Table 4-2). However, in the second case, the magnetic exchange angle through μ_2-O$_{phenoxo}$ bridging is slightly less than 97.51°. The observed changes in the magnetic exchange Cu-O-Cu angles and copper-copper separations in complex **chapt4-1**, from 96.9(2) to 130.6(2)° and 2.924(1)-3.696(5)Å respectively, suggest the presence of both ferromagnetic and antiferromagnetic competition. Consequently, it can be observed that complex **chapt4-1** exhibits a relatively low strength of antiferromagnetic interaction.

AC susceptibility experiments were conducted within the temperature range of 2-10 K, with frequencies of 10 Hz and 997 Hz, as depicted in Figure 4-3. There is no discernible frequency dependence observed between 2 and 10 K for both in-phase and out-of-phase ac susceptibility signals. The magnetic data obtained from many experiments consistently demonstrate that complex **chapt4-1** does not exhibit single-molecule magnet (SCM) behavior above a temperature threshold of 2 K.

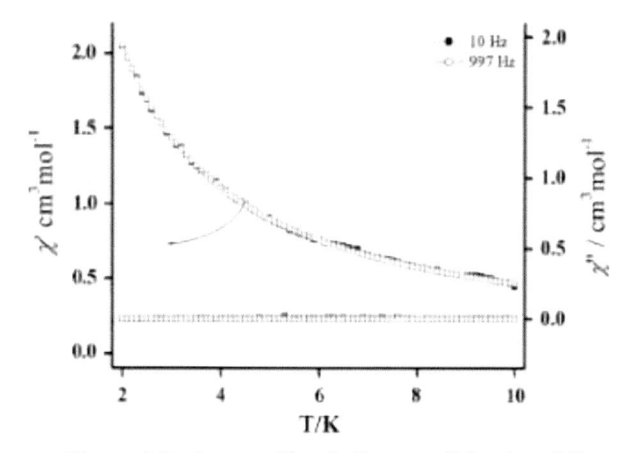

Figure 4-3. χ' versus T and χ'' versus T for chapt4-1

A new decanuclear Cu(II) cluster was produced and further analyzed. The solid-state structure was effectively characterized through the implementation of various analytical techniques, including infrared spectroscopy, elemental analysis, and single crystal X-ray diffractometry. The examination of the magnetic characteristics of complex **chapt4-1** indicates the presence of a rivalry between ferromagnetic and antiferromagnetic interactions. Complex **chapt4-1** ultimately develops a feeble antiferromagnetic contact among a total of 10 Cu II ions. The ligand L demonstrates three distinct coordination patterns.

References

1. Zhao, Y.; Wang, Y. J.; Wang, N.; Zheng, P.; Fu, H. R.; Han, M. L.; Ma, L. F.; Wang, L. Y. Tetraphenylethylene-Decorated Metal-Organic Frameworks as Energy-Transfer Platform for the Detection of Nitro-Antibiotics and White-Light Emission. Inorg. Chem., 2019, 58, 12700.
2. Xiao, Y.; Zhang, C.; Qin, Y.; Wu, C. C.; Zheng, X. Highly Efficient Removal of As(V) from Aqueous Solutions Using a Novel Octanuclear Zn(II)-Based Polymer: Synthesis, Structure, Properties and Optimization Using a Response Surface Methodology. J. Solid. State. Chem., 2018, 264, 6-14.
3. Zhang, C.; Xiao, Y.; Qin, Y.; Sun, Q. C.; Zhang, S. H. A Novel Highly Efficient Adsorbent $\{[Co_4(L)_2(\mu_3\text{-}OH)_2(H_2O)_3(4,4'\text{-}bipy)_2]\cdot(H_2O)_2\}_n$: Synthesis, Crystal Structure, Magnetic and Arsenic (V) Absorption Capacity. J. Solid. State. Chem., 2018, 261, 22-30.
4. Xiao, Y.; Liu, Y. Q.; Li, G.; Huang, P. Microwave-Assisted Synthesis, Structure and Properties of a Co-Crystal Compound with 2-Ethoxy-6-Methyliminomethyl-Phenol. Supramol. Chem., 2015, 27(3), 161-166.
5. Ma, L. F.; Han, M. L.; Qin, J. H.; Wang, L. Y.; Du, M. MnII Coordination Polymers Based on Bi-, Tri-, and Tetranuclear and Polymeric Chain Building Units: Crystal Structures and Magnetic Properties. Inorg. Chem., 2012, 51, 9431-9442.
6. Zhang, S. H.; Li, N.; Ge, C. M.; Feng, C.; Ma, L. F. Structures and Magnetism of $\{Ni_2Na_2\}$, $\{Ni_4\}$ and $\{Ni_6^{II}Ni^{III}\}$ 2-Hydroxy-3-Alkoxy-Benzaldehyde Clusters. Dalton Trans., 2011, 40, 3000-3007.
7. Wu, Y. P.; Tian, J. W.; Liu, S.; Li, B.; Zhao, J.; Ma, L. F.; Li, D. S.; Lan, Y. Q.; Bu, X. Bi-Microporous Metal–Organic Frameworks with Cubane $[M_4(OH)_4]$ (M=Ni, Co) Clusters and Pore-Space Partition for Electrocatalytic Methanol Oxidation Reaction. Angew. Chem. Int. Edit., 2019, 58, 12185-12189.
8. Chen, Z. H.; Zhang, S. H.; Zhang, S. M.; Sun, Q. C.; Xiao, Y.; Wang, K. Cadmium-Based Coordination Polymers from 1D to 3D: Synthesis, Structures, and Photoluminescent and Electrochemiluminescent Properties. Chempluschem, 2019, 84, 190-202.
9. Zhang, S. M.; Zhang, H. Y.; Qin, Q. P.; Fei, J. W.; Zhang, S. H. Syntheses, Crystal Structures and Biological Evaluation of Two New Cu(II) and Co(II) Complexes Based on (E)-2-(((4H-1,2,4-Triazol-4-Yl)Imino)Methyl)-6-Methoxyphenol. J. Inorg. Biochem., 2019, 193, 52-59.
10. Ahamad, M. N.; Sama, F.; Akhtar, M.; Chen, Y. C.; Tong, M. L.; Ahmad, M.; Shahid, M.; Sahid, H.; Khan, K. A Disc-like Co7 Cluster with a Solvent Dependent Catecholase Activity. New J. Chem., 2017, 41, 14057-14061.
11. Raizada, M.; Sama, F.; Ashafaq, M.; Shahid, M.; Ahmad, M.; Siddiqi, Z. A. New Hybrid Polyoxovanadate-Cu Complex with V⋯H Interactions and Dual Aqueous-Phase Sensing Properties for Picric Acid and Pd2+: X-ray Analysis, Magnetic and

Theoretical Studies, and Mechanistic Insights into the Hybrid's Sensing Capabilities. J. Mater. Chem. C., 2017, 5, 9315-9330.

12. Zhang, S. H.; Zhang, Y. D.; Zou, H. H.; Guo, J. J.; Li, H. P.; Song, Y.; Liang, H. A Family of Cubane Cobalt and Nickel Clusters: Syntheses, Structures and Magnetic Properties. Inorg. Chim. Acta., 2013, 396, 119-125.

13. Li, J.; Gómez-Coca, S.; Dolinar, B. S.; Yang, L.; Yu, F.; Kong, M.; Zhang, Y. Q.; Song, Y.; Dunbar, K. R. Hexagonal Bipyramidal Dy(III) Complexes as a Structural Archetype for Single-Molecule Magnets. Inorg. Chem., 2019, 58, 2610-2617.

14. Fetoh, A.; Cosquer, G.; Morimoto, M.; Irie, M.; El-Gammal, O.; Abu El-Reash, G. M.; Breedlove, B. K.; Yamashita M. Synthesis, Structures, and Magnetic Properties of Two Coordination Assemblies of Mn(III) Single Molecule Magnets Bridged Via Photochromic Diarylethene Ligands. Inorg. Chem., 2019, 58, 2307-2314.

15. Jia, J. H.; Li, Q. W.; Chen, Y. C.; Liu, J. L.; Tong, M. L. Luminescent Single-Molecule Magnets Based on Lanthanides: Design Strategies, Recent Advances and Magneto-Luminescent Studies. Coordin. Chem. Rev., 2019, 378, 365-381.

16. Long, J.; Guari, Y.; Ferreira, R. A. S.; Carlos, L. D.; Larionova, J. Recent Advances in Luminescent Lanthanide Based Single-Molecule Magnets. Coordin. Chem. Rev., 2018, 363, 57-70.

17. Sessoli, R.; Tsai, H. L.; Schake, A. R.; Sheyi, S.; Vincent, J. B.; Folting, K.; Gatteschi, D.; Christou, G.; Hendrickson, D. N. High-Spin Molecules: [Mn$_{12}$O$_{12}$(O$_2$CR)$_{16}$(H$_2$O)$_4$]. J. Am. Chem. Soc., 1993, 115(5), 1804-1816.

18. Sessoli, R.; Gatteschi, D.; Caneschi, A.; Novak, M. A. Magnetic Bistability in a Metal-Ion Cluster. Nature, 1993, 365, 141-143.

19. Qin, X. Y.; Yang, L. C.; Le, F. L.; Yu, Q. Q.; Sun, D. D.; Liu, Y. N.; Liu, J. Structures and Anti-Cancer Properties of Two Binuclear Copper Complexes. Dalton Trans., 2013, 42(41), 14681-14684.

20. Kalinowska-Lis, U.; Szewczyk, E. M.; Chęcińska, L.; Wojciechowski, J. M.; Wolf, W. M.; Ochocki, J. Synthesis, Characterization, and Antimicrobial Activity of Silver(I) and Copper(II) Complexes of Phosphate Derivatives of Pyridine And Benzimidazole. Chemmedchem, 2014, 9, 169-176.

21. Ng, N. S.; Leverett, P.; Hibbs, D. E.; Yang, Q. F.; Bulanadi, J. C.; Wu, M. J.; Aldrich-Wright, J. R. The Antimicrobial Properties of Some Copper(II) and Platinum(II) 1,10-Phenanthroline Complexes. Dalton Trans., 2013, 42(9), 3196-3209.

22. Ambika, S.; Arunachalam, S.; Arun, R.; Premkumar, K. Synthesis, Nucleic Acid Binding, Anticancer and Antimicrobial Activities of Polymer-Copper(II) Complexes Containing Intercalative Phenanthroline Ligand(DPQ). Rsc. Adv., 2013, 3(37), 16456-16468.

23. Pelosi, G.; Bisceglie, F.; Bignami, F.; Ronzi, P.; Schiavone, P.; Re, M. C.; Casoli, C.; Pilotti, E. Antiretroviral Activity of Thiosemicarbazone Metal Complexes. J. Med. Chem., 2010, 53(24), 8765-8769.

24. Katsarou, M. E.; Efthimiadou, E. K.; Psomas, G.; Karaliota, A.; Vourloumis, D. Novel Copper(II) Complex of N-Propyl-Norfloxacin and 1,10-Phenanthroline with Enhanced Antileukemic and DNA Nuclease Activities. J. Med. Chem., 2008, 51(3), 470-478.

25. Liu, W. K.; Gust, R. Metal N-Heterocyclic Carbene Complexes as Potential Antitumor Metallodrugs. Chem. Soc. Rev., 2013, 42(2), 755-773.
26. Huang, Q. P.; Zhang, S. N.; Zhang, S. H.; Wang, K.; Xiao, Y. Solvent and Copper Ion-Induced Synthesis of Pyridyl-Pyrazole-3-One Derivatives: Crystal Structure, Cytotoxicity. Molecules, 2017, 22(11), 1813.
27. Qin, X. Y.; Wang, Y. N.; Yang, X. P.; Liang, J. J.; Liu, J. L.; Luo, Z. H. Synthesis, Characterization, and Anticancer Activity of Two Mixed Ligand Copper(II) Complexes by Regulating the VEGF/VEGFR2 Signaling Pathway. Dalton Trans., 2017, 46(47), 16446-16454.
28. Zhao, X. F.; Ouyang, Y.; Liu, Y. Z.; Su, Q. J.; Tian, H.; Xie, C. Z.; Xu, J. Y. Two Polypyridyl Copper(II) Complexes: Synthesis, Crystal Structure and Interaction with DNA and Serum Protein in Vitro. New. J. Chem., 2014, 38(3), 955-965.
29. Zhang, P. L.; Hou, X. X.; Liu, M. R.; Huang, F. P.; Qin, X. Y. Two Novel Chiral Tetranucleate Copper-Based Complexes: Crystal Structures, Nanoparticles, and Inhibiting Angiogenesis and the Growth of Human Breast Cancer by Regulating the VEGF/VEGFR2 Signal Pathway in Vitro. Dalton Trans., 2020, 49(18), 6043-6055.
30. Psomas, G.; Kessissoglou, D. P. Quinolones and Non-Steroidal Anti-Inflammatory Drugs Interacting with Copper(II), Nickel(II), Cobalt(II) and Zinc(II): Structural Features, Biological Evaluation and Perspectives. Dalton Trans., 2013, 42(18), 6252-6272.
31. Brown, D. H.; Smith, W. E.; Teape, J. W.; Lewis, A. J. Antiinflammatory Effects of Some Copper Complexes. J. Med. Chem., 1980, 23(7), 729-734.
32. Fernández-Bachiller, M. I.; Pérez, C.; González-Muñoz, G. C.; Conde, S.; López, M. G.; Villarroya, M.; García, A. G.; Rodríguez-Franco, M. I. Novel Tacrine-8-Hydroxyquinoline Hybrids as Multifunctional Agents for the Treatment of Alzheimer's Disease, with Neuroprotective, Cholinergic, Antioxidant, and Copper-Complexing Properties. J. Med. Chem., 2010, 53(13), 4927-4937.
33. Griffith, D.; Parker, J. P.; Marmion, C. J. Enzyme Inhibition as a Key Target for the Development of Novel Metal-Based Anti-Cancer Therapeutics. Anti-Cancer Agent. Me., 2010, 10(5), 354-370.
34. Zhang, C., Yang, L., Chen, H., Zhang, S. H. A Novel Dinuclear Copper(II) Complex: Synthesis, Crystal Structure, Properties and Hirshfeld Surface Analysis. Chin. J. Struct. Chem., 2017, 36, 1904–1911.
35. Zhang, C.; Ma, X. D.; Chen, Z. H.; Zhang, S. H.; Hai, H. Synthesis, Structure and Properties of a Novel Tetranuclear Copper Cluster-Based Polymer with Di-Schiff-Base. J. Clust. Sci., 2017, 28(6), 3241-3252.
36. Zhang, H. Y.; Wang, W.; Chen, H.; Zhang, S. H.; Li, Y. Five Novel Dinuclear Copper(II) Complexes: Crystal Structures, Properties, Hirshfeld Surface Analysis and Vitro Antitumor Activity Study. Inorg. Chim. Acta., 2016, 453, 507-515.
37. Liu, X.; Hamon, J. R. Recent Developments in Penta-, Hexa- and Heptadentate Schiff Base Ligands and Their Metal Complexes. Coordin. Chem. Rev., 2019, 389, 94-118.
38. Kaczmarek, M. T.; Zabiszak, M.; Nowak, M.; Jastrzab, R. Lanthanides: Schiff Base Complexes, Applications in Cancer Diagnosis, Therapy, and Antibacterial Activity. Coordin. Chem. Rev., 2018, 370, 42-54.

39. Ojea, M. J. H.; Hay, M. A.; Cioncoloni, G.; Craig, G. A.; Wilson, C.; Shiga, T.; Oshio, H.; Symes, M. D.; Murrie, M. Ligand-Directed Synthesis of {Mn_5^III} Twisted Bow-Ties. Dalton Trans., 2017, 46(34), 11201-11207.
40. Chen, Y.; Zhang, S.; Xiao, Y.; Zhang, S. Synthesis, Crystal Structures and Magnetic and Electrochemiluminescence Properties of Three Manganese(II) Com¬plexes. Acta. Cryst. C., 2020, 76(3), 236-243.
41. Sheldrick, G. M. Crystal Structure Refinement with SHELXL. Acta Cryst. C., 2015, 71(1), 3-8.
42. Dolomanov, O. V.; Bourhis, L. J.; Gildea, R. J.; Howard, J. A. K.; Puschmann, H. OLEX2: a Complete Structure Solution, Refinement and Analysis Program. J. Appl. Cryst., 2009, 42(2), 339-341.
43. Alvarez, S.; Alemany, P.; Casanova, D.; Cirera, J.; Llunell, M.; Avnir, D. Shape Maps and Polyhedral Interconversion Paths in Transition Metal Chemistry. Coordin. Chem. Rev., 205, 249, 1693-1708.
44. Llunell, M.; Casanova, D.; Cirera, J.; Bofill, J.; Alemany, P.; Alvarez, S.; Pinsky, M.; Avnir, D. SHAPE v.2.1. Program for the Calculation of Continuous Shape Measures of Polygonal and Polyhedral Molecular Fragments (University of Barcelona, Barcelona, 2013).
45. Brown, I. D.; Altermatt, D. Bond-Valence Parameters Obtained from a Systematic Analysis of the Inorganic Crystal Structure Database. Acta. Cryst. B., 1985, 41, 244-247.
46. Brese, N. E.; O'Keeffe, M. Bond-valence Parameters for Solids. Acta Cryst. B., 1991, 47, 192-197.
47. Brown, I. D. Recent Developments in the Methods and Applications of the Bond Valence Model. Chem. Rev., 2009, 109(12), 6858-6919.
48. Kahn, O. Molecular magnetism (VCH Publications, New York, 1993).
49. Nandi, N. B.; Purkayastha, A.; Roy, S.; Kłak, J.; Ganguly, R.; Alkorta, I.; Misra, T. K. Tetranuclear Copper(II) Cubane Complexes Derived from Self-Assembled 1,3-Dimethyl-5-(O-Phenolate-Azo)-6-Aminouracil: Structures, Non-Covalent Interactions and Magnetic Property. New J. Chem., 2021, 45, 2742-2753.
50. Papadakis, R.; Rivière, E.; Giorgi, M.; Jamet, H.; Rousselot Pailley, P.; Réglier, M.; Simaan, A. J.; Tron, T. Structural and Magnetic Characterization of a Tetranuclear Copper(II) Cubane Stabilized by Intramolecular Metal Cation-π Interactions. Inorg. Chem., 2013, 52, 5824-5830.
51. Haddad, M. S.; Wilson, S. R.; Hodgson, D. J.; Hendrickson, D. N. Magnetic Exchange Interactions in Binuclear Copper(II) Complexes with Only a Single Hydroxo Bridge: the X-ray Structure of Mu.-Hydroxo-Tetrakis(2,2'-Bipyridine)Dicopper(II) Perchlorate. J. Am. Chem. Soc., 1981, 103, 384-391.
52. Xie, Y. S.; Ni, J.; Zheng, F.; Cui, Y.; Wang, Q. G.; Ng, S. W.; Zhu, W. H. Tetra- and Binuclear Complexes of Hydroxy-Rich Ligands: Supramolecular Structures, Stabilization of Unusual Water Clusters, and Magnetic Properties. Cryst. Growth Des., 2009, 9(1), 118-126.
53. Dias, S. S. P.; André, V.; Kłak, J.; Duarte, M. T.; Kirillov, A. M. Topological Diversity of Supramolecular Networks Constructed from Copper(II) Aminoalcohol Blocks and

2,6-Naphthalenedicarboxylate Linkers: Self-Assembly Synthesis, Structural Features, and Magnetic Properties. Cryst. Growth Des., 2014, 14(7), 3398-3407.

54. Sagar, S.; Sengupta, S.; Chattopadhyay, S. K.; Mota, A. J.; Ferao, A. E.; Riviere, E.; Lewis, W.; Naskar, S. Cubane-Like Tetranuclear Cu(II) Complexes Bearing a Cu_4O_4 Core: Crystal Structure, Magnetic Properties, DFT Calculations and Phenoxazinone Synthase Like Activity. Dalton Trans., 2017, 46(4), 1249-1259.

55. Patel, S. K.; Patel, R. N.; Singh, Y.; Singh, Y. P.; Kumhar, D.; Jadeja, R. N.; Roy, H.; Patel, A. K.; Patel, N.; Patel, N.; Banerjee, A.; ChoquesilloLazarte, D.; Gutierrez. A. Three New Tetranuclear Phenoxy-Bridged Metal(II) Complexes: Synthesis, Structural Variation, Cryomagnetic Properties, DFT Study and Antiprolifirative Properties. Polyhedron, 2019, 161, 198-212.

Chapter 5

Synthesis, Structures, and Properties of Heterometallic One-Dimensional Tetranuclear Cu–Na Cluster-Based Polymers at Room Temperature

Heterometallic complexes have garnered significant interest due to their capacity to amalgamate the characteristics of diverse metal ions, resulting in the development of synergistic systems. In recent times, a plethora of heterometallic complexes have been documented, encompassing combinations of transition metals with other transition metals, main group elements, or rare earth elements. These complexes exhibit a wide range of applications in several fields including optics, electrochemistry, magnetism, chemical sensing, luminescence, and catalysis.

The selection of suitable organic ligands capable of coordinating with multiple metal ions is a key method for the synthesis of heterometallic complexes. Furthermore, the self-assembly process of heterometallic complexes is subject to various influencing factors. These factors encompass the molar ratio between the metal and ligand, the coordination function exhibited by the ligands, the specific metal ions involved, the polarity of the solvent molecules, the pH value of the solution, the type of counterion present, the reaction temperature, and the sequence in which different metal ions are added. Thorough investigation of these elements is important in order to attain a comprehensive comprehension of the impact of ligands' coordination function on the formation of heterometallic complexes. In a recent publication, our research team documented the successful synthesis of $[Fe_5(\mu_3\text{-}O)_2L_3(Htmp)(ATZ)_4]\cdot 4H_2O$. The compound was prepared using H_2tmp, which is 2-(((1H-tetrazol-5-yl)imino)methyl)phenol, and HATZ, which is 5-Amino-1H-tetrazole. In this study, we sought to investigate the impact of incorporating a methoxide group into the H_2tmp ligand and providing an additional coordination site on the ligand's ability for coordination. Consequently, we formulated and produced two novel ligands, H_2L^1 and H_2L^2, and fabricated two distinct polymers based on heterometallic tetranuclear clusters, denoted as $[Cu_2Na_2(L^1)_2(AcO)_2(EtOH)_2]_n$ (**chapt5-1**) and $[Cu_2Na_2(L^2)_2(AcO)_2(H_2O)(CH_3OH)_2]_n$ (**chapt5-2**). The ligands H_2tmp and H_2L exhibit distinct coordination patterns. The coordination patterns of H_2tmp in Scheme 5-1a are $\mu_3\text{-}L\text{-}\kappa^4O^1, N^1,N^2,N^3$. On the other hand, the coordination patterns of H_2L in **chapt5-1** and **chapt5-2** in Scheme 5-1b are $\mu_5\text{-}L\text{-}\kappa^7O^1, O^2{:}O^2,N^1,N^2,N^3,N^4$.

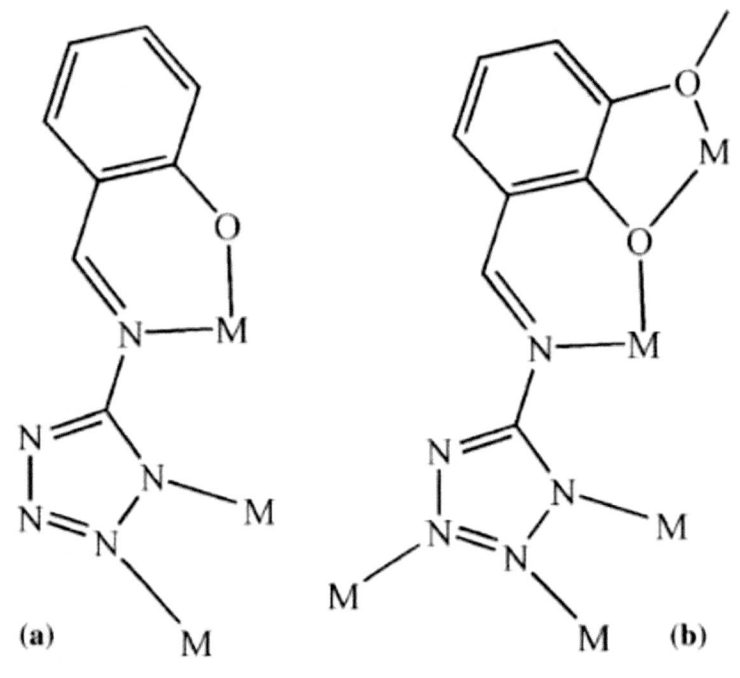

Scheme 5-1. Modes of coordination of H₂L and H₂tmp

Experimental

Substances and Physical Metrics

All of the compounds utilized in this study were readily obtainable from commercial sources and were employed in their original form without undergoing any purifying processes. The elemental studies for N-heterocyclic carbene (NHC) were conducted with a Perkin-Elmer 240 elemental analyzer. The preparation of samples for Fourier transform infrared (FTIR) spectroscopy involved the mixing of complex specimens with KBr and subsequent formation of pellets. The spectra were obtained by utilizing a Bio-Rad FTS-7 spectrometer, with measurements taken within the wavenumber range of 4000–400 cm^{-1}. The X-ray single crystal structures were found using the SuperNova diffractometer, which employs the Single source at offset, Eos technique. The crystal structures were further examined using the SHELXL program within the OLEX-2 graphical user interface for the purpose of modeling the molecular structures. The measurement of photoluminescence was conducted using a Hitachi F-4600 fluorescence spectrophotometer.

Syntheses

The synthesis of H₂L¹ and H₂L²

The ligands H₂L¹ and H₂L² were synthesized following a previously reported technique in the scientific literature.

Preparation of [Cu₂Na₂(L¹)₂(AcO)₂(EtOH)₂ (chapt5-1)

A solution containing Cu(AcO)₂·H₂O (0.5 mmol, 0.100 g), H₂L¹ (0.5 mmol, 0.110 g), NaOH (0.5 mmol, 0.020 g), ethanol (7 mL), and acetonitrile (3 mL) was subjected to stirring for a duration of 20 minutes at ambient temperature. In order to produce complex **chapt5-1**, the aforementioned mixture was transferred into a 20 mL container and left undisturbed at ambient temperature for a duration of 6 days. The filtration process was used to collect large, dark-red crystals of compound **chapt5-1**. These crystals were then subjected to three washes with 5 mL of ethanol each. Afterward, the crystals were left to dry in the air, resulting in a yield of around 0.105 g, which corresponds to approximately 51.2% based on the starting material H_2L^1. Analytical Calculations for Compound **chapt5-1**: $C_{26}H_{32}Cu_2N_{10}Na_2O_{10}$ (Molecular Weight = 817.68 g/mol). Calculated Percentages: C, 38.19%; H, 3.94%; N, 17.13%. The elemental composition of the sample was determined to be as follows: carbon (C) with a mass percentage of 38.13%, hydrogen (H) with a mass percentage of 3.95%, and nitrogen (N) with a mass percentage of 17.18%. The infrared (IR) data obtained for sample **chapt5-1** was collected using potassium bromide (KBr) as the medium. The observed wavenumbers (cm^{-1}) are as follows: a strong absorption peak at 3438 (m), a sharp absorption peak at 1605 (s), a weak absorption peak at 1546 (w), a sharp absorption peak at 1443 (s), a medium absorption peak at 1380 (m), a sharp absorption peak at 1209 (s), a medium absorption peak at 1100 (m), a weak absorption peak at 980 (w), and weak absorption peaks at 740 (w), 578 (w).

Preparation of $[Cu_2Na_2(L^2)_2(AcO)_2(H_2O)(CH_3OH)_2]_n$ (chapt5-2)

Complex **chapt5-2** was produced in a manner similar to that of **chapt5-1**, except H_2L^1 was substituted with H_2L^2 and ethanol was replaced with methanol. Red crystals of Complex **chapt5-2** were obtained (yield: 0.110 g, ca. 52.7% based on H_2L^2). Analytical Calculations for **chapt5-2**: $C_{26}H_{34}Cu_2Na_2N_{10}O_{11}$ (Mr = 835.69) Calculated: C 37.37; H 4.10; N 16.76. C, 37.29; H, 4.17; N, 16.91; discovered. IR data for molecule **chapt5-2** (KBr, cm^{-1}): 3436 s, 1607 s, 1546 w, 1444 m, 1322 w, 1212 m, 1102 w, 741 w, 584 w.

X-ray Single-Crystal Crystallography

The SuperNova diffractometer with graphite monochromated Mo-Kα radiation was used to collect single-crystal X-ray diffraction (XRD) data for compounds **chapt5-1** and **chapt5-2**. The data was obtained at a temperature of 16 ± 1 °C, using the x scan mode within the specified ranges: $3.40° \leq \theta \leq 26.37°$ for compound **chapt5-1**, and $3.48° \leq \theta \leq 25.00°$ for compound **chapt5-2**. The raw frame data was merged into the SAINT program. Structures **chapt5-1** and **chapt5-2** were determined by direct techniques employing the SHELXT software and subsequently refined using the full-matrix least-squares method on F^2 with the SHELXL-2018 program within the OLEX-2 graphical user interface. The researchers employed the SCALE3 ABSPACK scaling method to apply an empirical absorption correction using spherical harmonics. Anisotropic refinement was performed on all atoms except for hydrogen. The positions of all hydrogen atoms were determined using geometric methods and subsequently refined as riding. The software utilized in this study included CrysAlis PRO (Agilent Technologies), SHELXL (Sheldrick, 2015), and Olex2. The crystallographic information is presented in Table 5-1.

The calculation of Hirshfeld surfaces

The utilization of Hirshfeld surface calculations is a highly effective methodology for the examination and analysis of supramolecular interactions. The Crystal Explorer 3.1 application was utilized to do computations on molecular Hirshfeld surfaces. The bond lengths to hydrogen were adjusted to conform to the conventional default values, specifically C–H = 1.083 A°, N–H = 1.009 A°, and O–H = 0.983 A°. In this research, the generation of all Hirshfeld surfaces was conducted using a high standard resolution for the surface. The surfaces of the 3D dnorm were represented using a color scale ranging from 0.76 (red) to 2.4 (blue). The 2D fingerprint plots were acquired using the conventional 0.4–2.6 Å perspective, with the de and di distance scales clearly displayed on the graph axes.

Table 5-1. Crystallographic information on chapt5-1 and chapt5-2

Complex	**Chapt5-1**	**Chapt5-2**
Formula	$C_{26}H_{32}Cu_2N_{10}Na_2O_{10}$	$C_{26}H_{34}Cu_2N_{10}Na_2O_{11}$
M_r	817.68	835.69
Crystal size (mm)	0.19 × 0.16 × 0.08 mm	0.17 × 0.15 × 0.11 mm
Crystal system	Triclinic	Monoclinic
Space group	P-1	$P2_1/n$
a (Å)	8.991 (1)	8.807 (1)
b (Å)	9.406 (1)	21.349 (1)
c (Å)	10.699 (1)	10.784 (3)
a (°)	107.93 (1)	90.00
b (°)	98.16 (1)	107.27 (1)
c (°)	98.48 (1)	90.00
V (Å^3)	834.40 (13)	1936.03 (13)
$F(000)$	418	856
Z	1	2
D_c (g cm^{-3})	1.627	1.434
μ (mm^{-1})	1.370	1.184
θ range (°)	3.40–26.37	3.48–25.00
Ref. meas./indep.	5730, 3406	12,252, 3361
Obs. ref.[$I>2\theta(I)$]	2907	2713
R_{int}	0.0232	0.0295
R_1 [$I>2\theta(I)$][a]	0.0364	0.0478
xR_2 (all data)[b]	0.0895	0.1386
Goof	1.001	1.001
$\Delta\rho$(max, min) (e Å^{-3})	0.421, - 0.361	0.703, - 0.400

[a] $R_1 = R||F_o| - |F_c||/R|F_o|$, [b] $wR_2 = [Rw(|F^2|-|F^2|)^2/Rw(|F^2|)^2]^{1/2}$

Outcomes and Analysis

Structures crystalline of chapt5-1 and chapt5-2

The structures of complexes **chapt5-1** and **chapt5-2** were determined using single-crystal X-ray diffraction analysis. It was seen that these complexes exhibit similar structures, albeit with subtle variations in the coordination environments of metallic sodium and the ligands. This information is presented in Table 5-1 and Figure 5-1. Regarding the ligand aspect, it can be observed that the ligand present in complex **chapt5-1** is denoted as H$_2$L^1, whereas in compound **chapt5-2**, it is represented as H$_2$L^2. Hence, the focus of this analysis is solely on complex **chapt5-1**.

The triclinic crystal system in the $P\bar{1}$ space group is determined by the use of single-crystal X-ray diffraction, which indicates that **chapt5-1** belongs to this particular crystal system. Figure 5-1 illustrates the structural characteristics of a centrosymmetric heterotetranuclear cluster-based coordination polymer denoted as **chapt5-1**. This coordination polymer is composed of a centrosymmetric heterotetranuclear complex. The molecular structure can be described as a planar arrangement of Cu$_2$Na$_2$L$^1{}_2$, with two ethanol molecules and two acetate groups positioned both above and below the plane. The ligand L exhibits a coordination mode of μ_5 -

L-κ^7O^1,O^2:O^2,N^1,N^2,N^3,N^4, connecting two copper and three sodium atoms as shown in Scheme 5-1b. The copper atoms in the compound display a distorted tetragonal pyramidal [CuO3N2] geometry. This geometry is achieved through coordination with two acetate groups (Cu1-O3, 2.047(2) Å, Cu1-O4^i, 2.030 Å, where the symmetry code (i) represents the operation 1 - x, 1 - y, - z.), one oxygen atom, and one nitrogen atom from ligand L^1 (Cu1-N1, 1.972(2) Å, Cu1-O2, 2.058(2) Å), as well as one nitrogen atom from another ligand L^1 (Cu1-N2^i, 1.986(2) Å). The O2 atom occupies the apical position. The distances between Cu and X (where X represents either O or N) fall within the range of values previously documented in the academic literature. The τ_5 value was determined by computing the difference between the largest (b) and second-largest (a) X-Cu-X angles, and then dividing this difference by 60. This calculation method follows the approach described by Addison et al. in their study on five-coordinate structures. Typically, a molecular configuration exhibiting trigonal bipyramidal geometry and D$_{3h}$ symmetry possesses a τ_5 value of 1, whereas a molecular configuration displaying tetragonal pyramidal geometry and C$_{4v}$ symmetry has a τ_5 value of 0. In this case, the value of τ_5 is calculated as (169.10 - 164.51)/60 = 0.077, indicating a proximity to zero. Therefore, it was determined that Cu1 possessed a tetragonal pyramidal structure.

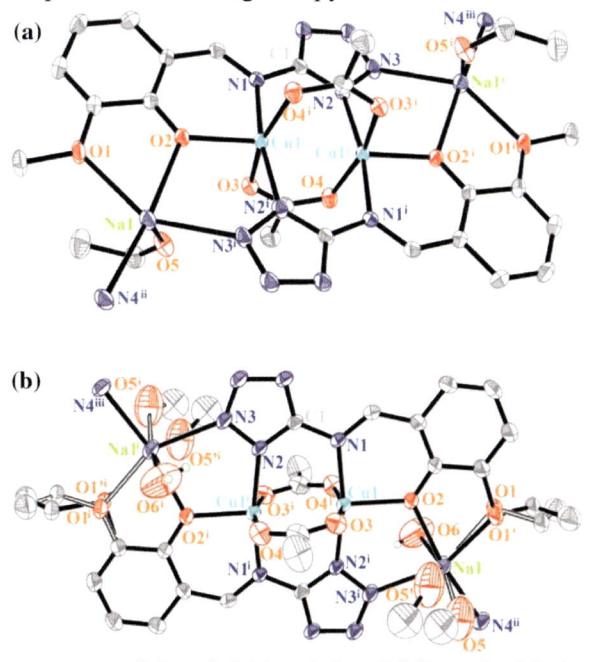

Figure 5-1: Molecule structures of chapt5-1 (a) and chapt5-2(b), omitted hydrogen atoms for clarity. symmetry code for chapt5-1: (i) 1 - x, 1 - y, - z; (ii) x, y, z + 1; (iii) 1 - x, 1 - y, - 1 - z. For chapt5-2: (i) - x, - y, - 1 - z; (ii) x, y, z + 1; (iii) - x, - y, - 2 - z

In sample **chapt5-1**, the intramolecular distance between Cu atoms is measured to be 2.769(2) Å. This distance is found to be shorter than the reported Cu···Cu distances in the copper complexes [Cu$_2$(bdhc)(CH$_3$OH)(NO$_3$)(DMF)$_2$] (H$_3$-bdhc = 1,5-bis(3,5-dibromosalicylidene)-carbohydrazide, Cu···Cu distance is 4.791 Å) and [Cu$_3$Na$_2$(ehbd)$_2$(N$_3$)$_6$]$_n$(Hehbd = 3-ethoxy-2-hydroxybenzaldehyde, Cu···Cu distances range from 3.142 to 3.739 Å). Nevertheless, the length of our value exceeded that which was published for [Cu$_2$(aba)$_4$(C$_3$H$_7$NO)$_2$], where Haba represents 4-azidobenzoic acid and the Cu-Cu distance is measured at 2.6366 (5) Å. Similarly, it also above the value given for [Cu$_2$(fluf)$_4$(DMF)$_2$], where Hfluf represents flufenamic acid and the Cu-Cu distance is measured at 2.618(1) Å. The Na1 ion exhibits a coordination number of five, being surrounded by two oxygen atoms (O1, O2) from a single L¹ ligand, two nitrogen atoms (N3^i, N4^{ii}, symmetry codes: (ii) $x, y, z + 1$) from two distinct L¹ ligands, and one oxygen atom (O5) from an ethanol molecule. This arrangement results in a noticeably deformed tetragonal pyramidal shape. The oxygen atom is situated in the apical position. The value of τ_5 can be calculated by subtracting 146.19 from 167.10 and dividing the result by 60. This yields a value of 0.349, which is in close proximity to zero. The [Cu$_2$Na$_2$(L¹)$_2$(AcO)$_2$(EtOH)$_2$] moiety undergoes further expansion in a one-dimensional chain through the coordination bond between Na1 and N4 (as seen in Figure 5-2). This expansion results in the construction of a two-dimensional network through interactions involving Na-H and C-H···π. The distances between Na1-H9B^i and Na1-H6^i (with symmetry code: (i) $1 - x, 2 - y, 1 - z$) were measured to be 3.665 Å and 3.593 Å, respectively. Similarly, the distances between C11 and π^g (C1-N2-N3-N4-N5) were found to be 3.5472 Å, with a symmetry code of (g) $- x, 1 - y, - z$. Furthermore, it should be noted that intramolecular hydrogen bonds are present in compound **chapt5-1**, specifically between the oxygen atom at position 5 (O5) and the hydrogen atom at position 5 (H5) with a bond length of 2.813 angstroms (Å).

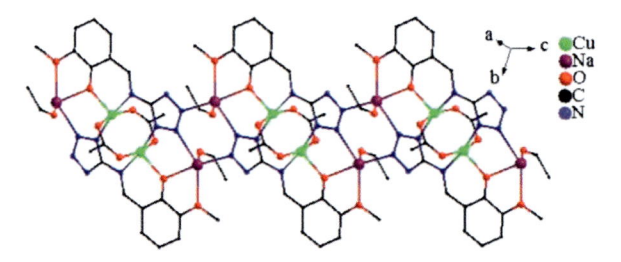

Figure 5-2: 1-D chain of chapt5-1, omitted hydrogen atoms for clarity

Attributes of Photoluminescence

In recent years, a number of studies have determined that the utilization of luminescent materials obtained from coordination polymers has garnered significant attention due to their wide-ranging potential in various fields. These applications include electrochemiluminescent immunosensing, the development of luminescent sensors, and photocatalysis. Notably, these materials have demonstrated particular efficacy in the detection and manipulation of Zn(II) ions, which possess closed d^{10} subshells. Therefore, an investigation was conducted on the photoluminescence properties of the polymer materials in order to showcase their potential for the aforementioned applications. The luminous properties of compounds **chapt5-1** and **chapt5-2**, which incorporate the H$_2$L ligand, were observed at ambient conditions (see Figure 5-3). The ligands H$_2$L¹ and H$_2$L² exhibited wide emission peaks at 626 nm and 632 nm, respectively, upon excitation with a wavelength of 420 nm. These emissions were ascribed to π–π* and σ–π* transitions. The emission centers of complexes **chapt5-1** and **chapt5-2** are situated at wavelengths of 634 nm and 648 nm, respectively, as depicted in Figure 5-3. These emissions occur when the complexes are stimulated at a wavelength of 420 nm. The solid-state luminescence of complexes **chapt5-1** and **chapt5-2** exhibited red-shifts of 8 nm and 16 nm, respectively, in comparison to the emission band observed in the absence of the H$_2$L¹ or H$_2$L² ligands. The emission wavelengths observed at 634 nm and 648 nm for complexes **chapt5-1** and **chapt5-2**, respectively, can be attributed to the paramagnetic effect of the Cu^{II} cation, which is a d⁹ ion. This effect likely contributes to the reduced fluorescence intensity observed in these complexes.

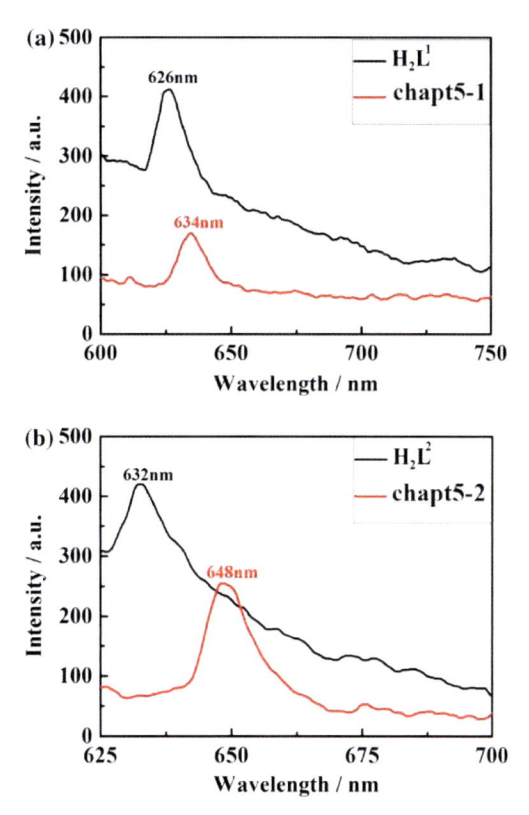

Figure 5-3: The solid-state fluorescence properties of HL$^{1\&2}$, chapt5-1 and chapt5-2

Infrared Spectrum

The Fourier Transform Infrared (FTIR) spectra of the ligands H$_2$L^1 and H$_2$L^2, as well as complexes **chapt5-1** and **chapt5-2**. The observed bands at 3223 (3212) cm^{-1} in the spectra of the ligands H$_2$L^1 (H$_2$L^2) can be attributed to the N–H bond of the ligand in its free form, H$_2$L^1 (H$_2$L^2). However, these bands were not observed in the spectra of complexes **chapt5-1** and **chapt5-2**, suggesting that the N-H bond has undergone deprotonation. The O-H stretching frequencies in the molecular structures of the ligands H$_2$L^1 and H$_2$L^2, as well as complexes **chapt5-1** and **chapt5-2**, were assigned to the bands seen at 3421, 3436, 3438, and 3436 cm^{-1}, respectively. The bands observed at 1603 (1600) cm^{-1} were assigned to the t(C=N) vibrations of the H$_2$L^1 (H$_2$L^2) ligands. These bands exhibited a hypochromatic shift to 1605 (1607) cm^{-1} for **chapt5-1** (**chapt5-2**), indicating their involvement in a six-membered chelation. The prominent peaks observed at 1461 (1464) cm^{-1} correspond to the C=C bond present in the benzene ring of the unbound H$_2$L^1 (H$_2$L^2) ligand. These peaks undergo a red-shift to 1443 (1444) cm^{-1} upon coordination with **chapt5-1** (**chapt5-2**), suggesting a decrease in the electron cloud density of the benzene ring following ligand coordination.

Surface Analysis Using the Hirshfeld Method

Hirshfeld surfaces analysis and two-dimensional fingerprint plots are frequently employed in order to ascertain factors associated with distinct proportions of intermolecular interactions. The molecular Hirshfeld surface, which represents the normalized distance between atoms (d_{norm}), employs a three-color scheme to depict the significant intermolecular interactions. In

Figure 5-4, the red, blue, and white surfaces correspond to intermolecular contacts that are closer, longer, or equal to the sum of their van der Waals radii, respectively. The regions exhibiting a deep red color on the dnorm surface correspond to locations where there are strong intermolecular interactions in close proximity. In order to analyze the dnorm (Figure 5-4i-1) data, we divided it into distinct categories based on the significant H-H, C-H, N-H, O-H, Na-O, and Cu-N interactions. These categories can be observed in Figure 5-4i-2 and Figure 5-4i-7, where i represents the values **chapt5-1** and **chapt5-2**. As depicted in Figure 5-4, the regions colored in deep red indicate the range of values observed for the interactions involving N-H, O-H, Na-O, and Cu-N in compound **chapt5-1**, which showed in Figure 5-4-1-4, 1-5, 1-6, 1-7, respectively. Similarly, compound **chapt5-2** exhibited values for N-H, Na-O, and Cu-N interactions which showed in Figure 5-4-2-4, 2-5, 2-7, respectively. Additional interactions, denoted by the blue regions, comprised of H-H and C-H for **chapt5-1**, and H-H, C-H, and O-H for **chapt5-2**. The 3D Hirshfeld surfaces of compound **chapt5-1**, as depicted in Figure 5-4, exhibit distinct red zones labeled as a-h. These red zones are a result of brief contacts. The N-H bond length for N3-H11^a is 2.753(2) Å, with a symmetry code of (a) - x, 1 - y, - z. The O-H bond length for H9b-O2^B and O2-H9b^B is 2.627 Å, with a symmetry code of (B) 1 - x, 2 - y, 1 - z. The Na-N bond lengths are as follows: N3-Na1^C is 2.454(2) Å, Na1-N3^C is 2.454(2) Å, and Na1-N4^D is 2.398(2) Å. The symmetry codes for these bonds are (C) 1 - x, 1 - y, - z and (D) x, y, 1 - z. The Cu-N bond length for Cu1-N2^C and N2-Cu1^C is 1.986(2) Å. In this study, the tetranuclear cluster [CuNa(L^1)(AcO)(EtOH)] was shown to form by intermolecular interactions involving zones e, g, and h. Additionally, these clusters subsequently assembled into one-dimensional chains through intermolecular interactions involving zones d and f. The formation of one-dimensional chains resulted in the creation of two-dimensional supramolecular networks in zones a-c and the blue zones characterized by H–H and C–H interactions. The Hirshfeld surface analysis of complex **chapt5-2** exhibited similarities to complex **chapt5-1**.

The utilization of a two-dimensional fingerprint plot is a highly advantageous method for the quantitative evaluation of intermolecular interactions, enabling a comprehensive analysis of their specific kind and characteristics. The process of simplifying to single atom pairs allows for a more detailed examination of tight interactions. In the context of the 2D fingerprint plot (Figure 5-4-1-2, 2-2), it was found that H-H contacts were present among the scattered spots located in the centre. The H-H interactions accounted for 36.9% and 43.9% of the total Hirshfeld surface interactions for compounds **chapt5-1** and **chapt5-2**, respectively. The shortest H-H distance observed was 2.572 Å (H6-H13^e, with a symmetry code of (e) - x, 2 - y, 1 - z) for compound **chapt5-1**, and 2.425 Å (H10a-H12f, with a symmetry code of (f) 1 + x, y, 1 + z) for compound **chapt5-2**. The intermolecular interactions involving carbon-hydrogen (C-H) bonds are depicted on the 2D fingerprint plot as sparrow and rabbit. These interactions account for roughly 14.1% and 15.0% of the total intermolecular interactions for compounds **chapt5-1** and **chapt5-2**, respectively. The observed interactions primarily arose from H···π, with the shortest H···π distance being 2.685 Å in case **chapt5-1** and 2.685 Å in case **chapt5-2**. These distances correspond to the H11c...π^g$_{(C1-N2-N3-N4-N5)}$ distance of 2.685 Å (symmetry code: (g) - x, 1 - y, - z) and the H10c...π^h$_{(C3-C4-C5-C6-C7-C8)}$ distance of 2.719 Å (symmetry code: (h) x - 0.5, 0.5 - y, z - 0.5.), respectively.

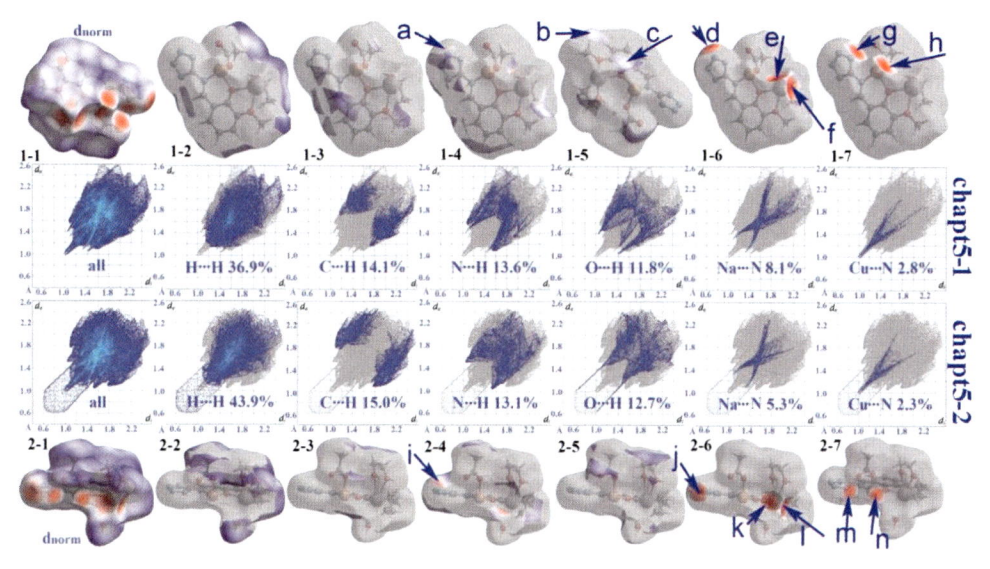

Figure 5-4: 3D Hirshfeld surfaces of d$_{norm}$, H···H, C···H, N···H, O···H, Na···O, Cu···N interactions and corresponding 2D fingerprints of various intermolecular forces in chapt5-1 and chapt5-2

Conclusion

At normal temperature, two heterometallic tetranuclear one-dimensional Cu-Na polymers, denoted as [Cu$_2$Na$_2$(L^1)$_2$(AcO)$_2$(EtOH)$_2$]$_n$ (**chapt5-1**) and [Cu$_2$-Na$_2$(L^2)$_2$(AcO)$_2$(H$_2$O)$_4$]$_n$ (**chapt5-2**), were successfully synthesized. The tetranuclear copper-sodium polymer units were synthesized using μ_5-L-κ^7O^1,O^2:O^2,N^1,N^2,N^3,N^4 bridges. Complexes **chapt5-1** and **chapt5-2** exhibited red fluorescence at wavelengths of 634 nm and 648 nm, respectively. This resulted in a minor red shift when compared to the emission band of the unbound H$_2$L^1 and H$_2$L^2 ligands, respectively. The Hirshfeld surface investigations conducted on compounds **chapt5-1** and **chapt5-2** revealed that interactions involving hydrogen atoms bonded to hydrogen, carbon, and nitrogen atoms are of considerable importance in facilitating the stabilization of the self-assembly process.

References

1. Lieberman, C. M.; Navulla, A.; Zhang, H.; Filatov, A. S.; Dikarev, E. V. Mixed-Ligand Approach to Design of Heterometallic Single-Source Precursors with Discrete Molecular Structure. *Inorg. Chem.*, 2014, *53(9)*, 4733-4738.
2. Feng, P. L.; Beedle, C. C.; Wernsdorfer, W.; Koo, C.; Nakano, M.; Hill, S.; Hendrickson, D. N. Heterometallic Cubane Single-Molecule Magnets. Inorg. Chem., 2007, 46(20), 8126-8128.
3. Niekerk, A. V.; Chellan, P.; Mapolie, S. F. Heterometallic Multinuclear Complexes as Anti-Cancer Agents-An Overview of Recent Developments. Eur. J. Inorg. Chem., 2019, 30, 3432-3455.
4. Hu, Z. G.; Zhao, R. X.; Zhang, S. H.; ChenSyntheses, S. L. Crystal Structure and Property of a Heterometallic Heptanuclear Cluster. J. Clust. Sci., 2016, 27(6), 1933-1943.
5. Zhang, S. H.; Zhao, R. X.; Li, G.; Zhang, H. Y.; Zhang, C. L.; Muller, G. Structural Variation from Heterometallic Heptanuclear or Heptanuclear to Cubane Clusters

Based on 2-Hydroxy-3-Ethoxy-Benzaldehyde: Effects of pH and Temperature. RSC. Adv., 2014, 4(97), 54837-54846.

6. Zhao, R. X.; Hai, H.; Li, G.; Zhang, H. Y.; Huang, Q. P.; Zhang, S. H.; Li, H. P. Room Temperature Syntheses, Structures and Magnetic Properties of Two Heterometallic Tetranuclear Clusters. J. Cluster. Sci., 2014, 25(6), 1541-1552.

7. Huebner, L.; Kornienko, A.; Emge, T. J.; Brennan, J. G. Heterometallic Lanthanide Group 12 Metal Iodides. Inorg. Chem., 2004, 43(18), 5659-5664.

8. Yang, Q.; Tang, J. Heterometallic Grids: Synthetic Strategies and Recent Advances. Dalton. T., 2019, 48(4), 769-778.

9. Beheshti, A.; Clegg, W.; Nobakht, V.; Harrington, R. W. Metal-to-Ligand Ratio as a Design Factor in the One-Pot Synthesis of Coordination Polymers with [MS4Cun] (M = W or Mo, n = 3 or 5) Cluster Nodes and a Flexible Pyrazole-Based Bridging Ligand. Cryst. Growth. Des., 2013, 13(3), 1023-1032.

10. Zhang, S. H.; Li, N.; Ge, C. M.; Feng, C.; Ma, L. F. Structures and Magnetism of {Ni$_2$Na$_2$}, {Ni$_4$} and {Ni$_6^{II}$Ni^{III}} 2-Hydroxy-3-Alkoxy-Benzaldehyde Clusters. Dalton Trans., 2011, 40(10), 3000-3007.

11. Yang, L.; Zhang, S. H.; Wang, W.; Guo, J. J.; Huang, Q. P.; Zhao, R. X.;Zhang, C. L.; Muller, G. Ligand Induced Diversification from Tetranuclear to Mononuclear Compounds: Syntheses, Structures and Magnetic Properties. Polyhedron., 2014, 74(28), 49-56.

12. Xin, L. Y.; Liu, G. Z.; Li, X. L; Wang, L. Y. Structural Diversity for a Series of Metal(II) Complexes Based on Flexible 1,2-Phenylenediacetate and Dipyridyl-Type Coligand. Cryst. Growth. Des., 2012, 12(1), 147-157.

13. Ma, L. F.; Li, X. Q.; Wang, L. Y.; Hou, H. W. Syntheses and Characterization of Nickel(II) and Cobalt(II) Coordination Polymers Based on 5-Bromoisophthalate Anion and Bis(imidazole) Ligands. Crystengcomm., 2011, 13(33), 4625-4634.

14. Toki, S.; Che, J.; Rong, L.; Hsiao, B. S.; Amnuaypornsri, S.; Nimpaiboon, A.; Sakdapipanich, J. Entanglements and Networks to Strain-Induced Crystallization and Stress-Strain Relations in Natural Rubber and Synthetic Polyisoprene at Various Temperatures. Macromolecules, 2013, 46(13), 5238-5248.

15. Yang, X. G.; Zhai, Z. M.; Lu, X. M.; Zhao, Y.; Chang, X. H.; Ma, L. F. Room Temperature Phosphorescence of Mn(II) and Zn(II) Coordination Polymers for Photoelectron Response Applications†. Dalton Trans., 2019, 48(29), 10785-10789.

16. Long, L. S. pH Effect on the Assembly of Metal-Organic Architectures. Crystengcomm., 2010, 12(9), 1354-1365.

17. Cheng, J. W.; Zheng, S. T.; Yang, G. Y. Diversity of Crystal Structure with Different Lanthanide Ions Involving in Situoxidation-Hydrolysis Reaction. Dalton Trans., 2007, 36, 4059-4066.

18. Zhang, S. H.; Ma, L. F.; Zou, H. H.; Wang, Y. G.; Liang, H.; Zeng, M. H. Anion Induced Diversification from Heptanuclear to Tetranuclear Clusters: Syntheses, Structures and Magnetic Properties. Dalton Trans., 2011, 40(32), 11402-11409.

19. Zhao, Y.; Zhai, L. L.; Fan, J.; Chen, K.; Sun, W. Y. Silver(I) Complexes of 4-(2-Oxazolinyl)Pyridine: Counteranion Dependent Structural Diversity. Polyhedron, 2012, 46(1), 16-24.

20. Chen, Z.; Fan, Y.; Wang, J.; Yang, L.; Zhang, S. Penta-Nuclear Fe(III) Cluster: Synthesis, Structure, Magnetic Properties and Hirshfeld Surface Analysis. ChemistrySelect, 2018, 3(34), 9841-9844.
21. Sheldrick, G. M. Crystal Structure Refinement with SHELXL. Acta Crystallogr. C., 2015, 71, 3-8.
22. Dolomanov, O. V.; Bourhis, L. J.; Gildea, R. J.; Howard, J. A. K.; Puschmann, H. OLEX2: A Complete Structure Solution, Refinement and Analysis Program. J. Appl. Crystallogr., 2009, 42, 339-341.
23. McKinnon, J. J.; Spackman, M. A.; Mitchell, A. S. Novel Tools for Visualizing and Exploring Intermol-Ecular Interactions in Molecular Crystals. Acta Crystallogr. B., 2004, B60, 627-668.
24. Allen, F. H.; Kennard,O.; Watson, D. G.; Brammer, L.; Orpen, A. G.; Taylor, R. Tables of Bond Lengths Determined by X-Ray and Neutron Diffraction. Part I. Bond Lengths in Organic Compounds. J. Chem. Soc. Perkin. Trans. II., 1987, 2, S1-S19.
25. Sun, W. W.; Qian, X. B.; Tian, C. Y.; Gao, E. Q. Synthesis, Structure and Ferromagnetic Properties of a Copper(II) Coordination Polymer with Azide and 4-pyridylacrylate. Inorg. Chim. Acta, 2009, 362(8), 2744-2748.
26. Zhang, H. Y.; Wang, W.; Chen, H.; Zhang, S. H.; Li, Y. Five Novel Dinuclear Copper(II) Complexes: Crystal Structures, Properties, Hirshfeld Surface Analysis and Vitro Antitumor Activity Study. Inorg. Chim. Acta, 2016, 453, 507-515.
27. Yang, L.; Powell, D. R.; Houser, R. P. Structural Variation in Copper(I) Complexes with Pyridylmethylamide Ligands: Structural Analysis with a New Four-Coordinate Geometry Index, τ4. Dalton. Trans., 2007, (9), 955-964.
28. Zhang, S. H.; Zhao, R. X.; Li, G.; Zhang, H. Y.; Huang, Q. P.; Liang, F. P. Room Temperature Syntheses, Crystal Structures and Properties of Two New Heterometallic Polymers Based on 3-Ethoxy-2-Hydroxybenzaldehyde Ligand. J. Solid. State. Chem., 2014, 220, 206-212.
29. Wang, A. Tetra¬kis(μ-4-Azidobenzoato-κ2O:O′)Bis[(N,N-Dimethylformamide-κO)Copper(II)]. Acta. Crystallogr. E., 2012, E68, m43.
30. Tolia, C.; Papadopoulos, A. N.; Raptopoulou, C. P.; Psycharis, V.; Garino, C.; Salassa, L.; Psomas G. Copper(II) Interacting with the Non-Steroidal Antiinflammatory Drug Flufenamic Acid: Structure, Antioxidant Activity and Binding to DNA and Albumins. J. Inorg. Biochem., 2013, 123, 53-65.
31. Heinke, L.; Tu, M.; Wannapaiboon, S.; Fischer, R. A.; Woell, C. Surface-Mounted Metal-Organic Frameworks for Applications in Sensing and Separation. Micropor. Mesopor. Mat., 2015, 216, 200-215.
32. Liu, W.; Yin, X. B. Metal-Organic Frameworks for Electrochemical Applications. Trac-Trend. Anal. Chem., 2016, 75, 86-96.
33. Ling, P.; Lei, J.; Jia, L.; Ju, H. Platinum Nanoparticles Encapsulated Metal–Organic Frameworks for the Electrochemical Detection of Telomerase Activity. Chem. Commun., 2016, 52, 1226-1229.
34. Lustig, W. P.; Mukherjee, S.; Rudd, N. D.; Desai, A. V.; Li, J.; Ghosh, S. K. Metal-Organic Frameworks: Functional Luminescent and Photonic Materials for Sensing Applications. Chem. Soc. Rev., 2017, 46, 3242-3285.

35. Wu, X. X.; Fu, H. R.; Han, M. L.; Zhou, Z.; Ma, L. F. Tetraphenylethylene Immobilized Metal-Organic Frameworks: Highly Sensitive Fluorescent Sensor for the Detection of Cr2O72- and Nitroaromatic Explosives. Cryst. Growth. Des., 2017, 17(11), 6041-6048.
36. Wen, G. X.; Han, M. L.; Wu, X. Q.; Wu, Y. P.; Dong, W. W.; Zhao, J.; Li, D. S.; Ma, L. F. A Multi-Responsive Luminescent Sensor Based on a Super-Stable Sandwich-Type Terbium(III)-Organic Framework. Dalton. Trans., 2016, 45(39), 15492-15499.
37. Kan, W. Q.; Liu, B.; Yang, J.; Liu, Y. Y.; Ma, J. F. A Series of Highly Connected Metal-Organic Frameworks Based on Triangular Ligands and d10 Metals: Syntheses, Structures, Photoluminescence, and Photocatalysis. Cryst. Growth. Des., 2012, 12(5), 2288-2298.
38. Cheng, Y. J.; Wang, R.; Wang, S.; Xi, X. J.; Ma, L. F.; Zang, S. Q. Encapsulating [Mo3S13]2− Clusters in Cationic Covalent Organic Frameworks: Enhancing Stability and Recyclability by Converting a Homogeneous Photocatalyst to a Heterogeneous Photocatalyst. Chem. Commun., 2018, 54, 13563-13566.
39. Johanna, H.; Klaus, M. B. Engineering Metal-Based Luminescence in Coordination Polymers and Metal-Organic Frameworks. Chem. Soc. Rev., 2013, 42(24), 9232-9242.
40. Javier, C.; Antonio, R. D. Tuning the Luminescence Performance of Metal-Organic Frameworks Based on d10 Metal Ions: from an Inherent Versatile Behaviour to Their Response to External Stimuli. Crystengcomm., 2016, 18(44), 8556-8573.
41. Mikhailov, I. E.; Vikrishchuk, N. I.; Popov, L. D.; Dushenko, G. A.; Beldovskaya, A. D.; Revinskii, Yu. V.; Minkin V. I. Absorption and Luminescence Spectra of 5-Aryl-3-Methyl-1,2,4-Oxadiazoles and Their Chelate Complexes with Zinc(II) and Copper(II). Russ. J. Gen. Chem+., 2016, 86(5), 1054-1063.
42. Shebl, M. Synthesis, Spectroscopic Characterization and Antimicrobial Activity of Binuclear Metal Complexes of a new Asymmetrical Schiff Base Ligand: DNA Binding Affinity of Copper(II) Complexes. Spectrochim. Acta. A., 2014, 117, 127-137.
43. Li, G.; Wang, W.; Zhang, S. H.; Zhang, H. Y.; Chen, F. Y. Synthesis, Structure and Properties of Linear Trinuclear Cobalt Cluster with 5-Fluoro-2-Hydroxy-Benzoic Acid. J. Clust. Sci., 2014, 25, 1589-1597.
44. Zhang, S. H.; Li, G.; Zhang, H. Y.; Li, H. P. Microwave-assisted Synthesis, Structure and Property of a Spin-Glass Heptanuclear Nickel Cluster with 2-Iminomethyl-6-Methoxy-Phenol. Z. Krist-Cryst. Mater, 2015, 230(7), 479-484.

Chapter 6

Analysis of the synthesis, crystal structures, fluorescence, electrochemiluminescent properties, and Hirshfeld surface of four Cu/Mn Schiff-basecomplexes

The present focus of research involves the development and production of new coordination polymer (CP) materials utilizing Schiff base as an organic ligand. These materials have garnered significant attention due to their diverse range of applications in fields such as optics, electromagnetism, adsorption, and catalysis. At now, the predominant coordination modes observed in Schiff bases include the binding of metal ions to oxygen (O) and nitrogen (N) atoms. Hence, the selection of an organic ligand plays a crucial role in determining the characteristics of coordination polymers (CPs). The utilization of the 1,2,4-triazole ligand and its derivatives in coordination chemistry enables the formation of high-nuclear compounds and their coordination polymers (CPs) by bridging transition metal ions through the N-M coordination mode. These compounds exhibit distinctive characteristics. Hyunsoo Park chose 3-Amino-1,2,4-triazole as an organic bridging ligand in order to synthesize four novel coordination polymers (CPs) using zinc (Zn). Yun Gong et al. employed 4-amine-4H-1,2,4-triazole and its derivative 3,5-dimethyl-4-amino-4H-1,2,4-triazole as primary ligands, which were further coupled with Cu and Ag to generate metal organic framework materials having 1D–3D structures. Copper compounds demonstrated superior electrocatalytic performance in the production of hydrogen gas from water. The present investigation involved the synthesis of a C=N bond using an aldehyde-amino-group condensation reaction, wherein 4-amine-4H-1,2,4-triazole was reacted with either 3,5-dichloro-2-hydroxybenzaldehyde or 3,5-dibromo-2-hydroxy-benzaldehyde. The coordination of ligands with metal ions (Cu^{II}, Mn^{II}) was carried out under specific conditions in order to synthesize coordination polymers (CPs). Four coordination polymers (CPs) were produced, whereby the metal centers consisted of Cu^{II} and Mn^{II}. The structures of the samples were analyzed by several techniques including single crystal X-ray diffraction, elemental analysis, infrared (IR) spectroscopy, and thermogravimetric analysis.

The utilization of electrochemical luminescence (ECL) materials has gained prominence in various professional domains owing to their advantageous characteristics, such as little background noise and exceptional sensitivity to electrochemical response signals. The ECL (Electrochemiluminescence) technique employs a specific sequence of electrical signals to induce excitation energy in the material, subsequently resulting in the emission of energy radiation through an electrical signal of specific characteristics. One commonly employed approach involves the utilization of composite materials, with Ru(II) and Ir(II) being frequently selected as appropriate metals for the synthesis of coordination polymers (CPs). All of the aforementioned methodologies are characterized by high costs and intricate experimental protocols. The synthetic Schiff-base raw materials and metal salts utilized in this study exhibit favorable cost-effectiveness and efficiency.

Hirshfeld surface analysis is a valuable approach that can provide insights into the underlying challenges encountered in the process of material creation. It is extensively employed as a distinctive technique for examining intermolecular interactions, utilizing a two-dimensional fingerprint map. The research has also focused on the analysis of Hirshfeld surfaces. Fluorescent composite polymer materials include robust and enduring fluorescent characteristics, substantial specific surface area, and controllable structure, rendering them suitable for discerning the selective identification of particular ions, organisms, or cancer cells. Furthermore, the remarkable fluorescent luminescent characteristics of conjugated polymers (CPs) are relatively unaffected by external factors and typically demonstrate strong fluorescence intensity at ambient circumstances.

An additional significant determinant is that the four newly formed complexes do not arise from the electron transfer that occurs during the original *d–d* transition, but rather from the electron transfer between the ligand and the metal, known as ligand-to-metal charge transfer (LMCT). The fluorescence analysis of the four complexes indicated that each complex exhibited varying degrees of red-shift compared to the maximum fluorescence intensity of the ligands. Specifically, complexes **chapt6-1** and **chapt6-2** displayed red-shifts ranging from 44 to 57 nm, while complexes **chapt6-3** and **chapt6-4** exhibited red-shifts of approximately 7 to 10 nm. Furthermore, it is plausible to hypothesize that the presence of halogen atoms in salicylaldehyde could lead to the quenching of fluorescence in the complexes due to the influence of the C=N bond on their fluorescent characteristics.

Experimentation
Components and Instrumentation
All compounds utilized in this study were obtained commercially and employed in their as-received state without undergoing any additional purifying procedures. The crystal structures were determined utilizing the SuperNova diffractometer (single source at offset, Eos, Agilent Technologies, Palo Alto, America) and the SHELXL crystallographic software for analyzing molecular structures. The FT-IR spectra were obtained by analyzing KBr pellets using a Nicolet Nexus 470 FT-IR infrared spectrometer (manufactured by Nicolet, an American company) within the wavelength range of 4000 to 400 cm^{-1}. The X-ray powder diffraction patterns (PXRDs) of compounds **chapt6-1-chapt6-4** were obtained using an X'Pert3 Powder X-ray diffractometer manufactured by Panaco in the Netherlands. Thermogravimetric analysis (TGA) was conducted using an SDT Q600 Thermogravimetric Analyzer (TA, American) to investigate the thermal behavior of the crystalline sample. The sample was heated from 25 to 900 $^{\circ}$C at a rate of 10 $^{\circ}$C·min^{-1} under a nitrogen (N$_2$) environment. The investigation involved

the examination of the electrochemiluminescence (ECL) characteristics and cyclic voltammetry (CV) of compounds **chapt6-1–chapt6-4**. This analysis was conducted in a solution of N,N-dimethylformamide (DMF) using the MPI-E Electrochemiluminescence Analysis System, manufactured by Xi'an Ruimai Analytical Instrument Co., Ltd. in Xi'an, China.

Syntheses

Synthesis of HL¹

In a 100 ml three-necked flask, a mixture of 3,5-dichloro-2-hydroxybenzaldehyde (1.91 g, 10 mmol), 4H-4-amino-1,2,4-triazole (taya, 0.84 g, 10 mmol), and ethanol (20 mL) was refluxed at 80°C for 120 minutes. At 80 degrees Celsius for two hours, the color of the solution changed to brown and it was enriched. By filtration, a brown powder was obtained, rinsed with hot ethanol (10 ml × 3), and dried in an oven at 50 °C for 24 hours (yield: 2.468 g, approximately 96%, based on taya). Analysis calculated (percent) for HL¹, $C_9H_6Cl_2N_4O$ (*Mr* = 257.08): C = 42.05; H = 2.35; N = 21.79. C, 41.98; H, 2.42; N, 21.85; discovered. 3438 m, 3130 m, 1660 w, 1597 s, 1515 s, 1465 s, 1377 m, 1327 s, 1245 s, 1176 m, 1056 s, 868 m, 723 m, 680 w.

Synthesis of HL²

The method of synthesis for HL² is analogous to that of HL¹, except 3,5-dibromosalicylaldehyde is substituted for 3,5-dichloro-2-hydroxybenzaldehyde. By filtration, a brown powder was obtained, washed with ethanol (10 milliliter × 3), and dried in an oven at 50 °C for 24 hours (yield: 3,356 g, approximately 97%, based on taya). C, 31.24; H, 1.75; N, 16.19; analysis calculated (%) for HL²: $C_9H_6Br_2N_4O$ (*Mr* = 345.98). C, 31.18; H, 1.82; N, 16.25; discovered. HL² IR data (KBr, cm⁻¹) 3450 s, 3124 m, 3067 m, 1634 w, 1515 s, 1452 m, 1364 s, 1307 s, 1232 s, 1176 s, 1062 s, 962 m, 868 s, 730 m, 634 w.

Synthesis of [Cu(L¹)₂]ₙ (chapt6-1)

HL¹ (0.051 g, 0.2 mmol) was added to a 25 ml vial of clean glass. Five milliliters of DMF were added to the glass vial. Cu(AcO)₂·H₂O (0.040 g, 0.2 mmol) was dissolved in 5 mL of deionized water at the same moment. The two solutions were then combined and stirred for 20 minutes in a glass vessel. The magneton was then extracted using a magnet, the glass container was sealed and baked at 90 degrees Celsius for three days, and blue block crystals were obtained. The reaction product was rinsed with 10 ml × 3 of heated DMF and 10 mL of double-distilled water. On the basis of HL¹, blue block crystals of **chapt6-1** were obtained (yield: 0.065 g, *ca* 56.3%). **chapt6-1**, $C_{18}H_{10}Cl_4CuN_8O_2$ (*Mr* = 575.68), analysis results (percent): C, 37.56; H, 1.75; N, 19.46. C, 37.48; H, 1.81; N, 19.53; discovered. 3111 m, 1597 s, 1509 m, 1440 s, 1314 m, 1314 m, 1214 m, 1157 m, 1069 s, 849 m, 668 m.

Synthesis of [Mn(L¹)₂]ₙ (chapt6-2)

The ratio of metal salt to ligand was **chapt6-1**, but Mn(AcO)₂·4H₂O was dissolved in dimethyl sulfoxide (DMSO) and agitated for twenty minutes. After adding 5 mL of double-distilled water, the reaction flask was sealed and deposited in an 80°C oven. Red block crystals of **chapt6-2** were obtained (yield: 0.066 g, ca 58.1%, based on HL¹). C, 38.13; H, 1.78; N, 19.76; analysis calculated (%) for **chapt6-2**, $C_{18}H_{10}Cl_4MnN_8O_2$ (*Mr* = 567.07). C, 38.10; H, 1.82; N, 19.79; discovered. The IR data for the molecule **chapt6-2** (KBr, cm⁻¹) are as follows: 3143 m, 1603 m, 1515 w, 1465 s, 1346 w, 1214 m, 1163 m, 1057 s, 855 w, 761 m, 661 w.

Synthesis of [Cu(L²)₂]ₙ (chapt6-3)

Compound **chapt6-3** was prepared similarly to compound **chapt6-1**, with the exception that HL^1 was substituted with HL^2. On the basis of HL^2, blue bulk crystals of **chapt6-3** were obtained (yield: 0.080 g, ca 51.2%). C, 28.69; H, 1.34; N, 14.82; analysis (%) for **chapt6-3**, C$_{18}$H$_{10}$Br$_4$CuN$_8$O$_2$ (M r = 753.49): C, 28.69; H, 1.34; N, 14.82. C, 28.66; H, 1.37; N, 14.85; discovered. Complex **chapt6-3** IR data (KBr, cm^{-1}): 3117 m, 1591 s, 1509 m, 1433 s, 1314 w, 1207 m, 1157 m, 1062 s, 962 w, 843 m, 761 s, 617 m.

Synthesis of [Mn(L^2)$_2$]$_n$ (chapt6-4)

Compound **chapt6-4** was prepared similarly to compound **chapt6-2**, with the exception that HL^1 was substituted with HL^2. On the basis of HL^2, red square crystals of **chapt6-4** were obtained (yield: 0.039 g, ca 52.4%). **chapt6-4**, C$_{18}$H$_{10}$Br$_4$MnN$_8$O$_2$ (Mr = 744.88): C = 29.03; H = 1.35; N = 15.04. Discovered C, 29.01; H, 1.38; N, 15.09. Complex **chapt6-4** IR data (KBr, cm^{-1}): 3130 m, 1591 s, 1509 m, 1459 s, 1370 w, 1226 m, 1151 m, 1056 s, 987 w, 855 w, 755 w, 704 m, 610 w.

Crystalline structure identification

The diffraction data were collected on a SuperNova using graphite monochromated Mo-K$_\alpha$ radiation (λ = 0.71073 Å) at 16 ± 1°C in the scan mode for the ranges 2.94° ≤ θ ≤ 25.24° (**chapt6-1**), 2.88 ≤ θ ≤ 25.01° (**chapt6-2**), 3.07° ≤ θ ≤ 25.24° (**chapt6-3**), and 2.86° ≤ θ ≤ 25.24° (**chapt6-4**). The program SAINT was incorporated with the raw frame data. The structures of **chapt6-1**–**chapt6-4** were determined by direct methods utilizing SHELXT and refined by full-matrix least-squares on F^2 utilizing SHELXL-2015 in the OLEX-2 GUI. The SCALE3 ABSPACK scaling algorithm incorporates an empirical absorption correction using spherical harmonics. All elements besides hydrogen were refined anisotropically. Using a riding model, all hydrogen atoms were arranged geometrically and further refined. Using SHELXTL, calculations and graphics were produced. CrysAlis PRO, Agilent Technologies, Version 1.171.37.35, SHELXL-15, and Olex2 were the computer programs utilized. The crystallographic information for 1 through 4 is given in Table 6-1. Table 6-2 lists selected bond lengths and angles for **chapt6-1**–**chapt6-4**.

Table 6-1. Crystallographic data for chapt6-1–chapt6-4

Complexes	**Chapt6-1**	**Chapt6-2**	**Chapt6-3**	**Chapt6-4**
Formula	C$_{18}$H$_{10}$Cl$_4$CuN$_8$O$_2$	C$_{18}$H$_{10}$Cl$_4$MnN$_8$O	C$_{18}$H$_{10}$Br$_4$CuN$_8$O$_2$	C$_{18}$H$_{10}$Br$_4$MnN$_8$O$_2$
M$_r$	575.68	567.07	753.49	744.88
Crystal size (mm)	0.19×0.20×0.13	0.21×0.17×0.12m	0.20×0.18×0.11m	0.21×0.18×0.14mm
Crystal system	Monoclinic	Tetragonal	Monoclinic	Tetragonal
Space group	$P2_1/c$	$P4_12_12$	$P2_1/c$	$P4_12_12$
a (Å)	12.173(1)	7.688(1)	12.699(1)	7.737(1)
b (Å)	8.504(1)	7.688(1)	8.706(1)	7.737(1)
c (Å)	10.447(1)	35.906(1)	10.440(1)	36.689(2)
α (°)	90.00	90.00	90.00	90.00
β (°)	101.328(4)	90.00	101.410(7)	90.00
γ (°)	90.00	90.00	90.00	90.00
V (Å^3)	1060.27(9)	2122.13(14)	1131.43(13)	2196.07(17)
$F(000)$	574	1132	718	1420
Z	2	4	2	4
D_c(g·cm^{-3})	1.803	1.775	2.212	2.253

μ (mm^{-1})	1.57	1.16	8.06	7.92
θ range (°)	2.94 – 25.24	2.88 – 25.24	3.07 – 25.24	2.86 – 25.24
Ref. meas. / indep.	4274/2164	21173/1984	4519/2332	4853/2161
Obs. ref.[$I > 2\sigma(I)$]	1435	1984	1733	1908
R_{int}	0.042	0.032	0.032	0.029
R_1 [$I \geq 2\sigma(I)$] [a]	0.056	0.052	0.045	0.037
ωR_2(all data) [b]	0.150	0.099	0.104	0.065
Goof	0.98	1.23	1.04	1.06
$\Delta\rho$(max, min) (e Å^{-3})	0.99 , –0.87	0.32 , –0.34	0.94 , –0.58	0.49 , –0.40

[a] $R_1 = \Sigma ||F_o| - |F_c||/\Sigma|F_o|$. [b] $wR_2 = [\Sigma w(|F_o^2|-|F_c^2|)^2/\Sigma w(|F_o^2|)^2]^{1/2}$.

Table 6-2. Selected bond length (Å) and bond angle (°) of chapt6-1–chapt6-4.

Complexes	Chapt6-1	Chapt6-2	Chapt6-3	Chapt6-4
M1–O1^i	1.947(3)	2.052(3)	1.941(5)	2.049(4)
M1–O1	1.947(3)	2.053(3)	1.941(5)	2.049(4)
M1–N4	2.344(4)	2.378(4)	2.384(6)	2.408(4)
M1–N4^i	2.344(4)	2.378(4)	2.384(6)	2.408(4)
M1–N2^{ii}	2.049(4)	2.248(5)	2.048(6)	2.252(5)
M1–N2^{iii}	2.049(4)	2.248(5)	2.048(6)	2.252(5)
O1–M1–O1^i	180.00(16)	165.0(2)	180.0(3)	164.5(2)
O1–M1–N4	82.08(13)	78.11(14)	80.7(2)	78.34(15)
O1^i–M1–N4	97.91(13)	92.67(15)	99.3(2)	92.02(15)
O1–M1–N4^i	97.91(13)	92.67(15)	99.3(2)	92.02(15)
O1^i–M1–N4^i	82.09(13)	78.11(14)	80.7(2)	78.34(15)
O1–M1–N2^{ii}	88.96(14)	86.02(15)	89.2(2)	87.80(16)
O1–M1–N2^{iii}	91.04(14)	105.41(16)	90.8(2)	103.99(16)
O1^i–M1–N2^{iii}	88.96(14)	86.02(15)	89.2(2)	87.80(16)
O1^i–M1–N2^{ii}	91.04(14)	105.41(16)	90.8(2)	103.99(16)
N4^i–M1–N4	180.0	104.9(2)	180.0	103.8(2)
N2^{iii}–M1–N4	93.88(15)	88.73(16)	94.5(2)	88.81(17)
N2^{ii}–M1–N4^i	93.88(15)	88.73(16)	94.5(2)	88.81(17)
N2^{ii}–M1–N4	86.12(15)	159.39(15)	85.5(2)	161.42(17)
N2^{iii}–M1–N4^i	86.12(15)	159.39(15)	85.5(2)	161.42(17)
N2^{ii}–M1–N2^{iii}	180.0	82.8(2)	180.0	82.6(3)
Symmetry codes:	(i)–x+1, –y, 1–z; (ii)x, –y–0.5, z+0.5; (iii)–x+1,y+0.5,0.5–z.	(i)y–1, x+1, –z–1; (ii)x, y+1, z; (iii) y, x+1, –z–1.	(i) 2–x, –y, 1–z; (ii)x, –y–0.5, z–0.5; (iii) –x+2, y+0.5, 1.5–z.	(i)y, x, 1–z; (ii)x–1, y, z; (iii)y, x–1, 1–z,

Outcomes and Analysis
Detailed description of crystal structures
Descriptions of the crystal structures of chapt6-1 and chapt6-3

The isomorphism of complexes **chapt6-1** and **chapt6-3** was confirmed through the utilization of single crystal X-ray diffraction research, as depicted in Figure 6-1. Moreover, it was determined that both complexes shared the same crystal system (monoclinic) and space group ($P2_1/c$). Consequently, solely complex **chapt6-1** was subjected to analysis.

Complex **chapt6-1** exhibited the monoclinic space group $P2_1/c$. As illustrated in Figure 6-1, Cu^{2+} coordinates with two oxygen atoms (O1, O1^i) and four nitrogen atoms (N4, N4^i, N2^{ii}, N2^{iii}) provided by four L^1 ligands to create a hexacoordinated octahedral CuN4O2 coordination structure. Cu1–O1, Cu1–N4, and Cu1–N2^{ii} (symmetry code: (ii) x, y 0.5, $z + 0.5$) had bond distances of 1.947(3), 2.344(4), and 2.049(4), respectively. Note that the difference in bond length around Cu1 may have resulted from the Jahn–Teller effect and that the L ligand exhibited the μ_2-L-$\kappa^3 O^1,N^1,N^2$ coordination mode (Figure 6-1), which is distinct from the coordination mode of [Cu(TMP)$_2$(H$_2$O)$_2$]. (HTMP is (E)-2-(((4H-1,2,4-triazol-4-yl) imino)methyl)-6-methoxyphenol with the coordination mode μ_1-TMP-$\kappa^2 O^1,N^1$. In addition, the L ligand's single coordination atom (N1) was not implicated in coordination. O1, O1^i, N4, N4^i, and Cu1 atoms were on the same plane in the ac plane (the plane equation is 1.6888 x + 7.0731 y + 5.2207 z = 7.8357) due to the fact that the bond angles between O1–Cu1–O1^i and N4–Cu1–N4^i were also 180 degrees. As the atoms in the Cu-coordinated octahedral environment were derived from four distinct ligand groups, the steric hindrance of each atom was unique, resulting in a twisted octahedral coordination configuration of copper ions.

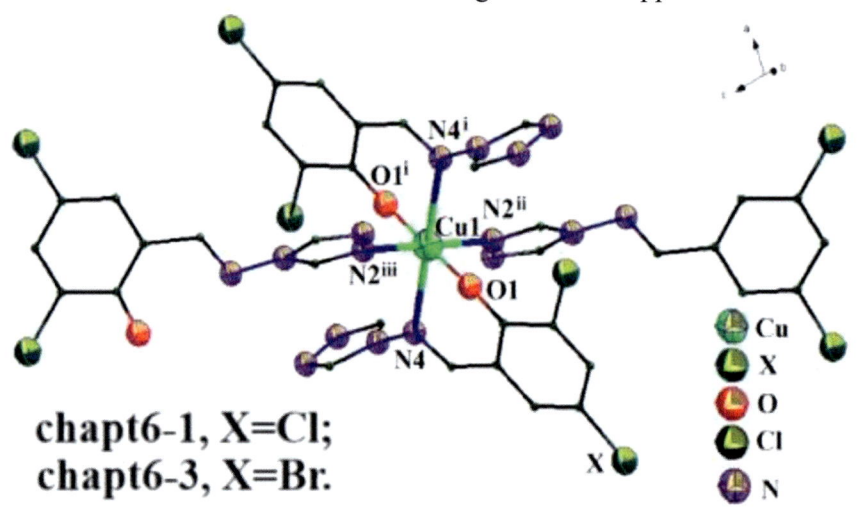

Figure 6-1. Molecular structures of chapt6-1 and chapt6-3

Each ligand functioned as a connector, facilitating the linkage between two neighboring Cu(II) ions, ultimately resulting in the formation of a chain with a distinctive staircase-like structure. The length of the step in the staircase-shaped chains was measured to be 10.96 and 10.94 Å for **chapt6-1** and **chapt6-3**, respectively. These chains were composed of two 4-amine-4H-1,2,4-triazole groups from the L ligands and one Cu ion. The vertical distance between steps in the staircase-shaped chains was measured to be 4.680 and 4.751 Å for steps **chapt6-1** and **chapt6-3**, respectively. This measurement corresponds to the distance between N4 atoms in the crystal structure, with symmetry codes (i) $1 - x, - y, 1 - z$ for **chapt6-1** and $2 - x, - y, 1 - z$ for **chapt6-3**. The angle between N4⋯N4^i⋯N4B was measured to be 112.4 and 114.08 for **chapt6-1** and **chapt6-3**, respectively. The symmetry code for **chapt6-1** was (B): $1 - x, -1 - y, -z$; and for **chapt6-3** it was: $x, 1 + y, z - 1$. Two-dimensional networks were constructed by the sharing of copper atoms, with one-dimensional chains extending in opposite directions. The N4⋯Cu1⋯N4^{iii} angle measured 84.40 and 85.26 for compounds **chapt6-1** and **chapt6-3**, respectively. The symmetry code (iii) for compound **chapt6-1** was $1 - x, 0.5 + y, 0.5 - z$, whereas for compound **chapt6-3** it was $2 - x, 0.5 + y, 1.5 - z$. Consequently, a rectangular void materialized within the two-dimensional plane. The 2D network structure was arranged in a stacked manner in the a-axis direction, resulting in a 3D structure. The layer spacing between the stacked layers was measured to be 12.439 Å. This 3D structure exhibited X···π interactions, specifically for the **chapt6-1**: Cl2···π^e with a distance of 3.428(1) Å (symmetry code: (e) 2 − x, y − 0.5, 1.5 − z.), and for the **chapt6-3**: Br2···π^f with a distance of 3.277(1) Å (symmetry code: (f) 1 − x, y − 0.5, 0.5 − z.).

Descriptions of the crystal structures of 2 and 4

The isomorphism of complexes **chapt6-2** and **chapt6-4** was determined through the examination of single crystal X-ray diffraction, as depicted in Figure 6-2. Furthermore, it was observed that both complexes shared the same crystal system (tetragonal) and space group (*P*4$_1$2$_1$2). Consequently, solely complex **chapt6-2** was subjected to analysis.

The metal coordination of compounds **chapt6-2** and **chapt6-4** exhibited similarities to those of compounds **chapt6-1** and **chapt6-3**. However, it should be noted that the ligands in compounds **chapt6-2** and **chapt6-4** displayed distinct spatial orientations. The bidentate ligands, μ_1-*L*-κ^2 O^1,N^1, in positions **chapt6-1** and **chapt6-3**, exhibit center symmetry with the copper atom serving as the point of symmetry. A plane was produced by five atoms, as depicted in Figure 6-3a. Nitrogen atoms in the N2^{ii} and N2^{iii} positions are coordinated with copper atoms located above and below the plane, respectively. The copper atoms exhibited a precise arrangement in the shape of an octahedron, as seen in Table 6-2. The bond angles between O1–Cu1–O1^i and N4–Cu1–N4^i were measured to be 180 degrees. In the case of **chapt6-2** and **chapt6-4**, the two μ_1 -*L*-κ^2O^1,N bidentate ligands attached to the Cu ion resulted in a noticeably deformed tetrahedral geometry, resembling a seesaw shape (Figure 6-3b). The bond angles between O1, Mn1, and O1 were determined to be 165.0(2) degrees, while the bond angles between N4, Mn1, and N4^i were found to be 104.9(2) degrees. These measurements were made using the symmetry code (i) y − 1, x + 1, −z − 1 for **chapt6-2**. In the deformed octahedron, the remaining two coordination sites in positions **chapt6-2** and **chapt6-4** were found to be near.

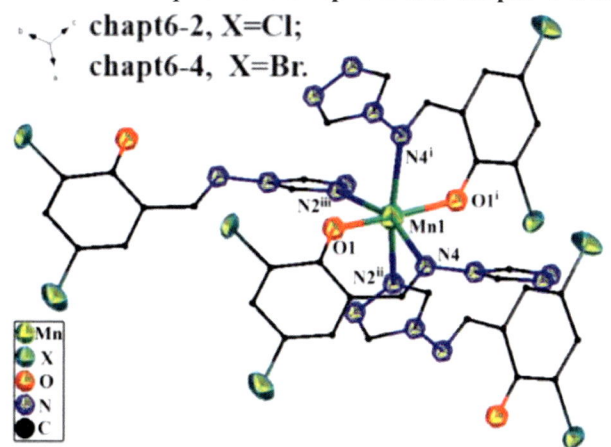

Figure 6-2. Molecular structures of chapt6-2 and chapt6-4

Manganese (Mn1) exhibits coordination with two oxygen atoms (O1, O1^i) and four nitrogen atoms (N4, N4^i, N2^{ii}, N3^{iii}) originating from four distinct ligands (*L*). This coordination results in the formation of a MnN$_4$O$_2$ coordination configuration, which is slightly deformed from an ideal octahedral geometry. The bond distances between Mn1 and O1, Mn1 and N4, and Mn1 and N2 (symmetry code: (ii) *x*, *y* + 1, *z*.) were measured to be 2.053(3), 2.378(4), and 2.248(5) Å, respectively. The 1D chain of the mononuclear Mn(L^1)$_2$ unit is formed through a Mn–N coordination bond, which distinguishes it from the staircase-shaped chain observed in compounds **chapt6-1** and **chapt6-3**. In the one-dimensional chain consisting of manganese atoms with atomic numbers **chapt6-2** and **chapt6-4**, the manganese atoms were arranged in a linear fashion. The distance between the Mn1 and Mn1a atoms, denoted as Mn1···Mn1a, was measured to be 7.688(1) Å, as shown in Figure 6-4. The 1D chain was extended to form a 2D lattice by means of Mn–N2 and N2–Mn bonding interactions. The distance neighboring the one-dimensional chain was measured to be 7.688(1) Å. Consequently, the plane exhibits a square lattice with dimensions of 7.668 × 7.688 Å and 7.737 × 7.737 Å for cases **chapt6-2** and **chapt6-4**, respectively. This is in contrast to the rectangular gap observed for cases **chapt6-1** and **chapt6-3**. The 2D lattice is formed by a 3D supramolecular network through the X···X interaction. Specifically, for compound **chapt6-2** (Cl2···Cl2^E), the distance between the chlorine atoms is 3.623(1) Å, with a symmetry code of (E) −1 − *y*, −1 − *x*, −1.5 − *z*. For compound **chapt6-4** (Br2···Br2^F), the distance between the bromine atoms is 3.738(1) Å, with a symmetry code of (F) 1 − *y*, 1 − *x*, 1.5 − *z*. Additionally, the network is stabilized by C–H···N^G hydrogen bonds. In compound **chapt6-2**, the distance between the carbon and nitrogen atoms is 3.388(1) Å, with a symmetry code of (G) *y* − 0.5, −0.5 − *x*, 1.75 + *z*. In compound **chapt6-4**, the distance between the carbon and nitrogen atoms is 3.419(1) Å. The symmetry code, denoted as G, can be represented as (0.5 - *y*, *x* - 0.5, 0.25 + *z*.).

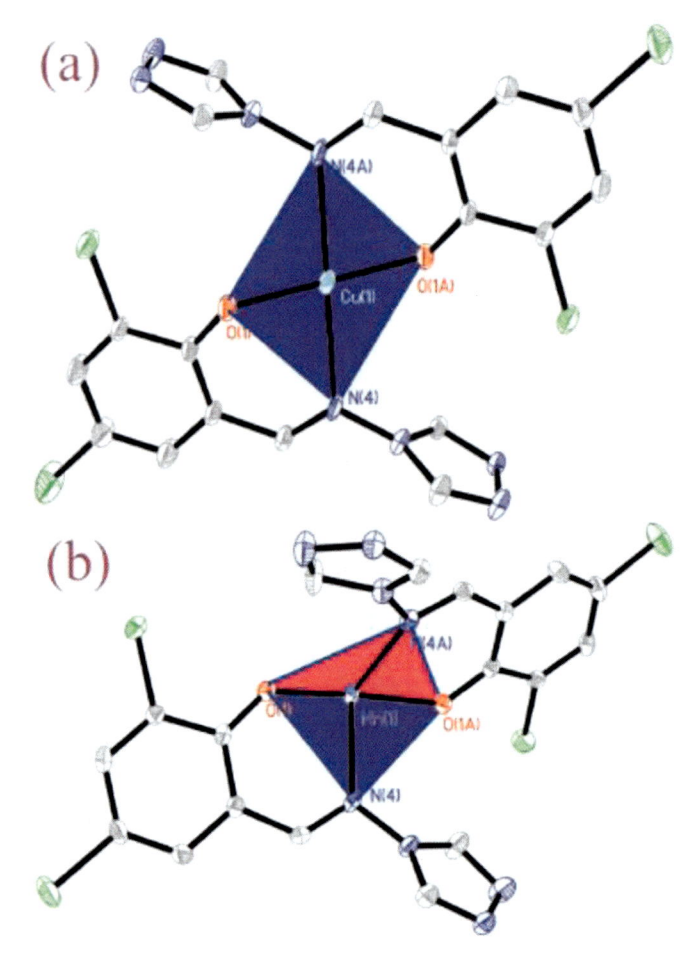

Figure 6-3. Compare the polyhedron of MO2N2 for (a) chapt6-1 and (b) chapt6-2.

The infrared spectrum clearly displayed distinct absorption peaks for each distinctive group included in the series of compounds. The ligands HL[1&2] exhibited a broad absorption band at 3448–3450 cm^{-1} (O–H), which can be attributed to the stretching vibration adsorption peak of crystal water molecules present in the surrounding atmosphere or within the complexes. The bands observed at 1660 and 1634 cm^{-1} can be attributed to the presence of the Schiff base imine group −CH=N− in the free HL[1] and HL[2] compounds, respectively. Upon complexes, these bands undergo a red-shift and are observed at 1597, 1603, 1591, and 1591 cm^{-1} for compounds **chapt6-1**–**chapt6-4**, respectively. The findings suggest that the nitrogen atom of the −CH=N− group in *L* ligands exhibited coordination. The C−O stretching vibrations seen at 1245 and 1232 cm^{-1} for free HL[1] and HL[2] ligands, respectively, exhibited a red-shift to 1214, 1214, 1207, and 1226 cm^{-1} for **chapt6-1**–**chapt6-4** complexes, respectively. This red-shift indicates the involvement of the ligands in chelation. The given text represents a numerical range between 35 and 40. The weak C−H stretching vibration of the benzene ring is responsible for the observed bands at 3130, 3124, 3111, 3143, 3117, and 3130 cm^{-1} in HL[1], HL[2], **chapt6-1**–**chapt6-4**, respectively. On the other hand, the C−X (X = Cl or Br) stretching vibration is attributed to the bands at 868, 868, 849, 855, 843, and 855 cm^{-1} in HL[1], HL[2], **chapt6-1**–**chapt6-4**, respectively. Through a comparative analysis of the infrared (IR) spectra of the HL[1] and HL[2] ligands in relation to the complexes **chapt6-1**–**chapt6-4**, it is shown that the alterations in the IR spectrum might potentially be attributed to variations in the electron cloud density around the ligand molecule subsequent to its coordination with the metal ions.

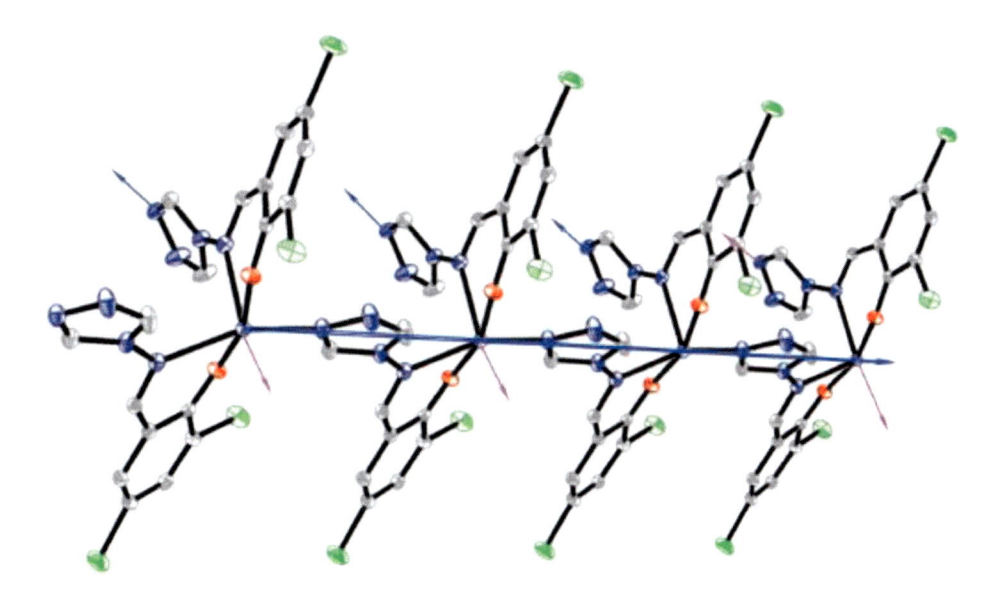

Figure 6-4. 1D chain of chapt6-2 and chapt6-4

Thermal stability examination

The thermal stability of complexes **chapt6-1**–**chapt6-4** was evaluated under controlled test circumstances, including a nitrogen (N$_2$) flow rate of 100.0 mL/min and a heating rate of 10 °C/min. The temperature range for testing ranged from room temperature to 900°C. It is worth noting that the purity of the samples was confirmed through the use of powder X-ray diffraction

(PXRD). Figure 6-5 displays the thermogravimetric curves of complexes **chapt6-1**–**chapt6-4**. The weightlessness behaviors of the four complexes were found to be quite similar, with complexes **chapt6-1** and **chapt6-3** displaying comparable characteristics, while complexes **chapt6-2** and **chapt6-4** revealed small distinctions. Complexes **chapt6-2** and **chapt6-4** exhibited decomposition at approximately 329°C, whereas complexes **chapt6-1** and **chapt6-3** shown degradation at around 220°C. This observation suggests that complexes **chapt6-2** and **chapt6-4** possess greater stability compared to complexes **chapt6-1** and **chapt6-3**. The temperature at which decomposition ceased was around 720 degrees Celsius, resulting in the formation of the respective metal oxides as the remaining products.

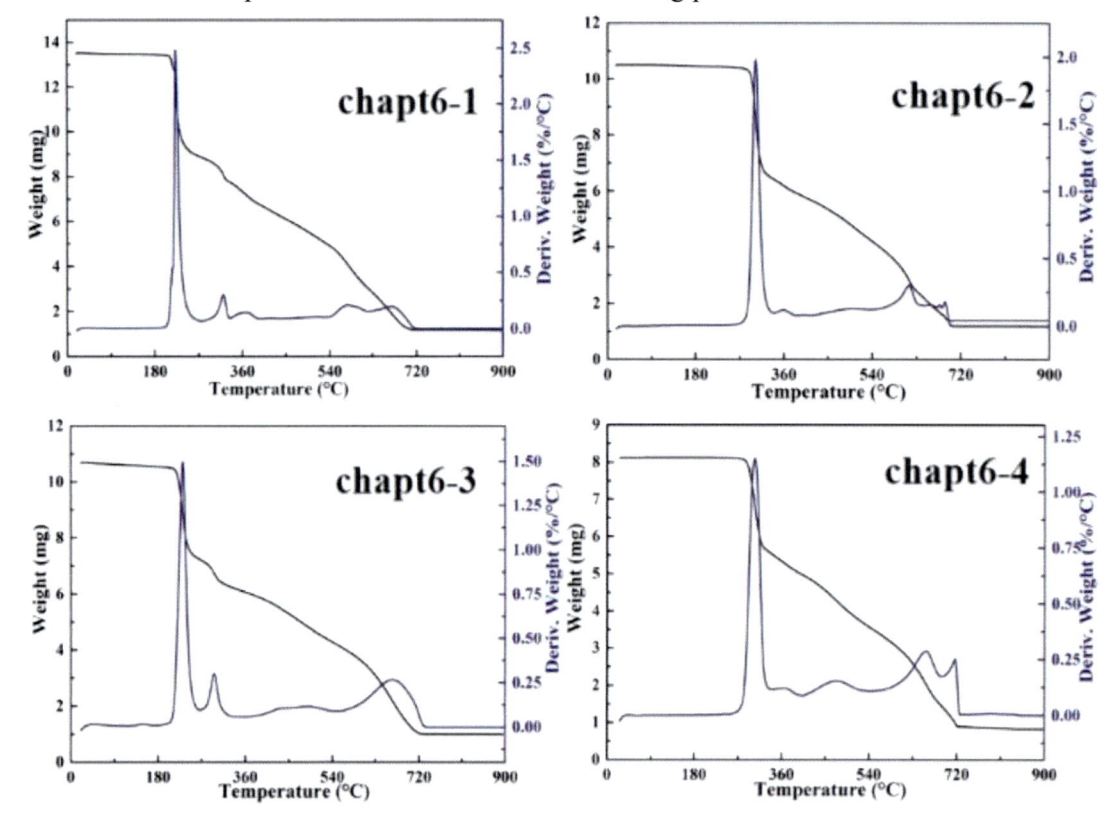

Figure 6-5. Thermogravimetric curves of chapt6-1-chapt6-4.

Hirshfeld surface examination

The 2D fingerprint acquired by the Hirshfeld analysis of the surface effect of the structural unit is depicted in Figure 6-6. The quantitative analysis of the properties and types of intermolecular interactions within the crystal was conducted, and the calculations for this aspect were performed using the CrystalExplorer 3.1 software. The intermolecular forces between distinct elements were examined individually inside the two-dimensional fingerprint, followed by an analysis of the relative magnitudes of these forces in different regions to investigate the structure. In the case of compounds **chapt6-1**–**chapt6-4**, the X (Cl and Br)–H interaction contributes significantly to the overall 2D fingerprint, with proportions of 21.2%, 16.5%, 20.9%, and 17.0%, respectively. The correlation between the intramolecular halogens (Cl and Br) and the extramolecular hydrogen (H) is observed in the fingerprint region located in the lower-left corner (donor) of the fingerprint. The positioning of hydrogen (H) within the molecule and its interaction with the external X elements (Cl and Br) occurred in the receptor region of the lower-right corner of the fingerprint area. This positioning suggests the presence of a distinct C–H⋯X (Cl and Br) nonconventional hydrogen bond in the crystal structure of compounds **chapt6-1–chapt6-4**. The involvement of the C–X (Cl and Br) interaction is significant in determining the overall 2D fingerprint. The compounds **chapt6-1–chapt6-4** exhibited C-X (Cl and Br) percentages of 12.7%, 13.4%, 12.8%, and 15.1%, respectively. The C⋯X distances for **chapt6-1–chapt6-4** were measured to be 3.501, 3.408, 3.533, and 3.397 Å, respectively. The H–H contact emerged as a significant intermolecular interaction in compounds **chapt6-1–chapt6-4**, as evidenced by its prominent presence in the central region of the scattering point within the 2D fingerprint. The H–H effect accounted for 13.4%, 10.7%, 12.7%, and 10.6% of the compounds **chapt6-1–chapt6-4**, respectively. Table 6-3 provides a comprehensive summary of the forces exhibited by various components.

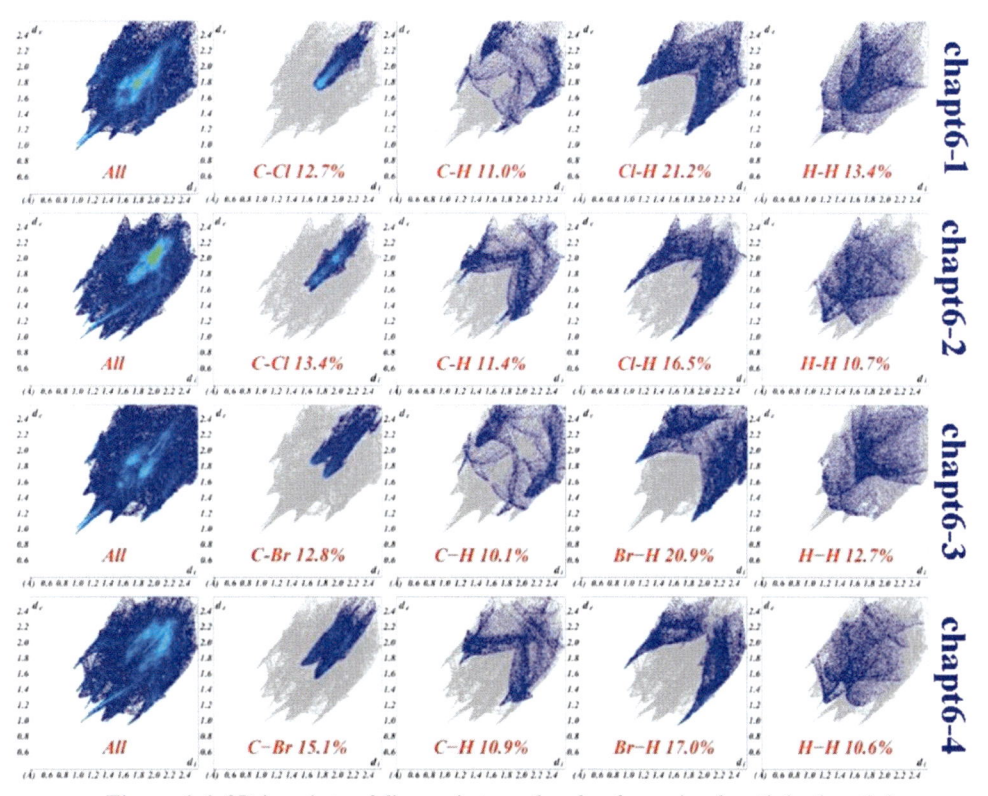

Figure 6-6. 2D imprints of diverse intermolecular forces in chapt6-1–chapt6-4

Table 6-3. Calculations of Hirshfeld surface (percent) for chapt6-1–chapt6-4.

Complex	X⋯H (X = Cl, Br)	H⋯H	C⋯X	C⋯H	N⋯X	N⋯H
Chapt6-1	21.2	13.4	12.7	11.0	4.3	8.5
Chapt6-2	16.5	10.7	13.4	11.4	8.3	8.6
Chapt6-3	20.9	12.7	12.8	10.1	4.1	8.4
Chapt6-4	17.0	10.6	15.1	10.9	8.4	7.9

Fluorescence characteristics of chapt6-1–chapt6-4

The investigation focused on the luminous characteristics of compounds **chapt6-1–chapt6-4** and the free $HL^{1\&2}$ ligands, which were conducted in a DMF solvent at a concentration of 5×10^{-5} mol/L (Figure 6-7). The excitation wavelength for testing the fluorescence spectra of the compounds was chosen to be the maximum absorption wavelength. A 438 nm wavelength was employed to stimulate the luminescent properties of a set of HL^1, **chapt6-1**, and **chapt6-2**, utilizing a slit width of 2.5 nm. When the HL^1 ligand was subjected to photoexcitation at a wavelength of 438 nm, it exhibited a blue luminescent property. The emission spectrum of this compound showed a peak at 470 nm, which can be mostly attributed to fluorescence resulting from π–π* transition. Under the conditions of a photoexcitation at a wavelength of 438 nm, both **chapt6-1** and **chapt6-2** demonstrated a green luminous emission band at 527 nm and 514 nm, respectively. In comparison to the unbound ligand HL^1, compounds **chapt6-1** and **chapt6-2** exhibit a red-shift of 57 and 44 nm, respectively. Additionally, the emission wavelengths of 527 and 514 nm, as well as the reduced fluorescence intensity, observed in compounds **chapt6-1** and **chapt6-2**, can likely be attributed to the paramagnetic effects of Cu^{II} and Mn^{II} cations. These cations possess d^9 and d^5 electron configurations, respectively.

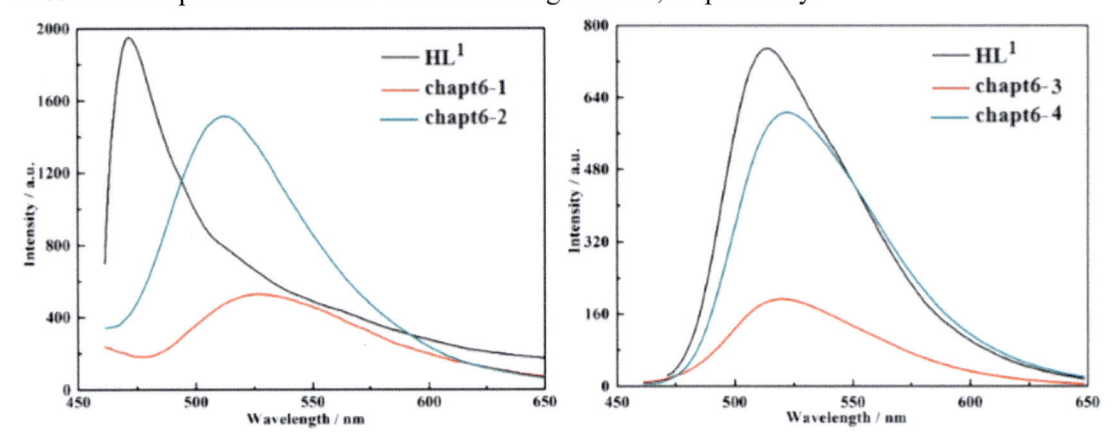

Figure 6-7. Fluorescent characteristics of HL$^{1\&2}$ and chapt6-1–chapt6-4

According to the data presented in Figure 6-7b, when the HL^2 ligand was subjected to photoexcitation at a wavelength of 450 nm, it emitted a luminescent peak at 512 nm, which was mostly attributed to fluorescence resulting from π–π* transition. Under the conditions of a 450 nm photoexcitation, it was observed that both **chapt6-3** and **chapt6-4** had a luminescent emission peak in the green region of the spectrum, namely at wavelengths of 519 nm and 522 nm, respectively. The emission peaks of compounds **chapt6-3** and **chapt6-4** exhibited a red-shift of approximately 7 and 10 nm, respectively, in comparison to the unbound HL^2 ligand. The observed decrease in fluorescence intensity and redshift in the case of compounds **chapt6-3** and **chapt6-4** can likely be attributed to the paramagnetic effects of Cu^{II} and Mn^{II} cations, which possess d^9 and d^5 electron configurations, respectively. Through a comparison of the fluorescence intensity between compounds **chapt6-1** and **chapt6-2**, as well as compounds **chapt6-3** and **chapt6-4**, it was observed that the fluorescence intensity of compounds **chapt6-1** and **chapt6-3** was comparatively lower than that of compounds **chapt6-2** and **chapt6-4**, respectively. This discrepancy can be attributed to the electronegativity of the substituents and the electron density of the ligand. Specifically, the lower fluorescence intensity of compounds **chapt6-1** and **chapt6-3** can be explained by the higher electronegativity of chlorine in comparison to bromine. Consequently, the electron density of ligand HL^1 exhibited a lower value compared to that of ligand HL^2, so detrimentally affecting the ligand-to-metal charge transfer process. The distinctive luminous characteristics exhibited by this group of compounds warrant further investigation as a prospective fluorescent substance.

ECL characteristics of chapt6-1–chapt6-4

Figure 6-8 displays the electrochemiluminescence (ECL) of the pure complexes **chapt6-1–chapt6-4**. The phase purity of complexes **chapt6-1–chapt6-4** has been verified by powder X-ray diffraction (PXRD). Cyclic voltammetry (CV) was employed as a method of investigation in order to obtain a deeper understanding of the redox characteristics exhibited by compounds **chapt6-1–chapt6-4**. The experimental results of cyclic voltammetry (CV) utilizing glassy carbon disk electrodes that have been treated with complexes **chapt6-1–chapt6-4** are depicted in Figure 6-9. In the first experiment, with the addition of $K_2S_2O_8$ to the solution, an oxidation peak at a cathodic current of -1.5 V and a reduction peak at a cathodic current of -0.95 V were detected. The cyclic voltammetry (CV) curves observed for the remaining three complexes exhibit a resemblance to that of complex **chapt6-1**.

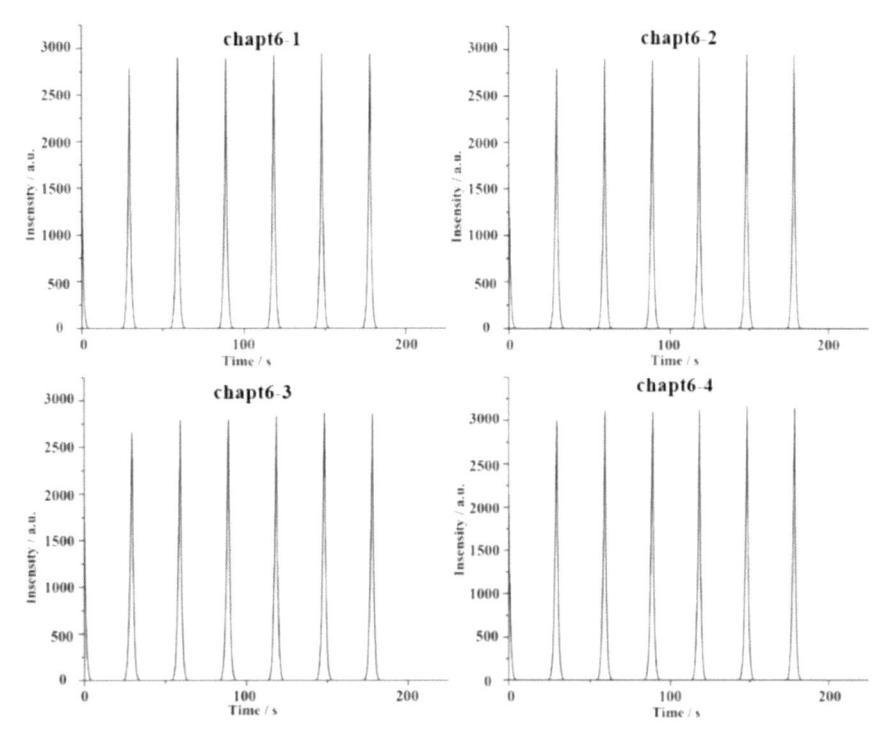

Figure 6-8. The electromagnetic emission spectrum of chapt6-1-chapt6-4

The maximum luminous intensity for complexes **chapt6-1–chapt6-4** was seen to be approximately 2850, 2960, 2850, and 3100 arbitrary units (a.u.), respectively. After undergoing seven cycles, the luminous intensities continued to exhibit consistent stability. In the various metal complexes formed by a common ligand, it is shown that the Mn(II) complex exhibits a greater maximum luminescence intensity compared to the Cu(II) complex. In a broader context, it can be observed that these four compounds exhibit robust and enduring luminous characteristics, rendering them highly valuable for possible applications in the field of electrochemical materials. Notably, compound **chapt6-4** stands out as particularly promising in this regard.

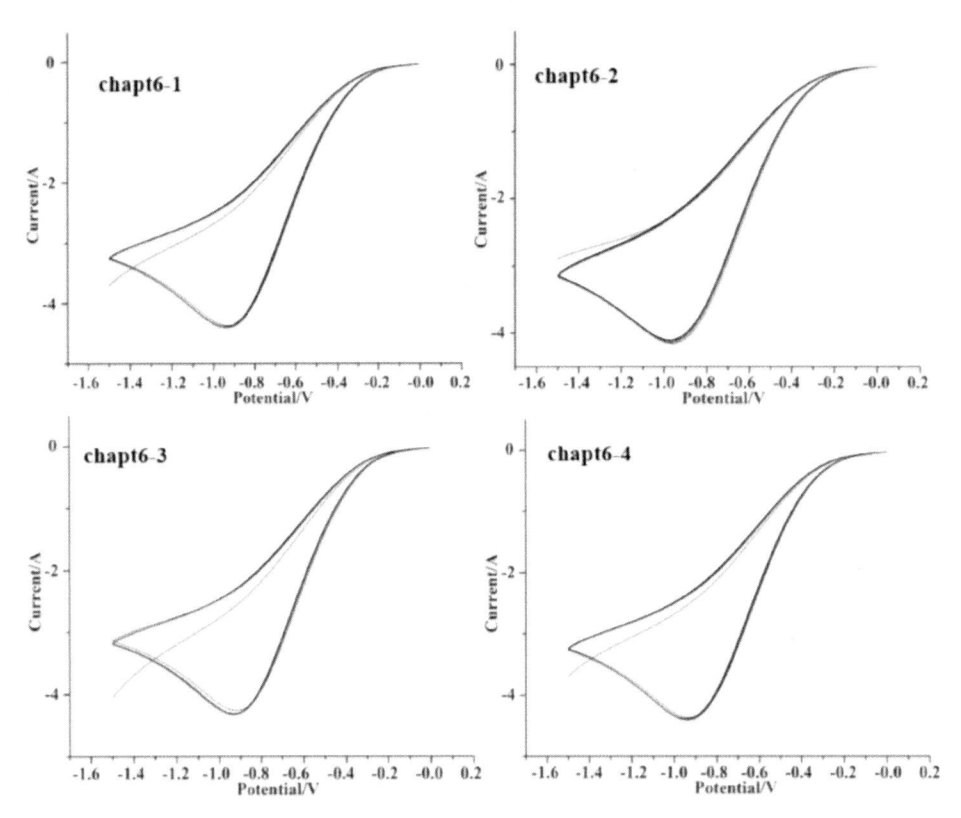

Figure 6-9. Curves of cyclic voltammetry for chapt6-1–chapt6-4

The complex $[Ru(bpy)_3]^{3+}$ has been utilized as a benchmark to assess the electrochemiluminescence (ECL) efficiency. The obtained ECL yields for complexes **chapt6-1–chapt6-4** were 0.63, 0.66, 0.63, and 0.69, respectively. The potential strengthening of the spin-orbit coupling effect and enhancement of the electrochemiluminescence (ECL) emission is tentatively proposed by the introduction of Cu and Mn ions, with a particular emphasis on the Mn ion. In comparison to previously published Ru-, Ir-, Pt-, Re-, Os-, and Cd-complexes, the four complexes presented in this study as novel polymer ECL materials demonstrate superior economic advantages and environmental compatibility due to the utilization of copper and manganese, which are metals with lower toxicity levels and more affordable prices.

Using two distinct $HL^{1\&2}$ ligands, four new 2D structures with Cu(II) and Mn(II) ions were effectively synthesized. According to the results of Hirshfeld surface analysis, XH (X = Br, Cl) interactions play a significant role in stabilizing the self-assembly process. The fluorescent properties of **chapt6-1–chapt6-4** can be investigated as a possible fluorescent material. In addition, complexes **chapt6-1–chapt6-4** exhibit greater stability and stronger ECL emissions, making them a valuable resource for the design of novel ECL materials.

References

1. Yuan, S.; Feng, L.; Wang, K.; Pang, J.; Bosch, M.; Lollar, C.; Sun, Y.; Qin, J.; Yang, X.; Zhang, P.; Wang, Q.; Zou, L.; Zhang, Y.; Zhang, L.; Fang, Y.; Li, J.;Zhou, H. C. Stable Metal-Organic Frameworks: Design, Synthesis, and Applications. Adv. Mater. 2018, 30(37), e1704303.

2. Xiao, J.; Chen, C. X.; Liu, Q. K.; Ma, J. P.; Dong, Y. B. Cd(II)-Schiff-Base Metal-Organic Frameworks: Synthesis, Structure, and Reversible Adsorption and Separation of Volatile Chlorocarbons. Cryst. Growth Des., 2011, 11(12), 5696-5701.
3. Chen, Y.; Zhang, S.; Xiao, Y.; Zhang, S. H. Synthesis, Crystal Structures and Magnetic and Electrochemiluminescence Properties of Three Manganese(II) Complexes. Acta. Crystallogr. C., 2020, 76(3), 236-243.
4. Zhao, Y.; Deng, D. S.; Ma, L. F.; Ji, B. M.; Wang, L. Y. A New Copper-Based Metal-Organic Framework as a Promising Heterogeneous Catalyst for Chemo- and Regio-Selective Enamination of β-ketoesters. Chem. Commun., 2013, 49(87), 10299-10301.
5. Zhang, E.; Ju, P.; Zhang, Z.; Yang, H.; Tang, L.; Hou, X.; You, J.; Wang, J. J. A Novel Multi-Purpose Zn-MOF Fluorescent Sensor for 2,4-dinitrophenylhydrazine, Picric Acid, La3+ and Ca2+: Synthesis, Structure, Selectivity, Sensitivity and Recyclability. Spectrochim. Acta. A., 2019, 222, 117207.
6. Zhao, G.; Wang, Y.; Li, X.; Yue, Q.; Dong, X.; Du, B.; Cao, W.; Wei, Q. Dual-Quenching Electrochemiluminescence Strategy Based on Three-Dimensional Metal-Organic Frameworks for Ultrasensitive Detection of Amyloid-β. Anal. Chem., 2019, 91(3), 1989-1996.
7. Falcaro, P.; Normandin, F.; Takahashi, M.; Scopece, P.; Amenitsch, H.; Costacurta, S.; Doherty, C. M.; Laird, J. S.; Lay, M. D. H.; Lisi, T.; Hill, A. J.; Buso, D. Dynamic Control of MOF-5 Crystal Positioning Using a Magnetic Field. Adv. Mater., 2011, 23(34), 3901-3906.
8. Tan, H.; Tang, G.; Wang, Z.; Li, Q.; Gao, J.; Wu, S. Magnetic Porous Carbon Nanocomposites Derived from Metal-Organic Frameworks as a Sensing Platform for DNA Fluorescent Detection. Anal. Chim. Acta, 2016, 940, 136-142.
9. Xiao, R.; Pan, Y.; Li, J.; Zhang, L.; Zhang, W. Layer-by-Layer Assembled Magnetic Bimetallic Metal-Organic Framework Composite for Global Phosphopeptide Enrichment. J. Chromatogr. A., 2019, 1601, 45-52.
10. Xie, M.; Tang, J.; Fang, G.; Zhang, M.; Kong, L.; Zhu, F.; Ma, L.; Zhou, D.; Zhan, J. Biomass Schiff Base Polymer-Derived N-Doped Porous Carbon Embedded with CoO Nanodots for Adsorption and Catalytic Degradation of Chlorophenol by Peroxymonosulfate. J. Hazard. Mater, 2020, 384, 121345.
11. Wang, Z.; Yu, H.; Han, J.; Xie, G.; Chen, S. Rare Co/Fe-MOFs Exhibiting High Catalytic Activity in Electrochemical Aptasensors for Ultrasensitive Detection of Ochratoxin A. Chem. Commun., 2017, 53(71), 9926-9929.
12. Paz, F. A. A.; Klinowski, J.; Vilela, S. M.; Tome, J. P.; Cavaleiro, J. A.; Rocha, J. Ligand Design for Functional Metal-Organic Frameworks. Chem. Soc. Rev., 2012, 41(3), 1088-1110.
13. Yang, X. G.; Lu, X. M.; Zhai, Z. M.; Zhao, Y.; Liu, X. Y.; Ma, L. F.; Zang, S. Q. Facile Synthesis of a Micro-Scale MOF Host-Guest with Long-Lasting Phosphorescence and Enhanced Optoelectronic Performance. Chem. Commun., 2019, 55(74), 11099-11102.
14. Ma, L.; Abney, C.; Lin, W. Enantioselective Catalysis with Homochiral Metal-Organic Frameworks. Chem. Soc. Rev., 2009, 38(5), 1248-1256.
15. Yang, D.; Gates, B. C., Catalysis by Metal Organic Frameworks: Perspective and Suggestions for Future Research. ACS. Catal., 2019, 9(3), 1779-1798.

16. Dhayabaran, V. V.; Prakash, T. D.; Renganathan, R.; Friehs, E.; Bahnemann, D. W. Novel Bioactive Co(II), Cu(II), Ni(II) and Zn(II) Complexes with Schiff Base Ligand Derived from Histidine and 1,3-Indandione: Synthesis, Structural Elucidation, Biological Investigation and Docking Analysis. J. Fluoresc., 2017, 27, 135-150.
17. Gong, Y.; Wu, T.; Jiang, P. G.; Lin, J. H.; Yang, Y. X. Octamolybdate-Based Metal-Organic Framework with Unsaturated Coordinated Metal Center As Electrocatalyst for Generating Hydrogen from Water. Inorg. Chem., 2013, 52(2), 777-784.
18. H. Liang, Y. Q. Zhou, P. W. Shen. The Structural Study on Metal Centre in Mn(II)-HSA and Mn(II)-BSA Complex. Chin. Sci. Bull., 1994, 39(17), 1452-1455.
19. Park, H.; Krigsfeld, G.; Teat, S. J.; Parise, J. B. Synthesis and Structural Determination of Four Novel Metal-Organic Frameworks in a Zn-3-Amino-1,2,4-Triazole System. Cryst. Growth Des., 2007, 7(7), 1343-1349.
20. Sun, L.; Chen, H.; Ma, C.; Chen, C. A New Topology of Hexanuclear Mn/Ln clusters: Synthesis, Structures and Magnetic Properties. Inorg. Chem. Commun., 2017, 77, 77-79.
21. Xu, Y.; Yin, X. B.; He, X. W.; Zhang, Y. K. Electrochemistry and Electrochemiluminescence from a Redox-active Metal-Organic Framework. Biosens. Bioelectron., 2015, 68, 197-203.
22. Feng, D.; Tan, X.; Wu, Y.; Ai, C.; Luo, Y.; Chen, Q.; Han, H. Electrochemiluminecence Nanogears Aptasensor Based on MIL-53(Fe)@CdS for Multiplexed Detection of Kanamycin and Neomycin. Biosens. Bioelectron., 2019, 129, 100-106.
23. Hu, G. B.; Xiong, C. Y.; Liang, W. B.; Zeng, X. S.; Xu, H. L.; Yang, Y.; Yao, L. Y.; Yuan, R.; Xiao, D. R. Highly Stable Mesoporous Luminescence-Functionalized MOF with Excellent Electrochemiluminescence Property for Ultrasensitive Immunosensor Construction. ACS. Appl. Mater. Inter., 2018, 10(18), 15913-15919.
24. Yang, X.; Yu, Y. Q.; Peng, L. Z.; Lei, Y. M.; Chai, Y. Q.; Yuan, R.; Zhuo, Y. Strong Electrochemiluminescence from MOF Accelerator Enriched Quantum Dots for Enhanced Sensing of Trace cTnI. Anal. Chem., 2018, 90(6), 3995-4002.
25. Wang, J. M.; Deng, Q. J.; Zhang, S. H. Micro-vial Synthesis, Structure, Magnetic Properties and Hirshfeld Surface Analysis of a Penta-Nuclear Fe (III) Cluster. Chinese. J. Struct. Chem+., 2020, 39(1), 118-125.
26. Shen, X.; Zhang, T.; Broderick, S.; Rajan, K. Correlative Analysis of Metal Organic Framework Structures Through Manifold Learning of Hirshfeld Surfaces. Mol. Syst. Des. Eng., 2018, 3, 826-838.
27. Zheng, X.; Yi, M.; Chen, Z.; Zhang, Z.; Ye, L.; Cheng, G.; Xiao, Y. Efficient Removal of As(V) from Simulated Arsenic-Contaminated Wastewater Via a Novel Metal-Organic Framework Material: Synthesis, Structure, and Response Surface Methodology. Appl. Organoment. Chem., 2020, 34(5), e5584.
28. Kojima, D.; Sanada, T.; Wada, N.; Kojima, K. Synthesis, Structure, and Fluorescence Properties of a Calcium-Based Metal-Organic Framework. RSC. Adv., 2018, 8, 31588-31593.
29. Chandrasekhar, P.; Mukhopadhyay, A.; Savitha, G.; Moorthy, J. N. Remarkably Selective and Enantiodifferentiating Sensing of Histidine by a Fluorescent Homochiral Zn-MOF Based on Pyrene-Tetralactic Acid. Chem. Sci., 2016, 7, 3085-3091.

30. Yanagimoto, T.; Nakagawa, A.; Komatsu, T.; Tsuchida, E. Photoreduction of a Self-Assembled (Lipidporphyrinato)iron(III) Complex in Saline by LMCT Excitation: Co-Aggregated Hyaluronic Acid Allows an Irreversible Electron Transfer. B. Chem. Soc. Jpn., 2001, 74(11), 2123-2128.
31. Dolomanov, O. V.; Bourhis, L. J.; Gildea, R. J.; Howard, J. A. K.; Puschmann, H. OLEX2: a Complete Structure Solution, Refinement and Analysis Program. J. Appl. Crystallogr., 2009, 42(2), 339-341.
32. Sheldrick, G. M. Crystal Structure Refinement with SHELXL. Acta Crystallogr., 2015, 71, 3-8.
33. Sheldrick, G. M. A Short History of SHELX. Acta. Crystallogr., 2008, A64, 112-122.
34. Zhang, S. H.; Zhao, R. X.; Li, G.; Zhang, H. Y.; Huang, Q. P.; Liang, F. P. Room Temperature Syntheses, Crystal Structures and Properties of Two New Heterometallic Polymers Based on 3-Ethoxy-2-Hydroxybenzaldehyde Ligand. J. Solid. State. Chem., 2014, 220, 206-212.
35. Halcrow, M. A. Jahn-Teller Distortions in Transition Metal Compounds, and their Importance in Functional Molecular and Inorganic Materials. Chem. Soc. Rev., 2013, 42, 1784-1795.
36. Zhang, S. M.; Zhang, H. Y.; Qin, Q. P.; Fei, J. W.; Zhang, S. H. Syntheses, Crystal Structures and Biological Evaluation of Two New Cu(II) and Co(II) Complexes Based on (E)-2-(((4H-1,2,4-Triazol-4-yl)Imino)Methyl)-6-Methoxyphenol. J. Inorg. Biochem., 2019, 193, 52-59.
37. Wu, C.; Zheng, Chen, X. G.; Chen, Z.; Xiao, Y. Solvothermal Syntheses, Crystal Structures and Magnetic Properties of Two Nickel Cubane-Type Cluster Complexes. J. Cluster Sci., 2019, 30, 1347-1354.
38. Zhang, H. Y. Xiao, Y. Zhu, Y. A Novel Copper(II) Complex Based on 4-Amino-1,2,4-Triazole Schiff-Base: Synthesis, Crystal Structure, Spectral Characterization, and Hirshfeld Surface Analysis. Chin. J. Struct. Chem., 2017, 36(5), 848–855.
39. Shebl, M. Synthesis, Spectroscopic Characterization and Antimicrobial Activity of Binuclear Metal Complexes of a New Asymmetrical Schiff Base Ligand: DNA Binding Affinity of Copper(II) Complexes. Spectrochim. Acta. A., 2014, 117, 127-137.
40. Richter, M. M. Electrochemiluminescence (ECL). Chem. Rev., 2004, 104(6), 3003-3036.
41. Huang, B. M.; Zhou, X. B.; Xue, Z. H.; Lu, X. Q. Quenching of the Electrochemiluminescence of Ru(bpy)$_3^{2+}$/TPA by Malachite Green and Crystal Violet. Talanta, 2013, 106, 174-180.
42. Zhou, Y.; Li, W.; Yu, L.; Liu, Y.; Wang, X.; Zhou, M. Highly Efficient Electrochemiluminescence from Iridium(III) Complexes with 2-Phenylquinoline ligand. Dalton. Trans., 2015, 44, 1858-1865.

Chapter 7

Synthesis, crystal structures, and investigation of the magnetic and electrochemiluminescent properties of three manganese (II) complexes

In recent decades, there has been significant interest in polynuclear metal compounds due to their diverse functional applications in science and technology. These compounds have garnered attention for their magnetic, fluorescent, optical, electronic, and catalytic properties. Additionally, they have shown promise in the treatment and diagnosis of various diseases, as well as in the development of sensors with unique properties. In the realm of transition polynuclear complexes, manganese complexes exhibit intriguing characteristics and diverse structures due to the larger spin ground states, flexible coordination modes, varying coordination numbers, and variable valence states of manganese. These valence states include +2, +3, +4, +5, +6, and +7. Furthermore, various synthesis parameters have the potential to influence the structure and nuclearity of transition polynuclear complexes. These parameters encompass metal ions, ligands, concentrations, counterions, templates, solvents, temperatures, and pH values.

On the contrary, electrogenerated chemiluminescence, also known as electrochemiluminescence (ECL), refers to a phenomenon wherein species produced using electrochemical means experience very energetic electron transfer processes, resulting in the emission of light from excited states. In recent years, numerous ECL active complexes have been documented by scientists, garnering significant interest for their possible use in chemical/biochemical sensors, molecular logic gates, molecular memory, and display displays. However, the majority of compounds employed as electrochemiluminescence (ECL) luminophores consist of elements such as iridium (Ir), ruthenium (Ru), platinum (Pt), rhenium (Re), osmium (Os), and cadmium (Cd). These compounds are composed of valuable metals or a very toxic heavy metal, namely Cadmium (Cd), which give rise to significant health and environmental risks as well as economic implications. Consequently, the utilization of the aforementioned chemicals in electrochemiluminescence (ECL) sensors would be constrained. The recent discovery of transition metal complexes that have both environmentally friendly characteristics and excellent electrochemiluminescence (ECL) activity is intriguing. Moreover, these complexes can also serve as ECL luminophores. In this study, we present the synthesis and characterization of three newly discovered manganese complexes. We investigate their electrochemiluminescence (ECL) and magnetic properties.

Experimental

Synthesis and crystallization

Synthesis of HL¹

The compound 2-Hydroxy-3-methoxy-benzaldehyde, also known as Hmbd, was used in this study. A quantity of 10 mmol (1.522 g) of Hmbd was employed. Additionally, (6-Chloro-pyridin-2-yl)Hydrazine (10 mmol, 1.44 g) and ethanol (20 mL) were subjected to reflux in a 100 mL three-necked flask at a temperature of 353 K for a duration of 2 hours. The solution underwent a color change to brown and was subjected to enrichment at a temperature of 353 K for a duration of 2 hours. The brown powder was acquired through the process of filtration, followed by three washes with ethanol (5 mL each). Subsequently, the powder was left to dry in ambient air conditions, resulting in a yield of 2.72 g, approximately 98% of the expected yield based on the initial amount of the starting material. The elemental composition of $C_{13}H_{12}C_{1}N_3O_2$ (molar mass = 277.71 g/mol) in terms of percentage is as follows: carbon (C) 56.13%, hydrogen (H) 4.28%, and nitrogen (N) 15.27%. The elemental composition of the compound is as follows: carbon (C) with a mass percentage of 56.21%, hydrogen (H) with a mass percentage of 4.32%, and nitrogen (N) with a mass percentage of 15.14%. The infrared (IR) data for HL¹, obtained using KBr as the medium and expressed in wavenumbers (cm^{-1}). The observed peaks are as follows: 3420 (sharp), 2918 (sharp), 1657 (sharp), 1617 (medium), 1581 (medium), 1534 (sharp), 1461 (sharp), 1417 (sharp), 1388 (sharp), 1303 (sharp), 1255 (sharp), 1215 (sharp), 1170 (sharp), 1147 (sharp), 998 (sharp), 777 (sharp), 724 (sharp), and 453 (sharp). The ^1H NMR spectrum was obtained using a 500 MHz instrument and $CDCl_3$ as the solvent. The chemical shifts (δ) and coupling constants (J) are as follows: a singlet (s) at δ 10.55 for one proton (^1H), another singlet at δ 8.27 for one proton (1H), a third singlet at δ 7.94 for one proton (^1H), a triplet (t) at δ 7.60 with a coupling constant of J = 7.9 Hz for one proton (^1H), a doublet (d) at δ 6.99 with a coupling constant of J = 8.2 Hz for one proton (^1H), a multiplet (m) in the range of δ 6.97-6.93 for one proton (^1H), a doublet of doublets (dd) at δ 6.91 with coupling constants of J = 6.6 Hz and 2.6 Hz for two protons (2H), a doublet (d) at δ 6.87 with a coupling constant of J = 7.6 Hz for one proton (^1H), and a doublet (d) at δ 3.96 with a coupling constant of J = 3.4 Hz for three protons (3H).

Synthesis of HL²

The preparation of HL² followed a similar procedure to that of HL¹, with the exception of substituting (6-Chloro-pyridin-2-yl)-hydrazine with (6-bromo-pyridin-2-yl)-Hydrazine, a yellow powder, was isolated through the process of filtration. The resulting product was subsequently washed with ethanol (5 mL × 3) and allowed to dry in ambient air. The yield of the hydrazine was determined to be 3.25 g, almost 97% of the theoretical yield based on the initial amount of starting material, Hmbd. The elemental composition of the compound $C_{13}H_{12}BrN_3O_2$ (molar mass = 322.15 g/mol) was determined using analytical calculations. The percentages of carbon (C), hydrogen (H), and nitrogen (N) were found to be 48.43%, 3.72%, and 13.07%, respectively. Upon experimental analysis, the measured percentages of C, H, and N were determined to be 48.45%, 3.73%, and 13.04%, respectively. The infrared (IR) data for HL² (KBr). The observed wavenumbers (cm^{-1}) are as follows: 3420 (strong), 2928 (strong), 1657 (medium), 1617 (weak), 1581 (weak), 1534 (weak), 1461 (weak), 1417 (weak), 1388 (medium), 1303 (strong), 1255 (strong), 1215 (strong), 1170 (medium), 1147 (medium), 998 (strong), 777 (strong), 724 (strong), and 453 (strong). The proton nuclear magnetic resonance

(^{1}H NMR) spectrum was obtained using a 500 MHz spectrometer with CDCl$_3$ as the solvent. The chemical shifts (δ) and corresponding multiplicities for the observed peaks are as follows: 10.53 (singlet, ^{1}H), 8.25 (singlet, ^{1}H), 7.92 (singlet, ^{1}H), 7.57 (triplet, J = 7.9 Hz, ^{1}H), 6.97 (doublet, ^{1}H), 6.93-6.91 (multiplet, ^{1}H), 6.89-6.88 (multiplet, ^{2}H), 6.85 (doublet, ^{1}H), and 3.94 (singlet, J = 3.4 Hz, 3H).

Synthesis of Mn$_4$(L^1)$_2$(CH$_3$COO)$_{5.17}$(HCOO)$_{0.83}$ (chapt7-1)

A mixture of HL^1 (0.5 mmol, 0.1385 g), Mn(CH$_3$COO)$_2$·4H$_2$O (0.5 mmol, 0.104 g), DMF (5 mL) and ethyl alcohol (5 mL) was put into a Teflon-lined autoclave (15 mL) and then heated at 353 K for 3 day and cooled to room temperature slowly. Yellow crystals of **chapt7-1** were obtained (Yield: 0.097 g, ca. 69 % based on Mn^{2+}) *Anal. Calc.* for **chapt7-1**: C$_{37.17}$H$_{38.34}$Cl$_2$Mn$_4$N$_6$O$_{16}$ (M_r = 1115.75): C, 40.01; H, 3.46; N, 7.53 %; Found: C, 40.53; H, 3.65; N, 7.52 %. IR data for **chapt7-1** (KBr, cm^{-1}): 3441, 3210, 2933, 1573, 1417, 1346, 1215, 1118, 1025, 1003, 856, 756, 734, 658.

Synthesis of Mn$_4$(L^2)$_2$(CH$_3$COO)$_6$ (chapt7-2). **chapt7-2** was prepared in the similar way to **chapt7-1**, except that HL^1 was taken place by HL^2. Yellow crystals of **chapt7-2** were obtained, Yield: 0.110 g, ca. 73 % based on Mn^{2+}). *Anal. Calc.* for **chapt7-2**: C$_{38}$H$_{40}$Br$_2$Mn$_4$N$_6$O$_{16}$ (M_r= 1216.32): C, 37.52; H, 3.31; N, 6.91 %; Found: C, 37.58; H, 3.39; N, 6.84 %. IR data for **chapt7-2** (KBr, cm^{-1}, Figure S2): 3413, 2933, 1572, 1415,1335, 1248, 1169, 1091, 1025, 856, 784, 732, 658, 614.

Synthesis of [Mn$_2$(L^1)(CH$_3$COO)$_3$H$_2$O]$_n$(chapt7-3). **chapt7-3** was prepared in the similar way to **chapt7-1**. When complex **chapt7-3** is synthesized, Mn(CH$_3$COO)$_2$·4H$_2$O is used twice as much as complex **chapt7-1**. Yellow crystals of **chapt7-3** were obtained, (Yield: 0.104 g, ca. 72 % based on Mn^{2+}). *Anal. Calc.* for **chapt7-3**: C$_{19}$H$_{22}$ClMn$_2$N$_3$O$_9$ (M_r = 581.72): C, 39.23; H, 3.81; N, 7.22 %; Found: C, 39.28; H, 3.72; N, 7.24 %. IR data for **chapt7-3** (KBr, cm^{-1}): 3441, 3210, 2933, 1573, 1474, 1346, 1215, 1170, 1118, 1089, 1025, 1003, 856, 756, 734, 658.

Refinement

The diffraction data for samples **chapt7-1**-**chapt7-3** were obtained using a SuperNova instrument with a Single source at offset, Eos configuration. The instrument utilized graphite monochromated Mo-Ka radiation with a wavelength of 0.71073 Å. The data was gathered using the ω–θ scan mode within the following angular ranges: 3.46° ≤ θ ≤ 25.1° for sample **chapt7-1**, 3.42° ≤ θ ≤ 25.01° for sample **chapt7-2**, and 3.41° ≤ θ ≤ 25.00° for sample **chapt7-3**. The raw frame data were processed using the SAINT program for integration. The structures **chapt7-1**-**chapt7-3** were resolved by direct approaches employing SHELXT and subsequently enhanced using full-matrix least-squares on F^2 with the aid of SHELXL-2018 within the OLEX-2 graphical user interface. The application of an empirical absorption adjustment was performed using spherical harmonics within the SCALE3 ABSPACK scaling method. Anisotropic refinement was performed on all atoms except for hydrogen. The hydrogen atoms were arranged in a geometric manner and subjected to refinement using the riding model. Several computer programs were utilized in this study, including CrysAlis PRO, Agilent Technologies (Version 1.171.37.35), SHELXL, and Olex2 (Dolomanov et al., 2009). The value of Rint is greater than 0.12 for a total of three instances. The summary of crystal data, data collecting, and structural refinement details may be found in Table 7-1.

Table 7-1 Experimental details

	chapt7-1	chapt7-2	chapt7-3
Complex Chemical formula	Mn$_4$(C$_{13}$H$_{11}$ClN$_3$O$_2$)$_2$-(C$_2$H$_3$O$_2$)$_{5.17}$(CHO$_2$)$_{0.83}$	Mn$_4$(C$_{13}$H$_{11}$BrN$_3$O$_2$)$_2$-(C$_2$H$_3$O$_2$)$_6$	[Mn$_2$(C$_{13}$H$_{11}$ClN$_3$O$_2$)$_2$-(C$_2$H$_3$O$_2$)$_3$(H$_2$O)]
M_r	1115.75	1216.32	581.72
Crystal system, Space group	Triclinic, P-1	Monoclinic, $P2_1/c$	Monoclinic, $P2_1/c$
Temperature(K)	293	289	293
a,b,c (Å)	8.550(1),11.055(1), 12.595(1)	14.602(1),19.188(1), 8.275(1)	8.529(1),31.32(1), 9.267(1)
$α,β,γ$ (°)	76.143(5),73.110(6),81.533(6)	90, 98.376 (3), 90	90, 110.631 (17), 90
V(Å^3)	1102.02 (14)	2293.58 (14)	2316.6 (6)
Z	1	2	4
$μ$ (mm^{-1})	1.32	2.89	1.26
Crystal size (mm)	0.25×0.22×0.18	0.23×0.19×0.15	0.20×0.18×0.15
Data collection			
T_{min}, T_{max}	0.726, 0.789	0.522, 0.649	0.777, 0.829
No. of measured, independent and observed [$I>2σ(I)$] reflections	6708, 3895, 2393	16303, 4024, 3225	16044, 4058, 1923
R_{int}	0.036	0.038	0.162
Refinement			
$R[F^2>2σ(F^2)], wR(F^2), S$	0.054, 0.136, 1.05	0.044, 0.123, 1.01	0.092, 0.286, 1.02
No. of reflections	3887	4024	4058
No. of parameters	306	302	307
No. of restraints	9	7	6
$Δρ_{max}, Δρ_{min}$ (eÅ^{-3})	0.57, -0.42	0.48, -0.97	1.17, -0.65

Electrochemical luminescence

The electrochemical luminescence studies were conducted with an MPI-A Electrochemical workstation manufactured in Xi An, China. All studies utilized a conventional three-electrode configuration consisting of a reference electrode (Ag/AgCl), an auxiliary electrode (platinum wire), and a working electrode (glassy carbon electrode with a diameter of 1 mm) for cyclic voltammetry in dimethylformamide (DMF). The electrolyte used for support in this experiment consisted of a solution containing 0.1 mol L^{-1} of potassium peroxydisulfate (K$_2$S$_2$O$_8$) dissolved in dimethylformamide (DMF).

Outcomes and Analysis

Synthetic aspects

Several factors can influence the structure, nuclear counts, and properties of transition polynuclear complexes during synthesis. These factors include metal ions, ligands, concentrations, counterions, templates, solvents, temperatures, the molar ratio of metal ion to ligand, and pH values. Initially, we conducted a high-level experiment using Mn(CH$_3$COO)$_3$·4H$_2$O in a mixed solution of DMF and ethanol, employing identical solvothermal reaction conditions as the reference study. Two tetranuclear manganese clusters, denoted as **chapt7-1** and **chapt7-2**, were synthesized. These clusters differ from the trinuclear manganese clusters previously reported in the literature. The observed phenomenon is hypothesized to be attributed to variations in the structures of the ligands. This study aims to conduct a comparative analysis of the ligands discussed in the present work with those documented in the existing literature. It was observed that the ligands discussed in the paper possess an additional oxygen atom in comparison to the ligands described in the existing literature. When the molar ratio of metal ions to ligands is increased to 2:1, compound **chapt7-3**, a tetranuclear manganese polymer, is produced under identical experimental conditions. The findings suggest that the stoichiometric ratio of metal ions to ligands has an impact on the structural characteristics of the complexes.

Description of the crystal structure

Description of the crystal structure chapt7-1

The triclinic space group $P\bar{1}$ is determined through the examination of single-crystal X-ray diffraction, indicating that **chapt7-1** belongs to this group. The tetranuclear cluster of compound **chapt7-1** consists of four manganese (II) ions, two L^1 ligands, 5.17 acetate groups, and 0.83 formate groups. The formate groups are produced via the oxidative breakdown of dimethylformamide (DMF), as shown in Figure 7-1 and Scheme 7-1. The central component of complex **chapt7-1** consists of a linear arrangement of four MnII ions. The disparity in coordination mode of acetate groups accounts for the discrepancy in the central metal-metal distance (Mn2···Mn2a), which is approximately 1.188 Å greater than the distances Mn1···Mn2 and Mn1a···Mn2a (symmetry code: (a) 1 - x, 1 - y, 1 - z). The structure of compound **chapt7-1** may be observed as consisting of two dinuclear units of $Mn_2(L^1)(CH_3COO)_2$, which are connected by two bridging groups of μ_2-acetate-κ^2O,O' in a *syn-anti* configuration. The coordination environment surrounding Mn1 and Mn2 exhibits distinct characteristics. The calculations of Continuous Shape Measures (CShM) reveal that the coordination environment of Mn1 is positioned at an intermediate point between a square pyramid and a trigonal bipyramid, as well suggested by the τ_5 values. The calculation of τ_5 values was performed using the approach developed by Anthony W. Addison et al. in the context of five-coordinate structures. These values were derived from the highest L-Mn-L angle (β) and the second-largest L-Mn-L angle (α), with τ_5 being defined as (β-α)/60. Therefore, it can be shown that a trigonal bipyramidal structure exhibiting D3h symmetry possesses a τ_5 value of **1**, but a square pyramidal structure with C_{4v} symmetry exhibits a τ_5 value of 0. In this context, the value of τ_5 can be calculated as (152.48-127.54)/60, resulting in a value of 0.42. This value is in proximity to the median value of 0.5. Manganese ion Mn1 is coordinated by two oxygen atoms and one nitrogen atom from a single L^1 ligand, with bond lengths of Mn1-N1 (2.233(5) Å) and Mn1-N3 (2.225(5) Å), as well as two oxygen atoms from different acetate groups, with bond lengths of Mn1-O6 (2.057(5) Å) and Mn1-O7 (2.062(5) Å). These atoms occupy the apical position relative to the O1 and N1 atoms. On the other hand, manganese ion Mn2 exhibits a distorted octahedral geometry, with *cis*-angles O–Mn–O ranging from 70.9(1)° to 106.1(2)°. The Mn-O bond lengths from four acetate groups and the μ_2-L^1-κ^5O1,O2:O2,N1,N2 ligand range from 2.094(4) Å to 2.328(4) Å. The tetranuclear manganese clusters were formed by the dinuclear unit, utilizing two *syn-anti* bridging acetates to connect the molecules in a linear chain along the z axis. This connection was achieved through the N-H···O hydrogen bonds (N2-H2A···O4i, with a bond length of 2.882(6)Å, where the symmetry code is specified as (i) $x, y, z - 1$).The length of the hydrogen bond is shorter than the published N-H···O hydrogen bond length of [Ni$_7$(immep)$_6$(MeO)$_6$](NO$_3$)$_2$, which measures 3.119Å. The compound Himmep, referred to as Himmep, is known as 2-iminomethyl-6-ethxoy-phenol according to the study conducted by Xiao et al. in 2013. The 1D chains in the system under study are strengthened by intrachain π···π interactions. Specifically, the distance between the benzene ring of L^1 and another pyridine ring of L^1 is measured to be 3.515(1)Å, as determined by the symmetry code (ii) 1 - x, 1 - y, - z. This distance is found to be shorter than the reported π···π distance of 3.733 Å observed between two parallel benzene rings in the complex {[Mn(timb)$_2$(H$_2$O)$_2$]·(Cl)$_2$·(H$_2$O)$_2$}$_n$ (timb = 1,3,5-tris-(imidazol-1-ylmethyl) benzene) (Yin, et al, 2010). It is important to mention that the one-dimensional chains were expanded into a two-dimensional supramolecular network by C-H···Cl hydrogen bonds (C15-H15B···Cl1^{iii} 3.100(1) Å, symmetry code: (iii) 1 - x, -y, 1 -z). Within the two-dimensional supramolecular network, it can be observed that the L^1 ligands are arranged in a parallel orientation to one another. The coordination mode of L^1 is μ_2-L^1-κ^5O^1,O^2:O^2,N^1,N^2, as reported by Dojer et al. (2015). Interestingly, the acetate groups exhibit two distinct coordination modes: *syn-syn*-acetate and *syn-anti*-acetate groups. In this context, it can be observed that the L^1 ligand's two nitrogen atoms, as well as the neighboring oxygen atom, are forming chelate bonds with one manganese (Mn) atom. Simultaneously, the two oxygen atoms are forming chelate bonds with the other Mn atom, while the central oxygen atom acts as a bridge between the two Mn atoms.

Scheme 7-1. Molecule structure of chapt7-1.

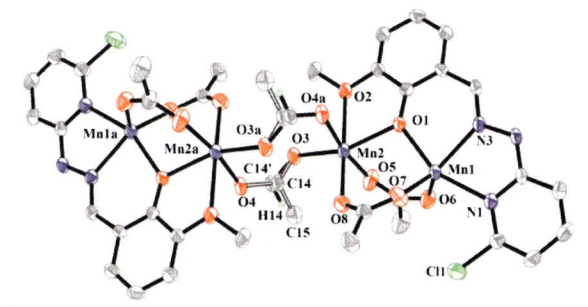

Figure 7-1 The molecular structure of chapt7-1, with some of the H atoms omitted for clarity. Displacement ellipsoids are drawn at the 30% probability level. [symmetry code: (a)1 - x, 1 - y, 1 - z.]

Description the crystal structure of chapt7-2

The monoclinic space group $P2_1/c$ was determined for **chapt7-2** via single-crystal X-ray diffraction research. The tetranuclear cluster of compound **chapt7-2** is composed of four manganese (II) ions, two L^2 ligands, and six acetate groups, as depicted in Figure 7-2 and Scheme 7-2. The central region of the intricate **chapt7-2** has a linear arrangement of four manganese (II) ions. The disparity in coordination mode of acetate groups accounts for the discrepancy in the central metal–metal distance (Mn2⋯Mn2a) being approximately 1.255 Å greater than Mn1⋯Mn2 and Mn1a⋯Mn2a (symmetry code: (a) -x, 1-y, 2-z.). The coordination environment surrounding Mn1 and Mn2 exhibits distinct characteristics. Manganese ion Mn1 is coordinated with two oxygen atoms and one nitrogen atom from one ligand L^2. The distances between Mn1 and the coordinating atoms are as follows: Mn1-N1, 2.257(3) Å; Mn1-N3, 2.240(3) Å; Mn1-O1, 2.092(4) Å. Additionally, Mn1 is coordinated with two oxygen atoms from different acetate groups, with distances of Mn1-O6, 2.107(5) Å and Mn1-O7, 2.038(3) Å. These acetate groups are located at the apical position relative to the O1 and N1 atoms. On the other hand, manganese ion Mn2 exhibits a distorted oxygen octahedral geometry. The *cis*-angles O–Mn2–O range from 70.55(11)° to 107.12(15)°, and the Mn2-O bond lengths vary from 2.066(3) Å to 2.344(3) Å. These bonds originate from four acetate groups and the ligands μ_2-L^2-$\kappa^5 O^1,O^2:O^2,N^1,N^2$. The results obtained from the Continuous Shape Measure (CShM) computations suggest that the coordination environment of Mn1 is positioned at an intermediate point between a square pyramid and a trigonal bipyramid. This finding is consistent with the observations made from the τ_5 values. The approach proposed by Anthony W. Addison et al was employed to compute τ_5 values based on the greatest (β) and second-largest (α) L-Mn-L angles in the five-coordinate structures. The formula used to determine τ_5 is given by ($\tau_5 = (\beta-\alpha)/60$), resulting in a determined value of 0.4925 for the specific case of ($\beta-\alpha$)/60 = (153.63-123.18)/60. This value is in close proximity to the median value of 0.5. The structural arrangement of **chapt7-2** can be seen as including two dinuclear units of Mn$_2$(L$_2$)(CH$_3$COO)$_2$, which are connected by two bridging groups of μ^2-acetate-$\kappa^2 O,O'$. The tetranuclear manganese clusters were created by the dinuclear unit through the utilization of two syn-anti-acetate bridges. These bridges facilitated the formation of a one-dimensional chain through N-H⋯O hydrogen bonds, namely N2-H2⋯O6[ii] with a bond length of 2.817(5)Å (symmetry code: (ii) 1 - x, 1 - y, 2 - z). The 1D chains are strengthened by intrachain π⋯π interaction, specifically the π⋯πii distance between L^2 and another L^2 is measured to be 3.455(2)Å. This interaction contributes to the formation of a 3D supramolecular network through O⋯Br interaction, with a distance of 3.027(3) Å between O7 and Br1iii (symmetry code: (iii) x, 0.5 - y, z - 0.5). Additionally, C-H⋯O hydrogen bonds, specifically C4-H4⋯O3[ii] with a distance of 3.240 (1) Å, are also involved in the network formation. The dihedral angle between the L^2 ligands in the next 1D chain inside the 3D supramolecular network is measured to be 74.5°, which contrasts with the corresponding angle observed in complex **chapt7-1**. In the first scenario, the ligands of the complexes are aligned in parallel fashion within adjacent one-dimensional chains.

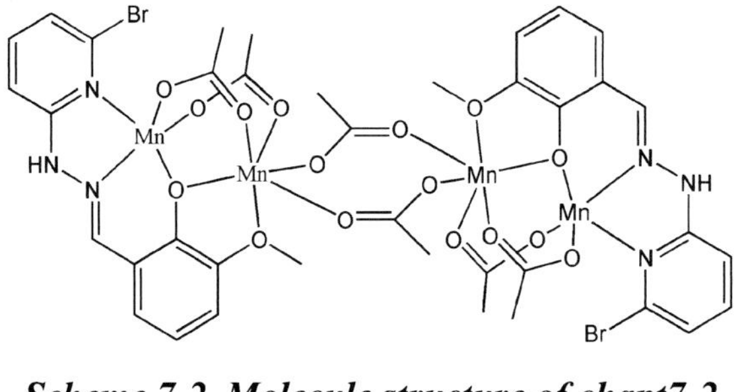

Scheme 7-2. Molecule structure of chapt7-2

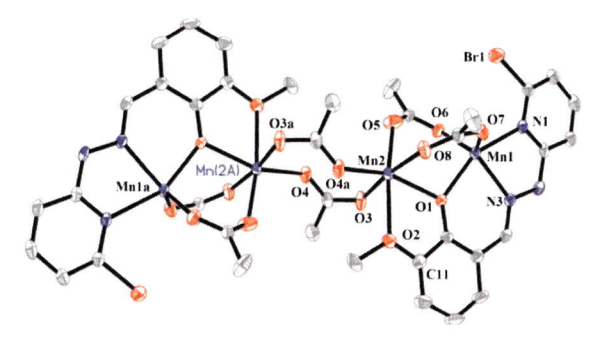

Figure 7-2 The molecular structure of chapt7-2, with some of the H atoms omitted for clarity. Displacement ellipsoids are drawn at the 30% probability level. [Symmetry code: (a) − x, 1 − y, 2 − z.]

Description the crystal structure of chapt7-3

The monoclinic system space group *P2₁/c* (Table 7-1, Scheme 7-3) is determined by the investigation of the single-crystal X-ray structure of compound **chapt7-3**. Figure 7-3 illustrates the presence of the CH_3COO^- anion bridged dinuclear-based 1-D chain, denoted as $[Mn_2(L^1)(CH_3COO)_3H_2O]_n$ (**chapt7-3**). The central region of the molecule consists of two separate manganese (II) ions that have produced tetranuclear secondary building blocks $[Mn_4(L^1)_2(CH_3COO)_6(H_2O)_2]$ by the use of *syn-anti*-acetate bridges. The coordination environment of two manganese ions (Mn^{II}) exhibits variation. In this case, Mn1 exhibits a distorted octahedral geometry, with coordination from two oxygen atoms originating from a μ_2-L^1-$\kappa^5 O^1,O^2:O^2,N^1,N^2$ ligand (Mn1-O4, 2.220(6)Å; Mn1-O5, 2.344(7)Å). Additionally, three oxygen atoms are coordinated to Mn1, originating from two syn-anti-acetate groups and one syn-syn-acetate group (Mn1-O9a, 2.101(6)Å; Mn1-O6, 2.113(8)Å; Mn1-O8, 2.174(6)Å; symmetry code: (a) *x*, 0.5 - *y*, 0.5 + *z*). Furthermore, one water molecule is coordinated to Mn1 (Mn1-O3, 2.191(6)Å). The Mn2 compound exhibits distorted octahedral geometries, with coordination from two nitrogen atoms and one oxygen atom originating from the L^1 ligand (Mn2-N1, 2.285(8); Mn2-N3, 2.252(7); Mn2-O4, 2.122(6)Å). Additionally, coordination occurs with two oxygen atoms from the μ_1-acetate-$\kappa^2 O,O'$ acetate group (Mn2-O1, 2.374(7)Å; Mn2-O2, 2.242(6)Å), as well as one oxygen atom from the *syn-syn*-acetate group (Mn2-O2, 2.067(7)Å). The formation of a 1D chain in the dinuclear unit was facilitated by the *syn-anti*-acetate group bridge (Figure 7-4). This chain then contributed to the construction of a 3D supramolecular network through N-H⋯O hydrogen bonds (N2-H2⋯O1b, 2.818(10)Å, symmetry code:(b) 1 - *x*, - *y*, - *z*.) and Cl⋯Cl interaction (Cl1⋯Cl1c, 3.454(10)Å, symmetry code:(c) 2 - *x*, 0.5 - *y*, 1 - *z*.). It is important to acknowledge that the acetate groups exhibit three distinct coordination modes: syn-syn symmetrically bridging acetate, syn-anti symmetrically bridging acetate with one oxygen forming a hydrogen connection with water molecules, and asymmetric chelating.

Scheme 7-3. Molecule structure of chapt7-3

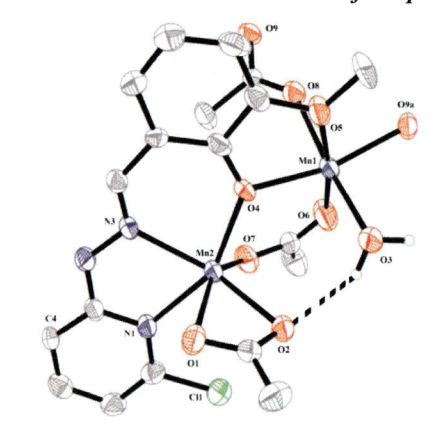

Figure 7-3 The molecular structure of chapt7-3, with some of the H atoms omitted for clarity. Displacement ellipsoids are drawn at the 30% probability level.

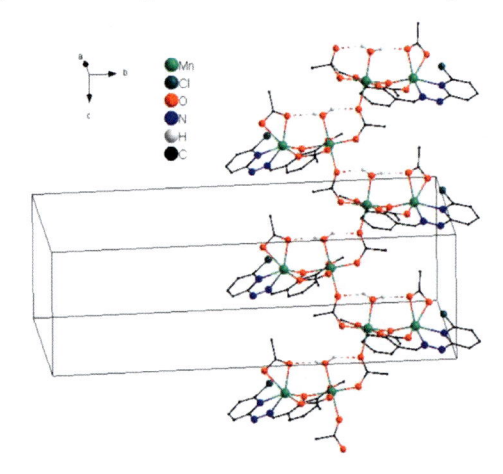

Figure 7-4 The 1D chain of chapt7-3.

Magnetic properties

The magnetic susceptibilities χ_M of samples **chapt7-1** - **chapt7-3** were determined through the utilization of crushed single crystalline specimens. The direct current susceptibilities of samples **chapt7-1** to **chapt7-3** were determined by subjecting them to an applied magnetic field of 1 kilo-Oersted at temperatures varying from 2 to 300 Kelvin.

Figure 7-5 displays the plots of χ_M and $\chi_M T$ as functions of temperature (T). The χ_M vs T curve exhibits a peak at around 2 K, 2.5 K, and 2.8 K for samples **chapt7-1** to **chapt7-3**, suggesting the presence of weak antiferromagnetic interaction (Pence, et al., 1996). At ambient temperature, the spin orbital coupling of the four Mn^{II} ions leads to $\chi_M T$ values of 8.06, 10.77, and 8.77 cm^{3}Kmol^{-1} for compounds **chapt7-1, chapt7-2, chapt7-3**, respectively. These values are significantly lower than the spin-only value of 17.5 cm^3 Kmol^{-1} for the four Mn^{II} ions with a non-interacting high-spin state of $S = 5/2$, assuming a g-factor of 2.0 (Liu, et al., 2011). However, the aforementioned values are significantly lower than the previously published value of 16.2 cm^{3}Kmol^{-1} for [Mn$_4$(DBA)$_4$(bix)]. In this context, H$_2$DBA refers to 4,4'-methylenedibenzoic acid, whereas bix represents 1,4-bis(imidazol-1-ylmethyl)benzene. The $\chi_M T$ product exhibits a consistent decline as temperature lowers and approaches zero at extremely low temperatures, indicating a predominant antiferromagnetic characteristic. Given that the spin carriers consist only of d^5 MnII ions, which are characterized as orbital singlet ions, our analysis solely accounted for the isotropic component of the exchange interaction, while disregarding the influence of the zero-field splitting. The compound [Mn$_4$(DBA)$_4$(bix)] had comparable magnetic properties.

The reciprocal susceptibility (χ_M^{-1}) above 15 K exhibits temperature dependence that can be described by the Curie-Weiss law ($\chi_M = C/(T - \theta)$). The Weiss constant (θ) values for samples **chapt7-1**, **chapt7-2**, and **chapt7-3** are -14.25 K, -21.85 K, and -36.478 K, respectively. The Curie constant (C) values for samples **chapt7-1**, **chapt7-2**, and **chapt7-3** are 8.44 cm^{3}K mol^{-1}, 11.677 cm^{3}K mol^{-1}, and 9.848 cm^{3}K mol^{-1}, respectively (refer to Figure 7-5). The presence of intramolecular antiferromagnetic interactions among the four MnII ions is further corroborated by the negative Weiss constant observed in this study.

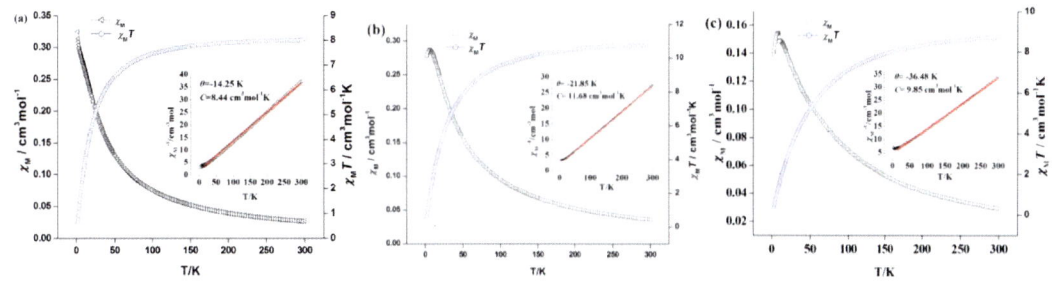

Figure 7-5 Plots of $\chi_M T$ and χ_M versus T measured in a 1000 Oe field for (a) chapt7-1, (b) chapt7-2 and (c) chapt7-3

ECL properties of chapt7-1–chapt7-3

The electrochemiluminescence (ECL) of the pure complexes **chapt7-1–chapt7-3** is depicted in Figure 7-6. The investigation of cyclic voltammetry (CV) was undertaken to acquire a deeper understanding of the redox characteristics shown by these complexes. The experimental results of cyclic voltammetry conducted using glassy carbon electrodes (GCE) modified with complexes **chapt7-1–chapt7-3** are presented in Figure 7-7. In the first experiment, upon the addition of K$_2$S$_2$O$_8$ to the solution, an oxidation peak is noticed in the cathodic current at a potential of -1.8 V, along with a reduction peak at -0.70 V in the same current. The cyclic voltammetry (CV) profiles of complexes **chapt7-2** and **chapt7-3** exhibit a resemblance to that of **chapt7-1**.

The complexes **chapt7-1**–**chapt7-3** exhibit respective maximum luminous intensities of approximately 2386, 1338, and 1270 arbitrary units (a.u.). After undergoing six or seven iterations, the light intensities of three entities exhibit consistent stability, whereas the luminous intensities of entities one and two noticeably diminish. It is posited that the stability of electrochemical luminescence is intricately linked to the stability of the complex present in the solution.

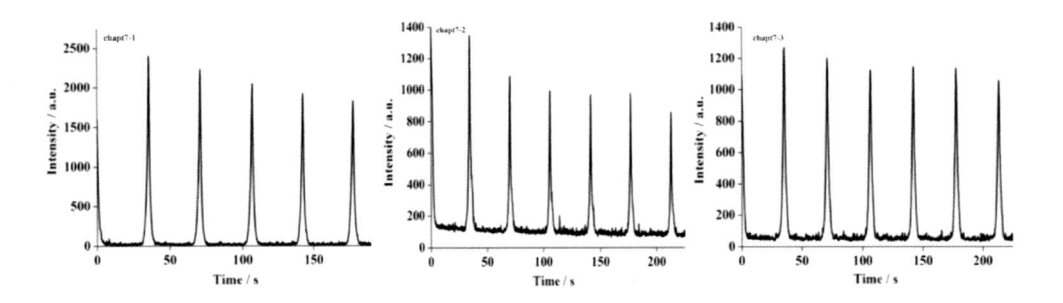

Figure 7-6 Electrochemical luminescence for chapt7-1-chapt7-3.

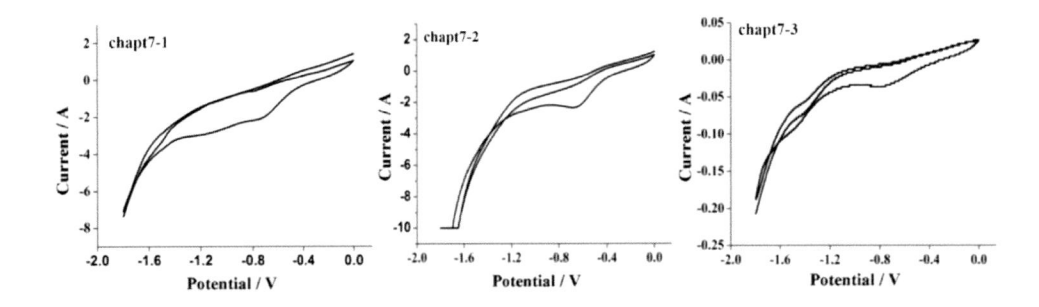

Figure 7-7. Cyclic voltammogram of chapt7-1-chapt7-3.

Conclusion

Three new complexes were synthesized using the solvothermal technique. The findings suggest that the stoichiometric ratio of metal ions to ligands has an impact on the structural characteristics of the complexes. Clusters **chapt7-1** and **chapt7-2** consist of tetranuclear manganese units, whereas **chapt7-3** has a one-dimensional network structure formed by tetranuclear [Mn$_4$(L^1)$_2$(CH$_3$COO)$_6$(H$_2$O)$_2$] building blocks. Complexes **chapt7-1**–**chapt7-3** exhibit prevalent antiferromagnetic interactions between MnII ions via μ2-O bridges. Simultaneously, compounds **chapt7-1**–**chapt7-3** exhibited favorable electrochemiluminescent (ECL) characteristics.

References

1. Addison, A. W.; Rao, T. N.; Reedijk, J.; Van Rijn, J.; Verschoor, G. C. Synthesis, Structure, and Spectroscopic Properties of Copper(II) Compounds Containing Nitrogen-Sulphur Donor Ligands; the Crystal and Molecular Structure of Aqua[1,7-Bis(N-Methylbenzimidazol-2′-Yl)-2,6-Dithiaheptane] Copper(II) Perchlorate. J. Chem. Soc., Dalton Trans., 1984, 7, 1349-1356.
2. Alvarez, S.; Alemany, P.; Casanova, D.; Cirera, J.; Llunell, M.; Avnir, D. Shape Maps and Polyhedral Interconversion Paths in Transition Metal Chemistry. Coordin. Chem. Rev., 2005, 249(17-18), 1693-1708.
3. Avila, J. R.; Emery, J. D.; Pellin, M. J.; Martinson, A. B. F.; Farha, O. K.; Hupp, J. T. Porphyrins as Templates for Site-Selective Atomic Layer Deposition: Vapor Metalation and in Situ Monitoring of Island Growth. ACS Appl. Mater. Inter., 2016, 8(31), 19853-19859.
4. Bao, S. S.; Zheng, L. M. Magnetic Materials Based on 3d Metal Phosphonates. Coordin. Chem. Rev., 2016, 319, 63-85.
5. Bertoncello, P.; Forster, R. J. Nanostructured Materials for Electrochemiluminescence (ECL)-Based Detection Methods: Recent Advances and Future Perspectives. Biosens. Bioelectron., 2009, 24(11), 3191-3200.
6. Davies, P. J.; Grove, D. M.; Van Koten, G.; Veldman, N.; Spek, A. L.; Lutz, B. T. Organoplatinum Building Blocks for One-Dimensional Hydrogen-Bonded Polymeric Structures. Angew. Chem. Int. Edit., 1996, 35(17), 1959-1961.
7. Dojer, B.; Pevec, A.; Belaj, F.; Kristl, M. Two New Zinc(II) Acetates with 3-and 4-Aminopyridine: Syntheses and Structural Properties. Acta Chim. Slov., 2015, 62(2), 312-318.
8. Dolomanov, O. V.; Bourhis, L. J.; Gildea, R. J.; Howard, J. A. K.; Puschmann, H. OLEX2: a Complete Structure Solution, Refinement and Analysis Program. J. Appl. Crystallogr., 2009, 42(2), 339-341.
9. Feng, C.; Ma, Y. H.; Zhang, D.; Li, X. J.; Zhao, H. Highly Efficient Electrochemiluminescence Based on Pyrazolecarboxylic Metal Organic Framework. Dalton Trans., 2016, 45(12), 5081-5091.
10. Guerra, W.; Silva-Caldeira, P. P.; Terenzi, H.; Pereira-Maia, E. C. Impact of Metal Coordination on the Antibiotic and Non-Antibiotic Activities of Tetracycline-Based Drugs. Coordin. Chem. Rev., 2016, 327, 188-199.
11. Gao, P.; Ma, H.; Wu, Q.; Qiao, L.; Volinsky, A. A.; Su, Y. Size-Dependent Vacancy Concentration in Nickel, Copper, Gold, and Platinum Nanoparticles. J. Phys. Chem. C., 2016, 120(31), 17613-17619.
12. Gwo, S.; Wang, C. Y.; Chen, H. Y.; Lin, M. H.; Sun, L.; Li, X.; Chen, W. L.; Chang, Y. M.; Ahn, H. Plasmonic Metasurfaces for Nonlinear Optics and Quantitative SERS. ACS Photonics, 2016, 3(8), 1371-1384.
13. Han, S. D.; Zhao, J. P.; Liu, S. J.; Bu, X. H. Hydro(Solvo)Thermal Synthetic Strategy towards Azido/Formato-Mediated Molecular Magnetic Materials. Coordin. Chem. Rev., 2015, 289, 32-48.
14. James, S. L.; Verspui, G.; Spek, A. L.; Van Koten, G. Organometallic Polymers: an Infinite Organoplatinum Chain in the Solid State Formed by (C CH···ClPt) Hydrogen Bonds. Chem. Commun., 1996, 1996, 1309-1310.

15. Kitchen, J. A. Lanthanide-Based Self-Assemblies of 2,6-Pyridyldicarboxamide Ligands: Recent Advances and Applications as Next-Generation Luminescent and Magnetic Materials. Coordin. Chem. Rev., 2017, 340, 232-246.
16. Kaushik, R.; Ghosh, A.; Jose, D. A. Recent Progress in Hydrogen Sulphide (H$_2$S) Sensors by Metal Displacement Approach. Coordin. Chem. Rev., 2017, 347, 141-157.
17. Lee, S. W.; Choi, B. J.; Eom, T.; Han, J. H.; Kim, S. K.; Song, S. J.; Lee, W.; Hwang, C. S. Influences of Metal, Non-Metal Precursors, and Substrates on Atomic Layer Deposition Processes for the Growth of Selected Functional Electronic Materials. Coordin. Chem. Rev., 2013, 257(23-24), 3154-3176.
18. Li, S.; Tao, H.; Li, J. Molecularly Imprinted Electrochemical Luminescence Sensor Based on Enzymatic Amplification for Ultratrace Isoproturon Determination. Electroanal., 2012, 24(7), 1664-1670.
19. Liu, G. X.; Cha, X. C.; Li, X. L.; Zhang, C. Y.; Wang, Y.; Nishihara, S.; Ren, X. M. An Unusual Two-Dimensional 2-Fold Interpenetrating Metal-Organic Framework Based on Tetranuclear Manganese(II) Clusters: Synthesis, Structure and Magnetic Properties. Inorg. Chem. Commun., 2011, 14(6), 867-872.
20. Liu, Y.; Xuan, W.; Cui, Y. Engineering Homochiral Metal-Organic Frameworks for Heterogeneous Asymmetric Catalysis and Enantioselective Separation. Adv. Mater., 2010, 22(37), 4112-4135.
21. Llunell, M., Casanova, D., Cirera, J., Bofill, J., Alemany, P., Alvarez, S., Pinsky, M., Avnir, D. Program for the Calculation of Continuous Shape Measures of Polygonal and Polyhedral Molecular Fragments; University of Barcelona: Barcelona, Spain. SHAPE v.2.1., 2013.
22. Oszajca, M.; Franke, A.; Brindell, M.; Stochel, G.; Van Eldik, R. Redox Cycling in the Activation of Peroxides by Iron Porphyrin and Manganese Complexes. 'Catching' Catalytic Active Intermediates. Coordin. Chem. Rev., 2016, 306, 483-509.
23. Pence, L. E.; Caneschi, A.; Lippard, S. J. Synthesis, Structural Studies, and Magnetic Exchange Interactions in Low-Valent Manganese Alkoxide Cubes. Inorg. Chem. Front, 1996, 35(10), 3069-3072.
24. Qin, J. H.; Ma, L. F.; Hu, Y.; Wang, L. Y. Syntheses, Structures and Photoluminescence of Five Zinc(II) Coordination Polymers Based on 5-Methoxyisophthalate and Flexible N-Donor Ancillary Ligands. Crystengcomm, 2012, 14(8), 2891-2898.
25. Sheldrick, G. M. Crystal Structure Refinement with SHELXL. Acta Crystallogr. C., 2015, 71(1), 3-8.
26. Sheldrick, G. M. SHELXT-Integrated Space-Group and Crystal-Structure Determination. Acta Crystallogr. B., 2015, 71(1), 3-8.
27. Soldatova, A. V.; Romano, C. A.; Tao, L.; Stich, T. A.; Casey, W. H.; Britt, R. D.; Tebo, B. M.; Spiro, T. G. Mn(II) Oxidation by the Multicopper Oxidase Complex Mnx: a Coordinated Two-Stage Mn(II)/(III) and Mn(III)/(IV) Mechanism. J. Am. Chem. Soc., 2017, 139(33), 11381-11391.
28. Suess, R. J.; Winnerl, S.; Schneider, H.; Helm, M.; Berger, C.; De Heer, W. A.; Murphy, T. E.; Mittendorff, M. Role of Transient Reflection in Graphene Nonlinear Infrared Optics. ACS Photonics, 2016, 3(6), 1069-1075.

29. Wang, Q. L.; Chen, M. M.; Zhang, H. Q.; Wen, W.; Zhang, X. H.; Wang, S. F. Selective and Sensitive Determination of Ochratoxin A Based on a Molecularly Imprinted Electrochemical Luminescence Sensor. Anal. Methods Accid. R., 2015, 7(24), 10224-10228.

30. Wen, G. X.; Han, M. L.; Wu, X. Q.; Wu, Y. P.; Dong, W. W.; Zhao, J.; Li, D. S.; Ma, L. F. A Multi-Responsive Luminescent Sensor Based on a Super-Stable Sandwich-Type Terbium(III)-Organic Framework. Dalton Trans., 2016, 45(39), 15492-15499.

31. Xiao, Y.; Huang, P.; Wang, W. Ligand Structure Induced Diversification from Dinuclear to 1D Chain Compounds: Syntheses, Structures and Fluorescence Properties. J. Clust. Sci., 2015, 26, 1091-1102.

32. Xiao, Y.; Liu, Y. Q.; Li, G. Microwave-Assisted Synthesis, Structure and Properties of a Co-Crystal Compound with 2-Ethoxy-6-Methyliminomethyl-Phenol. Supramol. Chem., 2015, 27(3), 161-166.

33. Xiao, Y.; Qin, Y.; Yi, M.; Zhu, Y. A Disc-Like Heptanuclear Nickel Cluster Based on Schiff Base: Synthesis, Structure, Magnetic Properties and Hirshfeld Surface Analysis. J. Clust. Sci., 2016, 27, 2013-2023.

34. Xuan, W.; Zhu, C.; Liu, Y.; Cui, Y. Mesoporous Metal-Organic Framework Materials. Chem. Soc. Rev., 2012, 41(5), 1677-1695.

35. Yin. X. J.; Zhang, S. H.; Zhou, X. H.; Zuo, J. L. A Mn(II) Coordination Polymer with the Flexible Tripodal Ligand 1,3,5-Tris-(Imidazol-1-Ylmethyl)Benzene. Chin. J. Sruct. Chem., 2010, 29(2), 302-306.

36. Zhang, H. Y.; Wang, W.; Chen, H. L.; Zhang, S. H.; Li, Y. Five Novel Dinuclear Copper(II) Complexes: Crystal Structures, Properties, Hirshfeld Surface Analysis and Vitro Antitumor Activity Study. Inorg. Chim. Acta, 2016, 453, 507-515.

37. Zhang, S. H.; Wang, J M.; Zhang, H. Y.; Fan, Y. P.; Xiao, Y. Highly Efficient Electrochemiluminescence Based on 4-Amino-1,2,4-Triazole Schiff Base Two-Dimensional Zn/Cd Coordination Polymers. Dalton Trans., 2017, 46(2), 410-419.

38. Zhang, S.; Hua, Y.; Chen, Z.; Zhang, S.; Hai, H. Manganese Trinuclear Clusters Based on Schiff Base: Synthesis, Characterization, Magnetic and Electrochemiluminescence Properties. Inorg. Chim. Acta, 2018, 471, 530-536.

39. Zhang, S. H.; Zhao, R. X.; Li, G.; Zhang, H. Y.; Zhang, C. L.; Muller, G. Structural Variation from Heterometallic Heptanuclear or Heptanuclear to Cubane Clusters Based on 2-Hydroxy-3-Ethoxy-Benzaldehyde: Effects of pH and Temperature. RSC Adv., 2014, 4(97), 54837-54846.

40. Zhang, S. H.; Zhang, Y. D.; Zou, H. H.; Guo, J. J.; Li, H. P.; Song, Y.; Liang, H. A Family of Cubane Cobalt and Nickel Clusters: Syntheses, Structures and Magnetic Properties. Inorg. Chim. Acta, 2013, 396, 119-125.

41. Zhang, Y.; Yuan, S.; Day, G.; Wang, X.; Yang, X.; Zhou, H. C. Luminescent Sensors Based on Metal-Organic Frameworks. Coordin. Chem. Rev., 2018, 354, 28-45.

42. Zhao, Y.; Chang, X. H.; Liu, G. Z.; Ma, L. F.; Wang, L. Y. Five Mn(II) Coordination Polymers Based on 2,3′,5,5′-Biphenyl Tetracarboxylic Acid: Syntheses, Structures, and Magnetic Properties. Cryst. Growth Des., 2015, 15(2), 966-974.

43. Zheng, L.; Chi, Y.; Dong, Y.; Lin, J.; Wang, B. Electrochemiluminescence of Water-Soluble Carbon Nanocrystals Released Electrochemically from Graphite. J. Am. Chem. Soc., 2009, 131(13), 4564-4565.

Chapter 8

Synthesis, characterization, and anticancer evaluation of hydrazylpyridine salicylaldehyde-copper(II)-1,10-phenanthroline complexes as possible anticancer agents

Platinum-based chemotherapeutic agents, commonly employed in the treatment of many cancer types, have limited selectivity and pose significant risks of neurotoxicity and nephrotoxicity. Therefore, there is an urgent demand for the development of novel medicinal molecules that do not rely on platinum metals. Copper (Cu(II)) is a crucial metal ion found in diverse cellular environments, playing a fundamental role in numerous biological processes and metalloenzymes. Copper(II) compounds have garnered significant interest owing to their limited adverse effects and favorable biocompatibility, rendering them highly utilized as advanced chemotherapeutic agents. Several copper(II) metal-coordination compounds have been investigated as potential antiproliferation drugs. These compounds encompass a range of ligands, such as benzyldipicolylamine, pyridyl- and aliphatic-amino- derivatives, thiosemicarbazone, fluoroquinolones, indolo[3,2-d][2]benzazepine, phenanthroline, tropolone, dasatinib, tryptanthrin derivatives, β-carboline, coumarin-amide ligand, and terpyridine, each exhibiting different coordination geometries. However, the efficacy of this inhibitory action is constrained in the context of clinical treatment.

Several copper(II)-based compounds, particularly complexes of salicylaldehyde derivatives, have exhibited potential as metallodrugs. The copper(II)-salicylaldehyde complexes mentioned, such as benzimidazole-salicylaldehyde, pyridine-salicylaldehyde, 1,2-phenylene-diamine-aniline-salicylaldehyde, coumarin-salicylaldehyde, 4-methoxybenzohydrazide-salicylaldehyde, bis(2-methoxyethyl)amine-salicylaldehyde, and 4-aminopyrimidine-salicylaldehyde-based copper(II) compounds, exhibit significant characteristics including high reactive oxygen species (ROS) generation, induction of mitophagy, impairment of mitochondrial function, and strong affinity for DNA binding. To date, there is a lack of research documenting the synthesis and evaluation of the anticancer properties of hydrazylpyridine salicylaldehyde-copper(II)-1,10-phenanthroline complexes(Table 8-1).

In this study, we present the synthesis, characterization, and assessment of the antiproliferation activity of a series of copper complexes, namely [Cu-(L^{1a})(phen)] (**Cugdupt1**), [Cu-(L^{2a})(phen)]·(CH$_3$CN) (**Cugdupt2**), [Cu-(L^{3a})(phen)] (**Cugdupt3**), [Cu-(L^{4a})(phen)]·(CH$_3$CN) (**Cugdupt4**), [Cu-(L^{5a})(phen)] (**Cugdupt5**), [Cu-(L^{6a})(phen)] (**Cugdupt6**), [Cu-(L^{7a})(phen)] (**Cugdupt7**), [Cu-(L^{8a})(phen)] (**Cugdupt8**), and [Cu-(L^{9a})(phen)]·0.5(H$_2$O) (**Cugdupt9**). These complexes consist of hydrazylpyridine salicylaldehyde ligands (L^{1}H$_2$–L^{9}H$_2$, Table 8-1) and 1,10-phenanthroline (phen). The copper (II) compounds were initially studied using several analytical techniques, including infrared spectroscopy, elemental analysis, electrospray ionization mass spectrometry (ESI-MS), X-ray crystallography, UV-visible spectroscopy, and nuclear magnetic resonance (NMR) spectroscopy. In addition, we conducted an investigation on the inhibitory impact of **Cugdupt1–Cugdupt9** on the A549, A549cis, and HL-7702 cell lines. Subsequently, an examination was conducted to explore the anticancer characteristics of **Cugdupt1** and **Cugdupt8**, focusing on their impact on ATP reduction and mitophagy pathways. It was observed that Cugdupt8 exhibited significant effectiveness in mice with A549 tumors.

Experimental

Materials and physical measurements

All compounds were procured from commercial sources and employed immediately upon their acquisition. The elemental analyses (CHN) were conducted using a Perkin-Elmer 240 elemental analyzer. The Fourier-transform infrared (FT-IR) spectra were obtained using a Bio-Rad FTS-7 spectrometer, with the measurements conducted in the 4000–400 cm^{-1} range. The spectra were recorded by placing KBr pellets on the spectrometer. The X-ray crystal structures were determined using the SHELXL crystallographic program and an Agilent G8910A CCD diffractometer. The Hitachi F-4600 fluorescence spectrophotometer was employed for conducting photoluminescence studies.

Synthesis of L^{1}H$_2$–L^{9}H$_2$

In this experiment, a solution containing either (6-chloro-pyridin-2-yl)-hydrazine (Hcph) or (6-bromo-pyridin-2-yl)- hydrazine (Hbph) (10 mmol), salicylaldehyde derivatives (10 mmol), and ethanol (20 mL) was subjected to reflux at a temperature of 80 °C for a duration of 1 hour. The reaction took place in a 100-mL flask. A precipitate of L^{n}H$_2$ with a beige coloration was seen and subsequently subjected to three rinses using 10 mL of fresh ethanol each time. The resulting precipitate was then dried at a temperature of 50°C for a duration of 24 hours.

Data of L^{1}H$_2$.

Yield: 3.5247 g, *ca.* 95% based on Hbph. *Anal. Calc.* for L^{1}H$_2$: C$_{12}$H$_9$Br$_2$N$_3$O, *calc.*: C, 38.84; H, 2.44; N, 11.32 %; Found: C, 38.82; H, 2.46; N, 11.34%. IR data for L^{1}H$_2$ (KBr, cm^{-1}, Figure 8-1): 3287s, 3046s, 1589s, 1525m, 1424m, 1252m, 825m, 689m, 633s, 571w. ^{1}H NMR (DMSO-d$_6$, 500 MHz, Figure 8-2) were as follows: δ 10.21 (s, 1H), 9.49 (s, 2H δ = 11.38 - 11.30 (m, 1H), 10.48 - 10.37 (m, 1H), 8.27 - 8.19 (m, 1H), 7.73 - 7.61 (m, 2H), 7.25 - 7.10 (m, 2H), 6.93 - 6.77 (m, 2H). The ESI-MS spectrum results were as follows: m/z = 371.9165 for [M+H]$^+$.

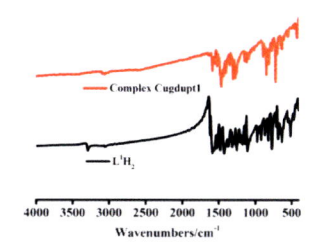

Figure 8-1. IR (KBr) spectra of Cugdupt1 and L¹H₂.

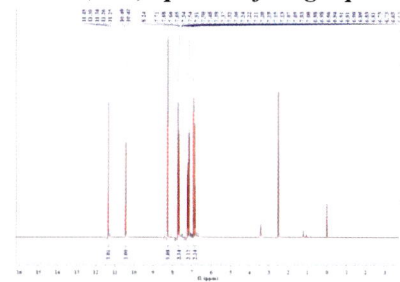

Figure 8-2. ¹H NMR (500MHz, DMSO-d6) for L¹H₂.

Data of L²H₂.

Yield: 3.3935 g, *ca.* 94 % based on Hbph; *Anal. Calc.* for L²H₂: C₁₂H₈BrCl₂N₃O , *calc.*: C, 39.92; H, 2.23; N, 11.63 %; Found: C, 39.90; H, 2.20; N, 11.60%. IR data for L²H₂ (KBr, cm⁻¹, Figure 8-3): 3236w, 3073s, 1596w, 1526w, 1429w, 1312w, 1113m, 970w, 859s, 690s, 568w. ¹H NMR (DMSO-d₆, 400 MHz, Figure 8-4) were as follows: δ 11.59 (s, 1H), 11.24 (s, 1H), 8.23 (s, 1H), 7.81 - 7.39 (m, 3H), 6.95 (dd, *J* = 48.5, 7.8 Hz, 2H). The ESI-MS spectrum results were as follows: m/z = 361.9277 for [M+H]⁺.

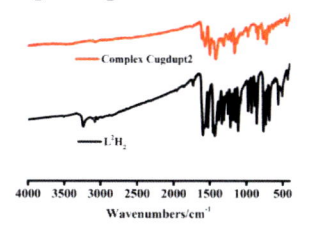

Figure 8-3. IR (KBr) spectra of Cugdupt2 and L²H₂.

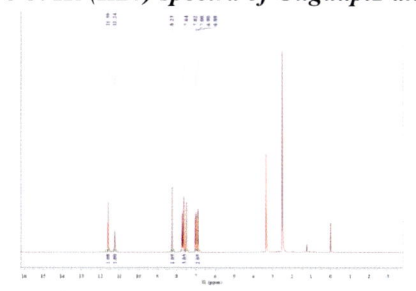

Figure 8-4. ¹H NMR (400MHz, DMSO-d6) for L²H₂.

Data of L³H₂.

Yield: 3.01892 g, *ca.* 94 % based on Hbph; *Anal. Calc.* for L³H₂: C₁₃H₁₂BrN₃O₂, *calc.*: C, 48.61; H, 3.76; N, 3.08 %; Found: C, 48.58; H, 3.78; N,13.10 %. IR data for L³H₂ (KBr, cm⁻¹, Figure 8-5): 3167w, 1594s, 1429w, 1244w, 1116m, 985w, 764s, 734s, 624w, 520w. ¹H NMR (DMSO-d₆, 500 MHz, Figure 8-6) were as follows: δ 11.27 (s, 1H), 9.69 (s, 1H), 8.32 (s, 1H), 7.66 (t, *J* = 7.9 Hz, 1H), 7.28 (d, *J* = 7.8 Hz, 1H), 7.06 (d, *J* = 8.2 Hz, 1H), 6.95 (d, *J* = 7.3 Hz,

1H), 6.81 (t, J = 7.7 Hz, 2H), 3.82 (s, 3H). The ESI-MS spectrum results were as follows: m/z = 322.0186 for [M+H]⁺.

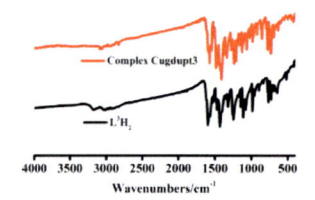

Figure 8-5. IR (KBr) spectra of Cugdupt3 and L³H₂.

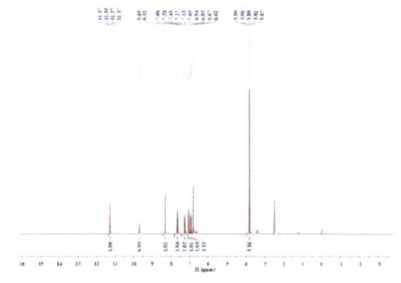

Figure 8-6. ¹H NMR (500MHz, DMSO-d6) for L³H₂.

Data of L⁴H₂.

Yield: 4.2292 g, *ca.* 94 % based on Hbph; *Anal. Calc.* for L⁴H₂: C₁₂H₈Br₃N₃O, *calc.*: C, 32.03; H, 1.79; N, 9.33 %; C, 32.00; H, 1.81; N, 9.35 %. IR data for L⁴H₂ (KBr, cm⁻¹, Figure 8-7): 3232w, 1587s, 1522w, 1436w, 1308w, 1115w, 980m, 857w, 770s, 680s, 558w. ¹H NMR (DMSO-d₆, 400 MHz, Figure 8-8) were as follows: δ 11.59 (s, 1H), 11.24 (s, 1H), 8.23 (s, 1H), 7.76 - 7.41 (m, 3H), 6.95 (dd, J=48.5, 7.8 Hz, 2H). The ESI-MS spectrum results were as follows: m/z = 449.827 for [M+H]⁺.

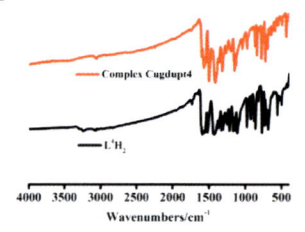

Figure 8-7. IR (KBr) spectra of Cugdupt4 and L⁴H₂.

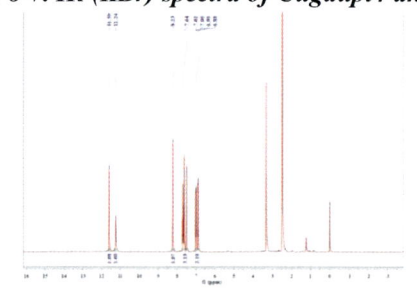

Figure 8-8. ¹H NMR (400MHz, DMSO-d6) for L⁴H₂.

Data of L⁵H₂.

Yield: 3.0511 g, *ca.* 94 % based on Hbph; *Anal. Calc.* for L⁵H₂: C₁₂H₉BrClN₃O, (Mr = 324.58), *calc.*: C, 44.40; H, 2.79; N, 12.94 %; Found: C, 44.43; H, 2.77; N, 12.92 %. IR data for L⁵H₂ (KBr, cm⁻¹, Figure 8-9): 3288w, 1557s, 1480w, 1374w,1316w, 1106w, 1106m, 975w, 830s, 775s, 694w, 643s, 520w. ¹H NMR (DMSO-d₆, 500 MHz, Figure 8-10) were as follows: δ 11.30 - 11.21 (m, 1H), 10.39 - 10.29 (m, 1H), 8.18 - 8.11 (m, 1H), 7.65 - 7.53 (m, 2H), 7.15 - 7.01

(m, 2H), 6.84 - 6.71 (m, 2H). The ESI-MS spectrum results were as follows: m/z = 325.9523 for [M-H]⁻.

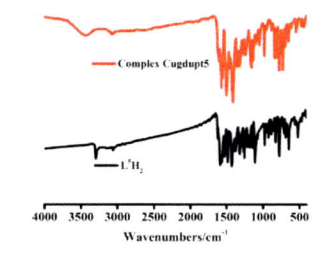

Figure 8-9. IR (KBr) spectra of Cugdupt5 and L⁵H₂.

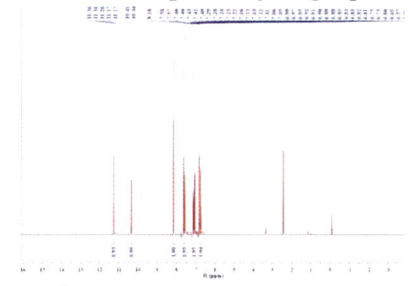

Figure 8-10. ¹H NMR (500MHz, DMSO-d6) for L⁵H₂.

Data of L⁶H₂.
Yield: 3.0073 g, *ca.* 95 % based on Hcph; *Anal. Calc.* for L⁶H₂: C₁₂H₈Cl₃N₃O, *calc.*: C, 45.53; H, 2.54; N, 13.27 %; Found: C, 45.55; H, 2.51; N, 13.25 %. IR data for L⁶H₂ (KBr, cm⁻¹, Figure 8-11): 3209w, 3086s, 1590w, 1529w, 1429w, 1225w, 1123m, 985w, 860s, 720s, 566w. ¹H NMR (DMSO-d₆, 400 MHz, Figure 8-12) were as follows: δ 11.59 (s, 1H), 11.24 (s, 1H), 8.23 (s, 1H), 7.74 - 7.56 (m, 2H), 7.51 (d, *J* = 2.6 Hz, 1H), 7.01 (d, *J* = 8.1 Hz, 1H), 6.89 (d, *J* = 7.6 Hz, 1H) The ESI-MS spectrum results were as follows: m/z = 315.9806 for [M+H]⁺.

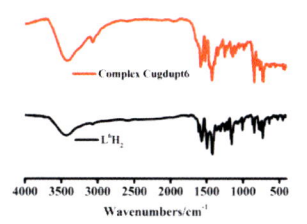

Figure 8-11. IR (KBr) spectra of Cugdupt6 and L⁶H₂

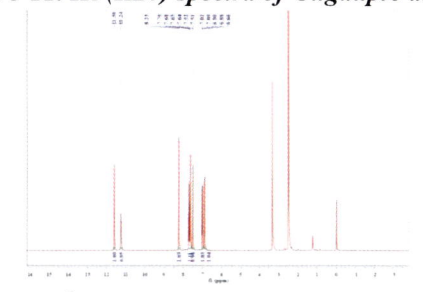

Figure 8-12. ¹H NMR (400MHz, DMSO-d6) for L⁶H₂.

Data of L⁷H₂.
Yield: 2.6518 g, *ca.* 94 % based on Hcph; *Anal. Calc.* for L⁷H₂: C₁₃H₁₂ClN₃O₂, *calc.*: C, 51.90; H, 4.35; N, 15.13 %; Found: C, 51.92; H, 4.33; N, 15.10 %; IR data for L⁷H₂ (KBr, cm⁻¹, Figure 8-13): 3289w, 2834s, 1598w, 1482w, 1439w, 1259w, 1070m, 909w, 777s, 721s, 598w. ¹H NMR (DMSO-d₆, 500 MHz, Figure 8-14) were as follows: δ 11.22 (d, *J* = 47.6 Hz, 1H),

9.69 (s, 1H), 8.24 (d, J = 83.5 Hz, 1H), 7.78 - 7.51 (m, 1H), 7.25 (dd, J = 26.3, 8.1 Hz, 1H), 7.06 (d, J = 8.2 Hz, 1H), 6.93 (t, J = 15.3 Hz, 1H), 6.81 (t, J = 7.7 Hz, 2H), 3.82 (s, 3H). The ESI-MS spectrum results were as follows: m/z = 278.0691 for [M+H]$^+$.

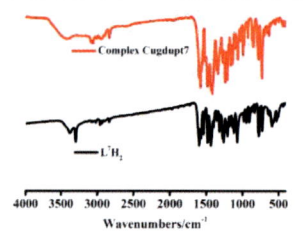

Figure 8-13. IR (KBr) spectra of Cugdupt7 and L^{7}H$_2$.

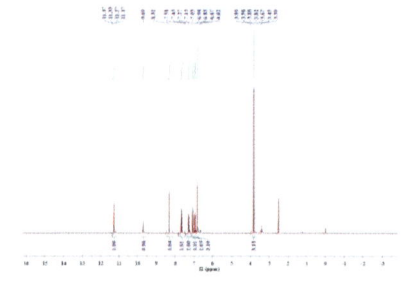

Figure 8-14. ^{1}H NMR (500MHz, DMSO-d6) for L^{7}H$_2$.

Data of L^{8}H$_2$.

Yield: 2.7511 g, *ca.* 94 % based on Hcph; *Anal. Calc.* for L^{8}H$_2$:C$_{12}$H$_9$ClN$_4$O$_3$, *calc.*: C, 49.24; H, 3.09; N, 19.14 %; *calc.*: C, 49.26; H, 3.06; N, 19.12 %; IR data for L^{8}H$_2$ (KBr, cm^{-1}, Figure 8-15): 3179w, 1631s, 1527w, 1486w, 1335w, 1130w, 986m, 827w, 700s, 525s. ^{1}H NMR (DMSO-d$_6$, 500 MHz, Figure 8-16) were as follows: δ 11.30 - 11.21 (m, 1H), 10.39 - 10.28 (m, 1H), 8.19 - 8.10 (m, 1H), 7.66 - 7.52 (m, 2H), 7.17 - 7.01 (m, 2H), 6.84 - 6.77 (m, 1H), 6.76 - 6.67 (m, 1H). The ESI-MS spectrum results were as follows: m/z = 293.0436 for [M+H]$^+$.

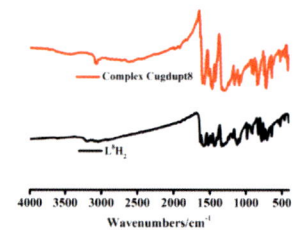

Figure 8-15. IR (KBr) spectra of Cugdupt8 and L^{8}H$_2$.

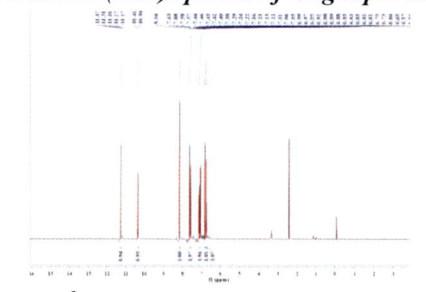

Figure 8-16. ^{1}H NMR (500MHz, DMSO-d6) for L^{8}H$_2$.

Data of L^{9}H$_2$.

Yield: 2.4600 g, *ca.* 94 % based on Hcph; *Anal. Calc.* for L^{9}H$_2$:C$_{13}$H$_{12}$ClN$_3$O, *calc.*: C, 59.66; H, 4.62; N, 16.05 %; Found: C, 59.68; H, 4.60; N, 16.03 %. IR data for L^{9}H$_2$ (KBr, cm^{-1}, Figure 8-17): 3271w, 2864s, 1500w, 1433w, 1317w, 1270w, 1228m, 1112w, 826w, 775s, 673s, 525s.

¹H NMR (DMSO-d₆, 500 MHz, Figure 8-18) were as follows: δ 11.27 (s, 1H), 9.69 (s, 1H), 8.32 (s, 1H), 7.66 (t, J = 7.9 Hz, 1H), 7.26 (t, J = 13.0 Hz, 1H), 7.06 (d, J = 8.2 Hz, 1H), 6.95 (d, J = 7.3 Hz, 1H), 6.81 (t, J = 7.7 Hz, 2H). The ESI-MS spectrum results were as follows: m/z = 262.0742 for [M+H]⁺.

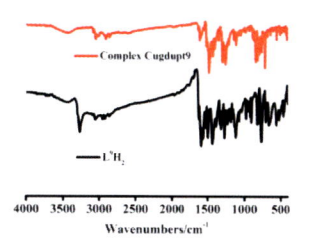

Figure 8-17. IR (KBr) spectra of Cugdupt9 and L⁹H₂.

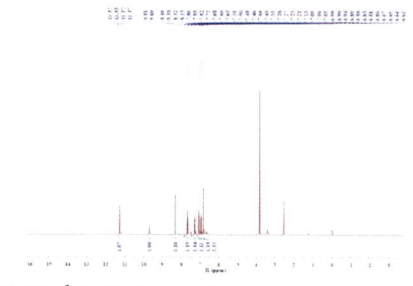

Figure 8-18. ¹H NMR (500MHz, DMSO-d6) for L⁹H₂.

Syntheses of Cugdupt1–Cugdupt9

The mixture containing LⁿH₂ (0.5 mmol), phen (2 mmol), ethanol (4 mL), and acetonitrile (6 mL) was subjected to stirring at ambient temperature for a duration of 30 minutes. The solution was further supplemented with 0.5 mmol of Cu(Ac)₂·H₂O until a red coloration was observed. Subsequently, the stirring process was ceased. The solution was transferred into a Teflon-coated autoclave with a volume of 15 mL and afterwards subjected to a temperature of 80°C for a duration of 72 hours. The black block crystals of Cugdupt1–Cugdupt9 were obtained through the process of filtration, followed by three washes with deionized water (10 mL each), and subsequent air drying.

Data of Cugdupt1.

Yield: 296 mg, *ca.* 30.2 % based on L¹H₂; *Anal. Calc.* for **Cugdupt1**: C₃₆H₂₂Br₄CuN₈O₂ (*M*r = 981.80), *calc.*: C, 44.08; H, 2.26; N, 11.42 %; Found: C, 44.10; H, 2.24; N, 11.40 %. IR data for **Cugdupt1** (KBr, cm⁻¹, Figure 8-1): 3049w, 1582s, 1462w, 1395w, 1112w, 848w, 719s, 629s, 547s.

Data of Cugdupt2.

Yield: 507 mg, *ca.* 50.6 % based on L²H₂; *Anal. Calc.* for **Cugdupt2**: C₃₈H₂₁Br₂Cl₄CuN₉O₂ (*M*r =1001.81), *calc.*: C, 45.55; H, 2.21; N, 12.58 %; Found: C, 45.57; H, 2.19; N, 12.56 %. IR data for **Cugdupt2** (KBr, cm⁻¹, Figure 8-3): 3068w, 1561s, 1494w, 1425w, 1310w, 1160w, 979w, 843w, 725s, 628s.

Data of Cugdupt3.

Yield: 358 mg, *ca.* 40.5 % based on L³H₂; *Anal. Calc.* for **Cugdupt3**: C₃₈H₂₈Br₂CuN₈O₂ (*M*r =884.04), C, 39.91; H, 2.82; N, 12.03 %; Found: C, 39.93; H, 2.80;N, 11.99 %. IR data for **Cugdupt3** (KBr, cm⁻¹, Figure 8-5): 3084w, 2823s, 1567w, 1405w, 1237w, 1126w, 982w, 774w, 724s, 641s. 548s.

Data of Cugdupt4.

Yield: 498 mg, *ca.* 42.3 % based on L⁴H₂; *Anal.Calc.* for **Cugdupt4**: C₃₈H₂₂Br₆CuN₉O₂ (*Mr* = 1179.65), *calc.*: C, 38.69; H, 1.87; N, 10.68 %;. Found: C, 38.69; H, 1.87; N, 10.68 %. IR data for **Cugdupt4** (KBr, cm⁻¹, Figure 8-7): 3057w, 1574s, 1500w, 1409w, 1319w, 1150w, 974w, 838s, 778s, 696s, 592s.

Data of Cugdupt5.

Yield: 275 mg, *ca.* 30.9 % based on L⁵H₂; *Anal. Calc.* for **Cugdupt5**: C₃₆H₂₂Br₂Cl₂CuN₈O₂ (*Mr* = 892.88), *calc.*: C, 48.37; H, 2.48; N, 12.53 %; Found: C, 48.39; H, 2.46; N, 12.50 %. IR data for **Cugdupt5** (KBr, cm⁻¹, Figure 8-9): 3071w, 1564s, 1501w, 1405w, 1358w, 1156w, 979w, 839w, 781s, 696s, 654s, 547w.

Data of Cugdupt6.

Yield: 362 mg, *ca.* 41.6 % based on L⁶H₂; *Anal.Calc.* for **Cugdupt6**: C₃₆H₂₀Cl₆CuN₈O₂ (*Mr* =872.84), *calc.*: C, 49.53; H, 2.30; N, 12.83 %; Found: C, 49.55; H, 2.28; N, 12.80 %. IR data for **Cugdupt6** (KBr, cm⁻¹, Figure 8-11): 3418w, 3059s, 1578w, 1518w, 1419w, 1252w, 1143w, 987w, 845s, 719s, 557s.

Data of Cugdupt7.

Yield: 340 mg, *ca.* 42.8 % based on L⁷H₂; *Anal. Calc.* for **Cugdupt7**: C₃₈H₂₈Cl₂CuN₈O₄ (*Mr* = 795.12), *calc.*: C, 57.40; H, 3.54; N, 14.09 %;. Found: C, 57.42; H, 3.52; N, 14.07 %. IR data for **Cugdupt7** (KBr, cm⁻¹, Figure 8-13): 3087w, 2831s, 1577w, 1469w, 1411w, 1238 w, 1206w, 1063w, 922s, 779s, 725w, 633s.

Data of Cugdupt8.

Yield: 290 mg, *ca.* 35.2 % based on L⁸H₂; *Anal. Calc.* for **Cugdupt8**: C₃₆H₂₂Cl₂CuN₁₀O₆ (*Mr* = 825.07), *calc.*: C, 52.40; H, 2.68; N, 16.97 %; Found: C, 52.42; H, 2.66; N, 16.95 %. IR data for **Cugdupt8** (KBr, cm⁻¹, Figure 8-15): 3060w, 1604s, 1516w, 1465w, 1341w, 1159w, 896w, 716w, 642s, 525s.

Data of Cugdupt9.

Yield: 240 mg, *ca.* 31.5 % based on L⁹H₂; *Anal. Calc.* for **Cugdupt9**: C₃₈H₂₈Cl₂CuN₈O₂.₅ (Mr =771.12), *calc.*: C, 59.80; H, 3.69; N, 14.68 %;. Found: C, 59.82; H, 3.67; N, 14.66 %.. IR data for **Cugdupt9** (KBr, cm⁻¹, Figure 8-17): 3083w, 2910s, 1479w, 1428w, 1352w, 1296w, 1253w, 1114w, 850s, 821s, 721s, 563w.

Crystal structure determination

The diffraction patterns of single crystals of complexes **Cugdupt1**, **Cugdupt2**, **Cugdupt4**–**Cugdupt7**, and **Cugdupt9** were acquired using a two-circle diffractometer equipped with a graphite monochromator and Mo-Kα radiation (λ = 0.71073 Å). The ω scan mode was employed to collect data within different ranges. The range of values for θ in the **Cugdupt1** dataset is between 2.61° and 27.58°. In the **Cugdupt2** dataset, the range is between 2.34° and 25.00°. The **Cugdupt4** dataset has a range of 2.33° to 25.53° for θ. For **Cugdupt5**, the range is between 2.04° and 27.54°. In the **Cugdupt6** dataset, the range is between 2.90° and 26.50°. The **Cugdupt7** dataset has a range of 3.09° to 25.00° for θ. Lastly, the **Cugdupt9** dataset has a range of 2.41° to 25.05° for θ. The experimental data for **Cugdupt3** and **Cugdupt8** were collected using a four-circle diffractometer equipped with a graphite monochromator and a micro-focus metal jet. The wavelength used for the measurements was 1.34050 Å. The data acquisition was performed in the ω scan mode within the following angular ranges: $2.91° \leq \theta \leq 60.29°$ for **Cugdupt3** and $2.13° \leq \theta \leq 60.14°$ for **Cugdupt8**. The integration of raw frame data was performed using the SAINT program. The structures were determined using direct approaches with the SHELXL software and further refined by full matrix least-squares on F^2 using the SHELXL-2015 program within the OLEX-2 graphical user interface. The program SADABS was utilized to implement empirical absorption corrections. Anisotropic refinement was performed on all non-hydrogen atoms. The hydrogen atoms were arranged in a geometric manner and their positions were refined using the riding model. The calculations and graphical representations were conducted using the SHELXTL software.

Table 8-1. The formula and name of $L^{1-9}H_2$ and phen

L^1H_2	$C_{12}H_9Br_2N_3O$	(E)-4-bromo-2-((2-(6-bromopyridin-2-yl)hydrazineylidene)methyl)phenol
L^2H_2	$C_{12}H_8BrCl_2N_3O$	(E)-2-((2-(6-bromopyridin-2-yl)hydrazineylidene)methyl)-4,6-dichlorophenol
L^3H_2	$C_{13}H_{12}BrN_3O_2$	(E)-2-((2-(6-bromopyridin-2-yl)hydrazineylidene)methyl)-6-methoxyphenol
L^4H_2	$C_{12}H_8Br_3N_3O$	(E)-2,4-dibromo-6-((2-(6-bromopyridin-2-yl)hydrazineylidene)methyl)phenol
L^5H_2	$C_{12}H_9BrClN_3O$	(E)-2-((2-(6-bromopyridin-2-yl)hydrazineylidene)methyl)-4-chlorophenol
L^6H_2	$C_{12}H_8Cl_3N_3O$	(E)-2,4-dichloro-6-((2-(6-chloropyridin-2-yl)hydrazineylidene)methyl)phenol
L^7H_2	$C_{13}H_{12}ClN_3O_2$	(E)-2-((2-(6-chloropyridin-2-yl)hydrazineylidene)methyl)-6-methoxyphenol
L^8H_2	$C_{12}H_9ClN_4O_3$	(E)-2-((2-(6-chloropyridin-2-yl)hydrazineylidene)methyl)-4-nitrophenol
L^9H_2	$C_{13}H_{12}ClN_3O$	(E)-2-((2-(6-chloropyridin-2-yl)hydrazineylidene)methyl)-4-methylphenol
Phen	$C_{12}H_8N_2$	1,10-Phenanthroline
$L^{1a}H_2$	$C_{24}H_{16}Br_4N_6O_2$	(E)-5-bromo-N'-((E)-5-bromo-2-hydroxybenzylidene)-N'',N''-bis(6-bromopyridin-2-yl)-2-hydroxybenzohydrazonohydrazide
$L^{2a}H_2$	$C_{24}H_{14}Br_2Cl_4N_6O_2$	(E)-N'',N''-bis(6-bromopyridin-2-yl)-3,5-dichloro-N'-((E)-3,5-dichloro-2-hydroxybenzylidene)-2-hydroxybenzohydrazonohydrazide
$L^{3a}H_2$	$C_{26}H_{22}Br_2N_6O_4$	(E)-N'',N''-bis(6-bromopyridin-2-yl)-2-hydroxy-N'-((E)-2-hydroxy-3-methoxybenzylidene)-3-methoxybenzohydrazonohydrazide
$L^{4a}H_2$	$C_{24}H_{14}Br_6N_6O_2$	(E)-3,5-dibromo-N'',N''-bis(6-bromopyridin-2-yl)-N'-((E)-3,5-dibromo-2-hydroxybenzylidene)-2-hydroxybenzohydrazonohydrazide
$L^{5a}H_2$	$C_{24}H_{16}Br_2Cl_2N_6O_2$	(E)-N'',N''-bis(6-bromopyridin-2-yl)-5-chloro-N'-((E)-5-chloro-2-hydroxybenzylidene)-2-hydroxybenzohydrazonohydrazide
$L^{6a}H_2$	$C_{24}H_{14}Cl_6N_6O_2$	(E)-3,5-dichloro-N'',N''-bis(6-chloropyridin-2-yl)-N'-((E)-3,5-dichloro-2-hydroxybenzylidene)-2-hydroxybenzohydrazonohydrazide
$L^{7a}H_2$	$C_{26}H_{22}Cl_2N_6O_4$	(E)-N'',N''-bis(6-chloropyridin-2-yl)-2-hydroxy-N'-((E)-2-hydroxy-3-methoxybenzylidene)-3-methoxybenzohydrazonohydrazide
$L^{8a}H_2$	$C_{24}H_{16}Cl_2N_8O_6$	(E)-N'',N''-bis(6-chloropyridin-2-yl)-2-hydroxy-N'-((E)-2-hydroxy-5-nitrobenzylidene)-5-nitrobenzohydrazonohydrazide
$L^{9a}H_2$	$C_{26}H_{22}Cl_2N_6O_2$	(E)-N'',N''-bis(6-chloropyridin-2-yl)-2-hydroxy-N'-((E)-2-hydroxy-5-methylbenzylidene)-5-methylbenzohydrazonohydrazide

Other methods

The experimental protocol for the in vivo assay of **Cugdupt8** was acquired from the Electronic Supporting Information Materials. Furthermore, the in vitro anticancer mechanisms employed for **Cugdupt1–Cugdupt9** were consistent with the technique previously documented by our research team.

Outcomes and Analysis

Synthesis and characterization

The synthesis involving the combination of hydrazine pyridine salicylaldehyde (L^1H_2–L^9H_2), 1,10-phenanthroline (phen), and Cu(Ac)$_2$ at a temperature of 80°C for a duration of 72 hours was conducted in the presence of 4.0 mL of CH$_3$CH$_2$OH and 6.0 mL of CH$_3$CN, as depicted in Scheme 8-1. The synthesis of copper (II) hydrazyl-pyridine-salicylaldehyde-phenanthroline **Cugdupt1-Cugdupt9** was performed. The crystals **Cugdupt1-Cugdupt9** exhibited high yields ranging from 30.2% to 50.6%, indicating their single-crystal nature. The samples underwent comprehensive characterization using various analytical techniques, including powder X-ray diffraction (XRD), elemental analysis, infrared spectroscopy (IR), UV-visible spectroscopy (UV-Vis), and X-ray crystallography.

The structures of **Cugdupt1-Cugdupt9** were confirmed using X-ray crystallography. The coordination geometry of the Cu(II) cation in the **Cugdupt1-Cugdupt9** combination underwent deformation. In all Cu (II) complexes, every Cu (II) ion is coordinated with one 1,10-phenanthroline (phen) ligand and two deprotonated hydrazyl pyridine salicylaldehyde (L^1H_2–L^9H_2) ligands.

Scheme 8-1. Synthetic routes for the copper(II) hydrazyl pyridine-1, 10-phenanthroline complexes Cugdupt1–Cugdupt9

The examination of X-ray single crystal diffraction data reveals that the structures of complexes **Cugdupt1-Cugdupt9** exhibit similarities, with the exception of variations in the halogen, methoxy, methyl, or nitro group substituents on the H_2L^{na} ligands (Figure 8-19). Hence, the analysis in this study focused solely on the complex **Cugdupt3**.

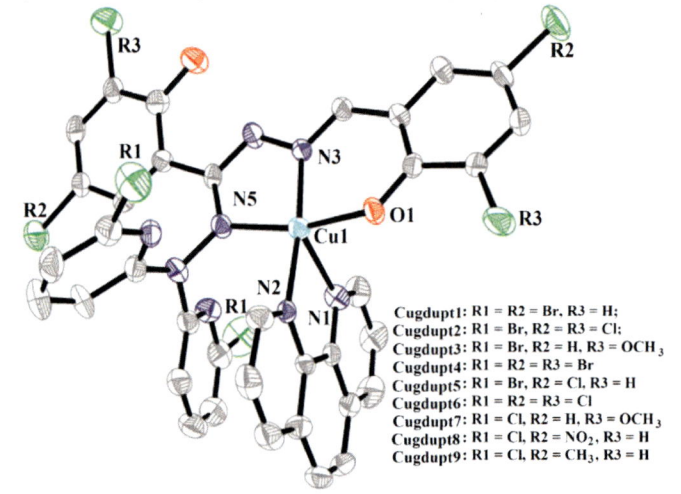

Figure 8-19. Molecule structures of Cugdupt1-Cugdupt9. Solvent molecules of Cugdupt2, Cugdupt4, Cugdupt9 were omitted for clarity

Cugdupt3 was produced using a solvothermal reaction involving the combination of $Cu(Ac)_2 \cdot H_2O$, phen, and L^3H_2 in a solution of ethanol and acetonitrile (4:6, v/v) at a temperature of 80°C for a duration of 72 hours. The monoclinic space group $P2_{1/c}$ was determined for **Cugdupt3** using single-crystal X-ray diffraction research. The compound is composed of one CuII atom, one phen molecule, and one L^{3a} ligand, which were produced using an in-situ process (Scheme 8-2). The Cu1 atom in **Cugdupt3** exhibits a coordination number of five, being coordinated to two N atoms (N3, N5) and one O atom (O1) in an L^{3a} ligand. The bond lengths are as follows: Cu1-N3 = 1.942(2) Å, Cu1-N5 = 1.945(2) Å, and Cu1-O1 = 1.940(2) Å. Additionally, Cu1 is coordinated to two N atoms (N1, N2) in a phen ligand, with bond lengths of Cu1-N1 = 2.012(2) Å and Cu1-N1 = 2.237(2) Å. Consequently, the resulting structure exhibits distorted tetragonal pyramid geometries.

The τ_5 value was used to indicate the calculations of Continuous Shape Measure (CShM). The τ_5 values were determined by applying the approach for five-coordinate structures, which involves calculating the difference between the biggest (β) and second-largest (α) L—Cu—L angles and dividing it by 60 [$\tau_5 = (\beta - \alpha)/60$]. Therefore, it can be shown that a molecular structure exhibiting trigonal bipyramidal geometry and possessing D_{3h} symmetry has a value of τ_5 equal to 1. Conversely, a molecular structure characterized by square-pyramidal geometry and possessing C_{4v} symmetry exhibits a value of τ_5 equal to 0. In the case of Cu1 in **Cugdupt3**, the value of τ_5 is calculated as (175.78-161.68)/60 = 0.235, which is in proximity to zero according to sources. The mononuclear complex **Cugdupt3** exhibits the formation of a three-dimensional network (Figure 8-20) via Cu$\cdots$H interactions (Cu1$\cdots$H2^i, with a distance of 2.988(2)Å, where the symmetry code is given as (i) 1 - x, y - 0.5, 0.5 - z). Additionally, hydrogen bonds (C13-H13B) are also involved in this network. The value of Br1^{ii} is determined to be 3.883(2)Å, whereas C26-H26A is also seen. The bond length between two bromine atoms (Br2) is determined to be 3.616(2)Å. Additionally, the distance between carbon atom The interatomic distances in the crystal structure are as follows: O3^{iv}-C8-H3$\cdots$O2^v with a distance of 3.191(2)Å, C3-H3A$\cdots$N4^{iv} with a distance of 3.383(2)Å. The symmetry codes for these distances are as follows: (ii) 1 + x, y, z; (iii) x, y - 1, z; (iv) x, y + 1, z; (v) 1 - x, 2 - y, 1 - z. Additionally, the **Cugdupt3** compound exhibits intramolecular $\pi\cdots\pi$ contacts between the pyridine ring (N7-C34-C35-C36-C37-C38) and the phen molecule, with a $\pi\cdots\pi$ distance of 3.420 (1) Å. The H$_2$L^{3a} compound was produced using an in situ process, as shown in Scheme 8-2.

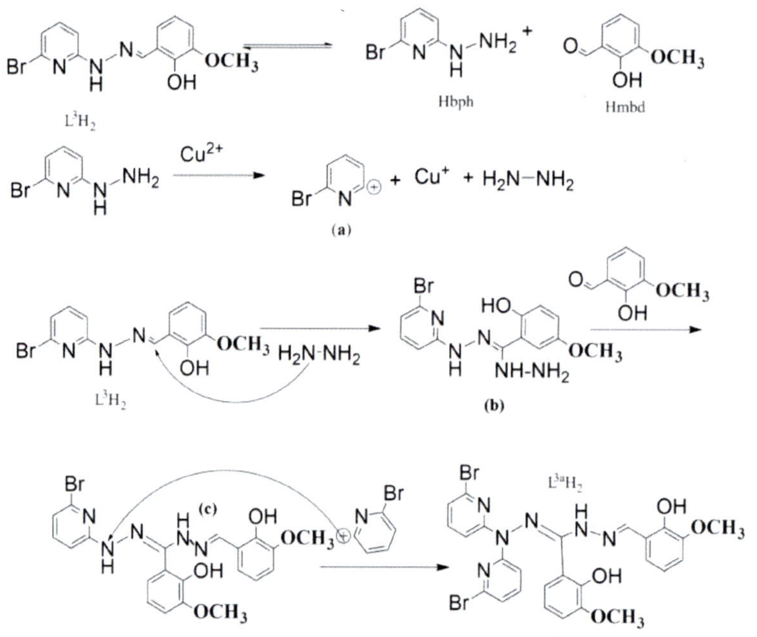

Scheme 8-2. Synthesis Mechanism of L³ᵃH₂.

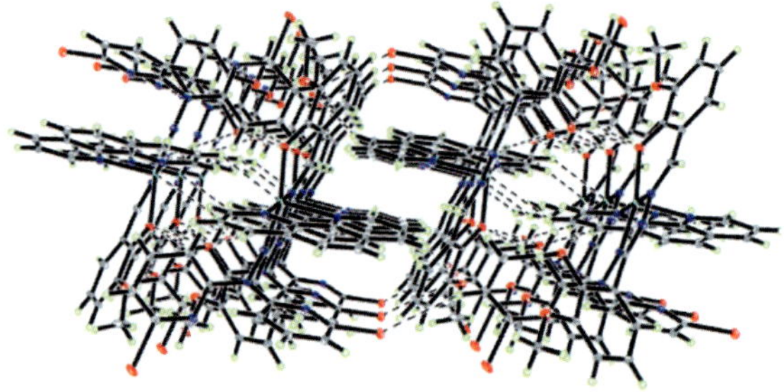

Figure 8-20. 3D network of Cugdupt3

Synthesis Mechanism

The ligands L¹ᵃH₂–L⁹ᵃH₂ were generated in **Cugdupt1–Cugdupt9** via a copper ion catalyzed in-situ process, as depicted in Scheme 8-2. L³ᵃH₂ was employed as a representative case study to facilitate the examination and exploration of its underlying reaction mechanism. The synthesis of Schiff base compounds is a reversible process, resulting in the presence of Hbph and 2-hydroxy-3-methoxybenzaldehyde (Hmbd) inside the reaction system. Under the catalytic oxidation of Cu^{2+}, Hbph undergoes decomposition to yield (**a**) and hydrazine. The chemical (**b**) is formed when hydrazine reacts with the carbon atom of the C=N double bond in the Schiff base L³H₂. The compounds Hmbd and **b** undergo a condensation process, resulting in the synthesis of compound **c**. Ultimately, an assault occurred, resulting in an electrophilic substitution reaction that produces L³ᵃH₂.

Cytotoxicity

The CCK-8 tests were employed to investigate the cytotoxic activity of **Cugdupt1–Cugdupt9** in A549, A549cis cancer cells, and HL-7702 normal cells, with the aim of determining the IC_{50} values (μM). The **Cugdupt1–Cugdupt9** compounds demonstrated a notably higher level of effectiveness against A549cis cells compared to A549 and HL-7702 cells, with varying levels of toxicity in comparison to cisplatin, as shown in Table 8-2. The cytotoxic action against A549cis is stronger in **Cugdupt1–Cugdupt9** compared to L¹H₂–L⁹H₂, Cu(Ac)₂·H₂O, phen, cisplatin, and Cu(II) complexes. Compound **Cugdupt8** possesses chlorine- and nitro-substituted groups, which are known to exhibit strong electron-absorbing properties. Consequently, it demonstrated significantly higher activity against A549cis cancer cells compared to **Cugdupt1–Cugdupt7** and **Cugdupt9**, with an enhancement ranging from 1.4 to 61.0 times. The findings of this study provide evidence that **Cugdupt8** exhibited a statistically significant superiority in its cytotoxicity against A549cis cells compared to L^1H_2–L^9H_2, $Cu(Ac)_2·H_2O$, **Cugdupt1–Cugdupt7**, phen, **Cugdupt9**, and cisplatin. **Cugdupt8** exhibited minimal cytotoxicity towards HL-7702 normal cells. **Cugdupt8** was subsequently chosen for additional examination and juxtaposed with **Cugdupt1**.

Table 8-2. IC$_{50}$ values (μM) of L^1H_2-L^9H_2, Cugdupt1–Cugdupt9, Cu(Ac)$_2$·H$_2$O, phen, and cisplatin for 24 h via CCK-8 assays.

	A549	A549cis	HL-7702
L^1H_2	>50	>50	>50
Cugdupt1	33.5±1.6	30.5±1.9	>50
L^2H_2	>50	>50	>50
Cugdupt2	24.4±0.7	18.3±1.6	>50
L^3H_2	>50	>50	>50
Cugdupt3	9.2±0.3	2.8±0.9	>50
L^4H_2	>50	>50	>50
Cugdupt4	31.1±0.8	28.0±0.6	>50
L^5H_2	>50	>50	>50
Cugdupt5	29.1±0.5	25.6±1.7	>50
L^6H_2	>50	>50	>50
Cugdupt6	20.0±0.2	15.4± 0.8	>50
L^7H_2	>50	>50	>50
Cugdupt7	6.0±1.4	0.7± 0.2	>50
L^8H_2	>50	>50	>50
Cugdupt8	3.7±0.1	0.5±0.1	>50
L^9H_2	>50	>50	>50
Cugdupt9	10.6±2.0	4.2±1.0	>50
$Cu(Ac)_2·H_2O$	>50	>50	>50
phen	>50	>50	>50
cisplatin	10.1±0.2	61.5±1.0	17.4±1.5

Cugdupt8 and Cugdupt1 induced apoptosis

Subsequently, the process of apoptosis in A549cis cells was assessed subsequent to their exposure to **Cugdupt8** at a concentration of 0.5 μM and **Cugdupt1** at a concentration of 10.0 μM. This evaluation was conducted by employing dual Annexin V-FITC/PI labeling, followed by flow cytometry analysis. Figure 8-21 illustrates that the untreated group exhibited a proportion of apoptotic cells amounting to 2.87±0.12%. The percentage of **Cugdupt8** (0.5 μM) at 24 hours was determined to be 17.38±0.80%. The experimental group treated with **Cugdupt1** at a concentration of 10.0 μM exhibited a relatively low percentage of apoptosis, specifically (3.10±0.21%). This finding indicates that the induction of cell death in A549cis cells by **Cugdupt8** primarily occurs through the process of apoptosis. The level of obviousness is greater in comparison to that of **Cugdupt1**.

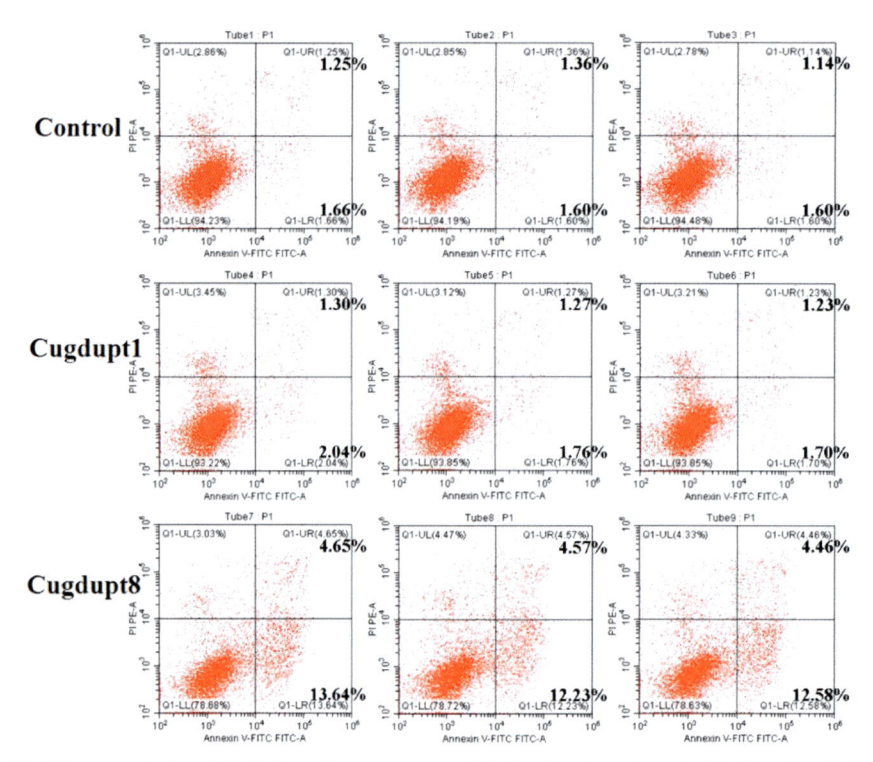

Figure 8-21. The apoptosis of A549cis cells was assessed following treatment with Cugdupt8 (0.5 μM) and Cugdupt1 (10.0 μM) for a duration of 24 hours.

In vivo antitumor effect

Subsequently, the effectiveness of **Cugdupt8** at a dosage of 5.0 mg per kg every 2 days was evaluated for a period of 21 days in a Balb/c nude model with A549 tumor cells, administered intraperitoneally. The experimental results presented in Figure 8-22 indicate that Cugdupt8 exhibited a tumor growth inhibition value (TGIV) of 56.9%. The observed value was notably greater compared to the 50.0% rate achieved with cisplatin in identical circumstances. Throughout the 21-day treatment period, there were no notable alterations in body weight (mean=21.3±0.8 g) detected in the **Cugdupt8** treatment group in comparison to the vehicle group (mean=21.1±0.5 g) (Figure 8-22).The findings of this study indicate that **Cugdupt8** had significant in vivo anticancer efficacy.

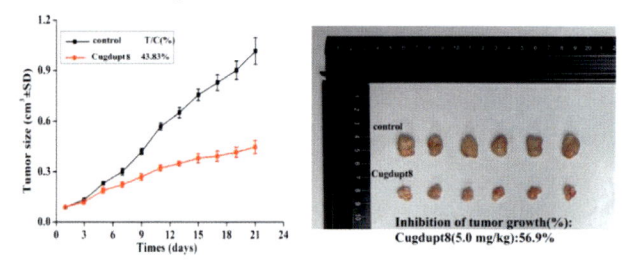

Figure 8-22. The effectiveness of a dosage of 5.0 mg/kg of Cugdupt8 in BABL/c nude mice with A549 tumors.

Cell death mechanism

Further investigation was conducted to elucidate the mechanism by which **Cugdupt8** exerts its enhanced anti-proliferative effects. The process of mitophagy has the potential to induce impairment in the function of mitochondrial respiratory chain complexes I and IV, thereby leading to a decrease in adenosine triphosphate (ATP) production. It exerted regulatory control over the production of the related proteins. The impact of **Cugdupt8** (0.5 μM) and Cugdupt1 (10.0 μM) on the MRCC-I/IV and ATP synthesis in A549cis cells was assessed following the guidelines provided by the manufacturer's kit. Tables 8-2–8-4 present data indicating that the application of **Cugdupt8** at a concentration of 0.5 μM resulted in reductions of 30.4%, 33.8%, and 31.1% in MRCC-I, MRCC-IV, and ATP levels, respectively, as compared to the control cells. Conversely, the inhibitory effects of **Cugdupt1** at a concentration of 10.0 μM on MRCC-I, MRCC-IV, and ATP generation were found to be less pronounced than those observed with **Cugdupt8** at 0.5 μM. The results of this study demonstrate that the administration of **Cugdupt8** at a concentration of 0.5 μM and Cugdupt1 at a concentration of 10.0 μM significantly impact the expression levels of MRCC-I, MRCC-IV, and ATP. Furthermore, these compounds have the potential to induce cell death in A549cis cells. Subsequently, the quantification of nine proteins linked with mitophagy was conducted by western blotting and immunofluorescence techniques. This investigation aimed to assess the extent of apoptosis in A549cis cells induced by **Cugdupt8** (0.5 μM) and **Cugdupt1** (10.0 μM). Figures 8-23 and 8-24 demonstrate that the presence of **Cugdupt8** at a concentration of 0.5 μM has a more pronounced effect on the synthesis or inhibition of proteins linked with the mitophagy pathway compared to both the **Cugdupt1** group at a concentration of 10.0 μM and the untreated groups. Cell death in A549cis cells was observed to be promoted by **Cugdupt8** and **Cugdupt1** through the activation of a pathway involving mitophagy and ATP dysfunction.

Table 8-2. ATP levels in A549cis cells treated for 24 hours with Cugdupt8 (0.5 μM) and Cugdupt1 (10.0 μM) (n = 3, p 0.05)

	Control	**Cugdupt1**	**Cugdupt8**
OD	43518	41482	29350
	41502	40926	29254
	43447	40017	29329
OD values after correction	43496	41460	29328
	41480	40904	29232
	43425	39995	29307
ATP values (μM)	3.95194	3.76870	2.69252
	3.77050	3.71866	2.66818
	3.94555	3.63685	2.67493
Mean	3.89	3.71	2.68
SD	0.10	0.07	0.01

Table 8-3. MRCC-I levels in A549cis cells after 24 hours of treatment with Cugdupt8 (0.5 μM) and Cugdupt1(10.0 μM) (n = 3, p 0.05).

Group	ΔA	Cpr	MRCC-I (U/mg prot)	Mean	SD
Control	0.033	0.567	93.54005314		
	0.031	0.598	83.37270768	85.23	7.56
	0.024	0.490	78.76509909		
Cugdupt1	0.031	0.612	81.39889574		
	0.022	0.464	76.21036957	80.48	3.89
	0.031	0.595	83.82440261		
	0.023	0.596	62.02428178	59.30	3.45

Group	ΔA	Cpr			
Cugdupt8	0.013	0.377	55.41884654		
	0.016	0.426	60.46146991		

Table 8-4. The levels of MRCC-IV in A549cis cells were assessed following a 24-hour treatment with Cugdupt8 (0.5μM) and Cugdupt1 (10.0μM). This experiment was conducted with a sample size of three, and statistical significance was determined at a p-value of less than 0.05.

Group	ΔA	Cpr	MRCC-IV (U/mg prot)	Mean	SD
Control	0.027	0.359	82.54416167		
	0.051	0.582	96.33979592	90.75	7.26
	0.033	0.388	93.35699843		
Cugdupt1	0.035	0.501	76.73976213		
	0.051	0.638	87.82824532	83.92	6.23
	0.05	0.630	87.20678800		
Cugdupt8	0.029	0.527	60.47468577		
	0.037	0.661	61.54359814	60.09	1.69
	0.038	0.717	58.23733674		

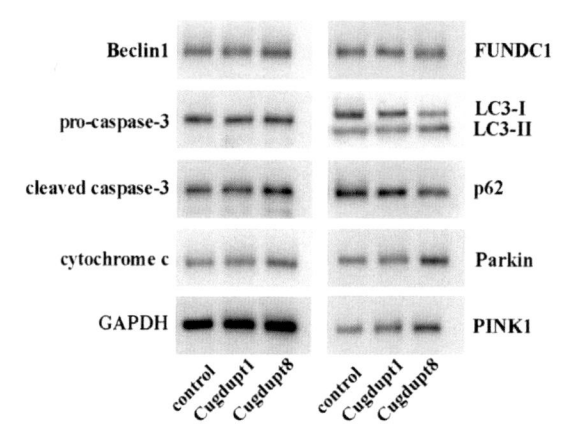

Figure 8-23. The impact of Cugdupt8 at a concentration of 0.5μM and Cugdupt1 at a concentration of 10.0μM on the levels of mitophagy-associated proteins in A549cis cells was assessed over a period of 24 hours.

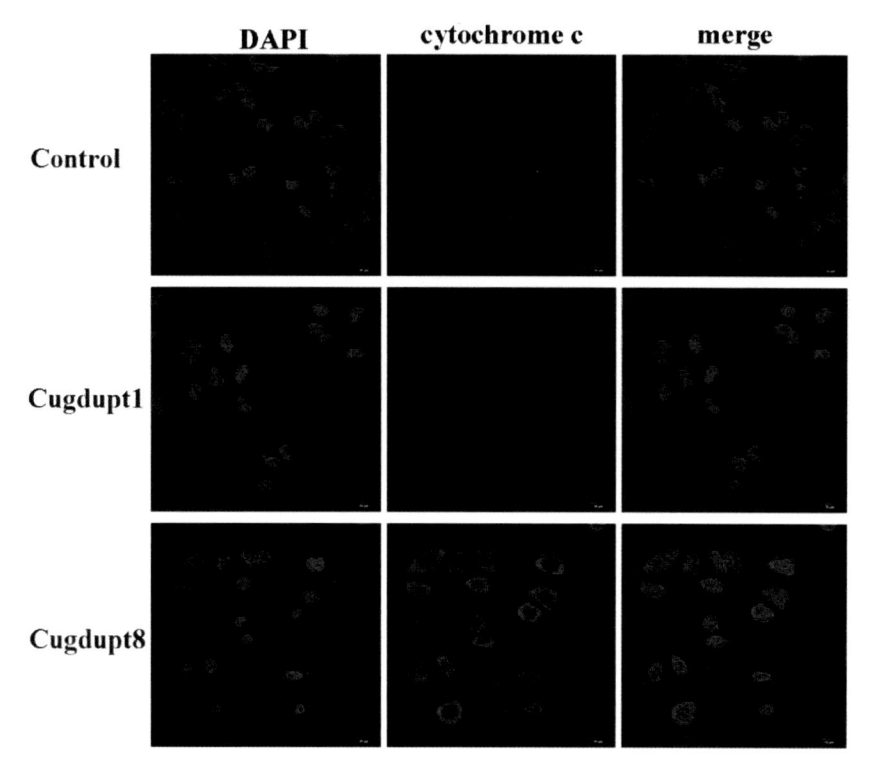

	DAPI	cytochrome c	merge
Control			
Cugdupt1			
Cugdupt8			

Figure 8-24. The present study investigated the impact of Cugdupt8 (0.5μM) and Cugdupt1 (10.0μM) on cytochrome c levels in A549cis cells after a 24-hour exposure period.

A total of nine new compounds, denoted as **Cugdupt1–Cugdupt9**, were synthesized and characterized using a range of spectroscopic techniques. These complexes are comprised of hydrazylpyridine salicylaldehyde ligands coordinated with copper(II) ions and 1,10-phenanthroline. **Cugdupt1–Cugdupt9** exhibited significant cytotoxicity against A549cis cancer cells, while demonstrating minimal cytotoxicity towards HL-7702 normal cells. Additionally, it was observed that the compounds **Cugdupt1** and **Cugdupt8** induced cell death in A549cis cells through the activation of a pathway involving mitophagy and malfunction of ATP. The experimental drug **Cugdupt8** had greater effectiveness in treating mice with A549 tumors compared to the standard chemotherapy drug cisplatin. The findings of this study indicate that **Cugdupt1–Cugdupt9** exhibit promising potential as pharmacological candidates for future applications in anticancer therapy.

References

1. Shen, W. Y.; Jia, C. P.; Liao, L. Y.; Chen, L. L.; Hou, C.; Liu, Y. H.; Liang, H.; Chen. Z. F. Copper(II) Complexes of Halogenated Quinoline Schiff Base Derivatives Enabled Cancer Therapy through Glutathione-Assisted Chemodynamic Therapy and Inhibition of Autophagy Flux. J. Med. Chem., 2022, 65(6), 5134-5148.
2. Wittmann, C.; Bacher, F.; Enyedy, E. A.; Dömötör, O.; Spengler, G.; Madejski, C.; Reynisson, J.; Arion. V. B. Highly Antiproliferative Latonduine and Indolo[2,3-c]Quinoline Derivatives: Complex Formation with Copper(II) Markedly Changes the Kinase Inhibitory Profile. J. Med. Chem., 2022, 65(3), 2238-2261.
3. Gasser, G.; Ott, I.; Metzler-Nolte, N. Organometallic Anticancer Compounds. J. Med. Chem., 2011, 54(1), 3-25.

4. Jung, Y.; Lippard, S. J. Direct Cellular Responses to Platinum-Induced DNA Damage., Chem. Rev., 2007, 107(5), 1387-1407.
5. Anthony, E. J.; Bolitho, E. M.; Bridgewater, H. E.; Carter, O. W. L.; Donnelly, J. M.; Imberti, C.; Lant, E. C.; Lermyte, F.; Needham, R. J.; Palau, M.; Sadler, P. J.; Shi, H.; Wang, F. X.; Zhang, W. Y.; Zhang, Z. Metallodrugs are Unique: Opportunities and Challenges of Discovery and Development. Chem. Sci., 2020, 11(48), 12888-12917.
6. Gourdon, L.; Cariou, K.; Gasser, G. Phototherapeutic Anticancer Strategies with First-Row Transition Metal Complexes: a Critical Review. Chem. Soc. Rev., 2022, 51(3), 1167-1195.
7. Kenny, R. G.; Marmion, C. J. Toward Multi-Targeted Platinum and Ruthenium Drugs—a New Paradigm in Cancer Drug Treatment Regimens?. Chem. Rev., 2019, 119(2), 1058-1137.
8. Cai, D. H.; Chen, B. H.; Liu, Q. Y.; Le, X. Y.; He, L. Synthesis, Structural Studies, Interaction with DNA/HSA and Antitumor Evaluation of New Cu(II) Complexes Containing 2-(1H-Imidazol-2-Yl)Pyridine and Amino Acids. Dalton Trans., 2022, 51(43), 16574-16586.
9. Novoa-Ramírez, C. S.; Silva-Becerril, A.; González-Ballesteros, M. M.; Gomez-Vidal, V.; Flores-Álamo, M.; Ortiz-Frade, L.; Gracia-Mora, J.; Ruiz-Azuara, L. Biological Activity of Mixed Chelate Cpper(II) Complexes, with Substituted Diimine and Tridentate Schiff Bases(NNO) and Their Hydrogenated Derivatives as Secondary Ligands: Casiopeína's Fourth Generation. J. Inorg. Biochem., 2023, 242, 112097.
10. Sen, S.; Won, M.; Levine, M. S.; Noh, Y.; Sedgwick, A. C.; Kim, J. S.; Sessler, J. L.; Arambula, J. F. Metal-Based Anticancer Agents as Immunogenic Cell Death Inducers: the Past, Present, and Future. Chem. Soc. Rev., 2022, 51(4), 1212-1233.
11. Gu, Y. Q.; Zhong, Y. J.; Hu, M. Q.; Li, H. Q.; Yang, K.; Dong, Q.; Liang, H.; Chen, Z. F. Terpyridine Copper(II) Complexes as Potential Anticancer Agents by Inhibiting Cell Proliferation, Blocking the Cell Cycle and Inducing Apoptosis in BEL-7402 Cells. Dalton Trans., 2022, 51(5), 1968-1978.
12. Shao, J.; Zhang, Q.; Wei, J.; Yuchi, Z.; Cao, P.; Li, S. Q.; Wang, S.; Xu, J. Y.; Yang, S.; Zhang, Y.; Wei, J. X.; Tian, J. L. Synthesis, Crystal Structures, Anticancer Activities and Molecular Docking Studies of Novel Thiazolidinone Cu(II) and Fe(III) Complexes Targeting Lysosomes: Special Emphasis on Their Binding to DNA/BSA. Dalton Trans., 2021, 50(38), 13387-13398.
13. Jiang, M.; Zhang, Z.; Li, W.; Man, X.; Sun, S.; Liang, H.; Yang, F. Developing a Copper(II) Agent Based on His-146 and His-242 Residues of Human Serum Albumin Nanoparticles: Integration to Overcome Cisplatin Resistance and Inhibit the Metastasis of Nonsmall Cell Lung Cancer. J. Med. Chem., 2022, 65(13), 9447-9458.
14. Gou, Y.; Chen, M. R.; Li, S.; Deng, J.; Li, J.; Fang, G.; Yang, F.; Huang, G. Dithiocarbazate-Copper Complexes for Bioimaging and Treatment of Pancreatic Cancer. J. Med. Chem., 2021, 64(9), 5485-5499.
15. Santini, C.; Pellei, M.; Gandin, V.; Porchia, M.; Tisato, F.; Marzano, C. Advances in Copper Complexes as Anticancer Agents. Chem. Rev., 2014, 114(1), 815-862.

16. Paterson, B. M.; Donnelly, P. S. Copper Complexes of Bis(Thiosemicarbazones): from Chemotherapeutics to Diagnostic and Therapeutic Radiopharmaceuticals. Chem. Soc. Rev., 2011, 40(5), 3005-3018.
17. Kant, R.; Maji, S. Recent Advances in the Synthesis of Piperazine Based Ligands and Metal Complexes and Their Applications. Dalton Trans., 2021, 50(3), 785-800.
18. Bhattacharyya, A.; Jameei, A.; Garai, A.; Saha, R.; Karande, A. A.; Chakravarty, A. R. Mitochondria-Localizing BODIPY-Copper(II) Conjugates for Cellular Imaging and Photo-Activated Cytotoxicity Forming Singlet Oxygen. Dalton Trans., 2018, 47(14), 5019-5030.
19. Massoud, S. S.; Louka, F. R.; Salem, N. M. H.; Fischer, R. C.; Torvisco, A.; Mautner, F. A.; Vančo, J.; Belza, J.; Dvořák, Z.; Trávníček, Z. Dinuclear Doubly Bridged Phenoxido Copper(II) Complexes as Efficient Anticancer Agents. Eur. J. Med. Chem., 2023, 246, 114992.
20. Massoud, S. S.; Louka, F. R.; Dial, M. T.; Malek, A. J.; Fischer, R. C.; Mautner, F. A.; Vančo, J.; Malina, T.; Dvořák, Z.; Trávníček, Z. Identification of Potent Anticancer Copper(II) Complexes Containing Tripodal Bis[2-Ethyl-Di(3,5-Dialkyl-1H-Pyrazol-1-Yl)]Amine Moiety. Dalton Trans., 2021, 50(33), 11521-11534.
21. Dankhoff, K.; Gold, M.; Kober, L.; Schmitt, F.; Pfeifer, L.; Dürrmann, A.; Kostrhunova, H.; Rothemund, M.; Brabec, V.; Schobert, R.; Weber, B. Copper(II) Complexes with Tridentate Schiff Base-Like Ligands: Solid State and Solution Structures and Anticancer Activity. Dalton Trans., 2019, 48(40), 15220-15230.
22. Qu, J. J.; Bai, P.; Liu, W. N.; Liu, Z. L.; Gong, J. F.; Wang, J.X.; Zhu, X.; Song, B.; Hao, X. Q. New NNN Pincer Copper Complexes as Potential Anti-Prostate Cancer Agents. Eur. J. Med. Chem., 2022, 244, 114859.
23. Perontsis, S.; Geromichalos, G. D.; Pekou, A.; Hatzidimitriou, A. G.; Pantazaki, A.; Fylaktakidou, K. C.; Psomas, G. Structure and Biological Evaluation of Pyridine-2-Carboxamidine Copper(II) Complex Resulting from N'-(4-Nitrophenylsulfonyloxy)2-Pyridine-Carboxamidoxime. J. Inorg. Biochem., 2020, 208, 111085.
24. Singh, N. K.; Kumbhar, A. A.; Pokharel, Y. R.; Yadav, P. N. Anticancer Potency of Copper(II) Complexes of Thiosemicarbazones. J. Inorg. Biochem., 2020, 210, 111134.
25. Mathuber, M.; Hager, S.; Keppler, B. K.; Heffeter, P.; Kowol, C. R. Liposomal Formulations of Anticancer Copper(II) Thiosemicarbazone Complexes. Dalton Trans., 2021, 50(44), 16053-16066.
26. Anjum, R.; Palanimuthu, D.; Kalinowski, D. S.; Lewis, K. W.; Park, K. C.; Kovacevic, Z.; Khan, I. U.; Richardson, D. R. Synthesis, Characterization, and in Vitro Anticancer Activity of Copper and Zinc Bis(Thiosemicarbazone) Complexes. Inorg. Chem. Front., 2019, 58(20), 13709-13723.
27. Bormio Nunes, J. H.; Hager, S.; Mathuber, M.; Pósa, V.; Roller, A.; Enyedy, É. A.; Stefanelli, A.; Berger, W.; Keppler, B. K.; Heffeter, P.; Kowol, C. R. Cancer Cell Resistance Against the Clinically Investigated Thiosemicarbazone COTI-2 Is Based on Formation of Intracellular Copper Complex Glutathione Adducts and ABCC1-Mediated Efflux. J. Med. Chem., 2020, 63(22), 13719-13732.
28. Zhang, Z.; Yu, P.; Gou, Y.; Zhang, J.; Li, S.; Cai, M.; Sun, H.; Yang, F.; Liang, H. Novel Brain-Tumor-Inhibiting Copper(II) Compound Based on a Human Serum

Albumin (HSA)-Cell Penetrating Peptide Conjugate. J. Med. Chem., 2019, 62(23), 10630-10644.
29. Carcelli, M.; Tegoni, M.; Bartoli, J.; Marzano, C.; Pelosi, G.; Salvalaio, M.; Rogolino, D.; Gandin, V. In Vitro and in Vivo Anticancer Activity of Tridentate Thiosemicarbazone Copper Complexes: Unravelling an Unexplored Pharmacological Target. Eur. J. Med. Chem., 2020, 194, 112266.
30. Gu, S.; Yu, P.; Hu, J.; Liu, Y.; Li, Z.; Qian, Y.; Wang, Y.; Gou, Y.; Yang, F. Mitochondria-Localizing N-Heterocyclic Thiosemicarbazone Copper Complexes with Good Cytotoxicity and High Antimetastatic Activity. Eur. J. Med. Chem., 2019, 164, 654-664.
31. Komarnicka, U. K.; Kozieł, S.; Pucelik, B.; Barzowska, A.; Siczek, M.; Malik, M.; Wojtala, D.; Niorettini, A.; Kyzioł, A.; Sebastian, V.; Kopel, P.; Caramori, S.; Bieńko, A. Liposomal Binuclear Ir(III)-Cu(II) Coordination Compounds with Phosphino-Fluoroquinolone Conjugates for Human Prostate Carcinoma Treatment. 2022, 61(48): 19261-19273. Inorg. Chem. Front., 2022, 61(48), 19261-19273.
32. Liu, Q. Y.; Qi, Y. Y.; Cai, D. H.; Liu, Y. J.; He, L.; Le, X. Y. Sparfloxacin-Cu(II)-Aromatic Heterocyclic Complexes: Synthesis, Characterization and in Vitro Anticancer Evaluation. Dalton Trans., 2022, 51(25), 9878-9887.
33. Kuznetcova, I.; Bacher, F.; Alfadul, S. M.; Tham, M. J. R.; Ang, W. H.; Babak, M. V.; Rapta, P.; Arion, V. B. Elucidation of Structure-Activity Relationships in Indolobenzazepine-Derived Ligands and Their Copper(II) Complexes: the Role of Key Structural Components and Insight into the Mechanism of Action. Inorg. Chem. Front., 2022, 61(26), 10167-10181.
34. Bacher, F.; Wittmann, C.; Nové, M.; Spengler, G.; Marć, M. A.; Enyedy, E. A.; Darvasiová, D.; Rapta, P.; Reiner, T.; Arion, V. B. Novel latonduine Derived Proligands and Their Copper(II) Complexes Show Cytotoxicity in the Nanomolar Range in Human Colon Adenocarcinoma Cells and in Vitro Cancer Selectivity. Dalton Trans., 2019, 48(28), 10464-10478.
35. Shi, X.; Chen, Z.; Wang, Y.; Guo, Z.; Wang, X. Hypotoxic Copper Complexes with Potent Anti-Metastatic and Anti-Angiogenic Activities Against Cancer Cells. Dalton Trans., 2018, 47(14), 5049-5054.
36. Naso, L. G.; Medina, J. J. M.; D'Alessandro, F.; Rey, M.; Rizzi, A.; Piro, O. E.; Echeverría, G. A.; Ferrer, E. G.; Williams, P. A. M. Ternary Copper(II) Complex of 5-Hydroxytryptophan and 1,10-Phenanthroline with Several Pharmacological Properties and an Adequate Safety Profile. J. Inorg. Biochem., 2020, 204, 110933.
37. Martínez-Valencia, B.; Corona-Motolinia, N. D.; Sánchez-Lara, E.; Noriega, L.; Sánchez-Gaytán, B. L.; Castro, M. E.; Meléndez-Bustamante, F.; González-Vergara, E. Cyclo-Tetravanadate Bridged Copper Complexes as Potential Double Bullet Pro-Metallodrugs for Cancer Treatment. J. Inorg. Biochem., 2020, 208, 111081.
38. Parsekar, S. U.; Velankanni, P.; Sridhar, S.; Haldar, P.; Mate, N. A.; Banerjee, A.; Antharjanam, P. K. S.; Koley, A. P.; Kumar, M. Protein Binding Studies with Human Serum Albumin, Molecular Docking and in Vitro Cytotoxicity Studies Using HeLa Cervical Carcinoma Cells of Cu(II)/Zn(II) Complexes Containing a Carbohydrazone Ligand. Dalton Trans., 2020, 49(9), 2947-2965.

39. Sharma, M.; Ganeshpandian, M.; Majumder, M.; Tamilarasan, A.; Sharma, M.; Mukhopadhyay, R.; Islam, N. S.; Palaniandavar, M. Octahedral Copper(II)-Diimine Complexes of Triethylenetetramine: Effect of Stereochemical Fluxionality and Ligand Hydrophobicity on CuII/CuI Redox, DNA Binding and Cleavage, Cytotoxicity and Apoptosis-Inducing Ability. Dalton Trans., 2020, 49(24), 8282-8297.

40. Mo, X.; Chen, Z.; Chu, B.; Liu, D.; Liang, Y.; Liang, F. Structure and Anticancer Activities of Four Cu(II) Complexes Bearing Tropolone. Metallomics, 2019, 11(11), 1952-1964.

41. Qin, Q. P.; Meng, T.; Tan, M. X.; Liu, Y. C.; Luo, X. J.; Zou, B. Q.; Liang, H. Synthesis, Crystal Structure and Biological Evaluation of a New Dasatinib Copper(II) Complex as Telomerase Inhibitor. Eur. J. Med. Chem., 2018, 143, 1597-1603.

42. [Qin, Q. P.; Zou, B. Q.; Tan, M. X.; Wang, S. L.; Liu, Y. C.; Liang, H. Tryptanthrin Derivative Copper(II) Complexes with High Antitumor Activity by Inhibiting Telomerase Activity, and Inducing Mitochondria-Mediated Apoptosis and S-Phase Arrest in BEL-7402. New J. Chem., 2018, 42(18), 15479-15487.

43. Lu, X.; Liu, Y. C.; Orvig, C.; Liang, H.; Chen, Z. F. Discovery of β-Carboline Copper(II) Complexes as Mcl-1 Inhibitor and in Vitro and in Vivo Activity in Cancer Models. Eur. J. Med. Chem., 2019, 181, 111567.

44. Lu, W.; Tang, J.; Gu, Z.; Su, L.; Wei, H.; Wang, Y.; Yang, S.; Chi, X.; Xu, L. Crystal Structure, in Vitro Cytotoxicity, DNA Binding and DFT Calculations of New Copper(II) Complexes with Coumarin-Amide Ligand. J. Inorg. Biochem., 2023, 238, 112030.

45. Kordestani, N.; Rudbari, H. A.; Fernandes, A. R.; Raposo, L. R.; Luz, A.; Baptista, P. V.; Bruno, G.; Scopelliti, R.; Fateminia, Z.; Micale, N.; Tumanov, N.; Wouters, J.; Kajani, A. A.; Bordbar, A. K. Copper(II) Complexes with Tridentate Halogen-Substituted Schiff Base Ligands: Synthesis, Crystal Structures and Investigating the Effect of Halogenation, Leaving Groups and Ligand Flexibility on Antiproliferative Activities. Dalton Trans., 2021, 50(11), 3990-4007.

46. Peña, Q.; Sciortino, G.; Maréchal, J. D.; Bertaina, S.; Simaan, A. J.; Lorenzo, J.; Capdevila, M.; Bayón, P.; Iranzo, O.; Palacios, Ò. Copper(II) N,N,O-Chelating Complexes as Potential Anticancer Agents. Inorg. Chem. Front., 2021, 60(5), 2939-2952.

47. Diz, M.; Durán-Carril, M. L.; Castro, J.; Alvo, S.; Bada, L.; Viña, D.; García-Vázquez, J. A. Antitumor Activity of Copper(II) Complexes with Schiff Bases Derived from N′-Tosylbenzene-1,2-Diamine. J. Inorg. Biochem., 2022, 236, 111975.

48. Mukherjee, S.; Hansda, S.; Nandi, S.; Chakraborty, T.; Samanta, D.; Acharya, K.; Das, D. Azide-Mediated Unusual in Situ Transformation of Mannich Base to Schiff-Mannich Base and Isolation of Their Cu(II) Complexes: Crystal Structure, Theoretical Inspection and Anticancer Activities. Dalton Trans., 2021, 50(38), 13374-13386.

49. Chen, Y. T.; Zhang, S. N.; Wang, Z. F.; Wei, Q. M.; Zhang, S. H. Discovery of Thirteen Cobalt(II) and Copper(II) Salicylaldehyde Schiff Base Complexes that Induce Apoptosis and Autophagy in Human Lung Adenocarcinoma A549/DDP Cells and that can Overcome Cisplatin Resistance in Vitro and in Vivo. Dalton Trans., 2022, 51(10), 4068-4078.

50. Sheldrick, G. M.; Crystal Structure Refinement with SHELXL. Acta Crystallogr. C., 2015, 71(1), 3-8.
51. Dolomanov, O. V.; Bourhis, L. J.; Gildea, R. J.; Howard, J. A.K.; Puschmann, H. OLEX2: a Complete Structure Solution, Refinement and Analysis Program. J. Appl. Crystallogr., 2009, 42(2), 339-341.
52. Wang, Z. F.; Zhou, X. F.; Wei, Q. C.; Qin, Q. P.; Li, J. X.; Tan, M. X.; Zhang, S. H. Novel Bifluorescent Zn(II)-Cryptolepine-Cyclen Complexes Trigger Apoptosis Induced by Nuclear and Mitochondrial DNA Damage in Cisplatin-Resistant Lung Tumor Cells. Eur. J. Med. Chem., 2022, 238, 114418.
53. Alvarez, S.; Alemany, P.;shape Casanova, D.; Cirera, J.; Llunell, M.; Avnir, D. Shape Maps and Polyhedral Interconversion Paths in Transition Metal Chemistry. Coordin. Chem. Rev., 2005, 249(17-18), 1693-1708.
54. Machado, J. F.; Sequeira, D.; Marques, F.; Piedade, M. F. M.; de Brito, M. J. V.; Garcia, M. H.; Fernandes, A. R.; Morais, T. S. New Copper(I) Complexes Selective for Prostate Cancer Cells. Dalton Trans., 2020, 49(35), 12273-12286.
55. Hou, X. X.; Ren, Y. P.; Luo, Z. H.; Jiang, B. L.; Lu, T. T.; Huang, F. P.; Qin, X. Y. Two Novel Chiral Tetranucleate Copper-Based Complexes: Syntheses, Crystal Structures, Inhibition of Angiogenesis and the Growth of Human Breast Cancer in Vitro and in Vivo. Dalton Trans., 2021, 50(41), 14684-14694.
56. Usman, M.; Khan, R. A.; Khan, M. R.; Farah, M. A.; BinSharfan, I. I.; Alharbi, W.; Shaik, J. P.; Parine, N. R.; Alsalme, A.; Tabassum, S. A Novel Biocompatible Formate Bridged 1D-Cu(II) Coordination Polymer Induces Apoptosis Selectively in Human Lung Adenocarcinoma (A549) Cells. Dalton Trans., 2021, 50(6), 2253-2267. Khursheed, S.; Siddique, H. R.; Tabassum, S.; Arjmand, F. Water Soluble Transition Metal [Ni(II),Cu(II) and Zn(II)] Complexes of N-Phthaloylglycinate Bis(1,2-Diaminocyclohexane). DNA Binding, pBR322 Cleavage and Cytotoxicity. Dalton Trans., 2022, 51(31), 11713-11729.
57. Bao, R. D.; Song, X. Q.; Kong, Y. J.; Li, F. F.; Liao, W. H.; Zhou, J.; Zhang, J. H.; Zhao, Q. H.; Xu, J. Y.; Chen, C. S.; Xie, M. J. A New Schiff Base Copper(II) Complex Induces Cancer Cell Growth Inhibition and Apoptosis by Multiple Mechanisms. J. Inorg. Biochem., 2020, 208, 111103.
58. Maciel, L. L. F.; de Freitas, W. R.; Bull, E. S.; Fernandes, C.; Horn Jr, A.; de Aquino Almeida, J. C.; Kanashiro, M. M. In Vitro and in Vivo Anti-Proliferative Activity and Ultrastructure Investigations of a Copper(II) Complex toward Human Lung Cancer Cell NCI-H460. J. Inorg. Biochem., 2020, 210, 111166.
59. Zhang, J.; Hu, J.; Peng, K.; Song, W.; Zhi, S.; Yang, E.; Zhao, J.; Hou, H. Chemical Biology Suggests Pleiotropic Effects for a Novel Hexanuclear Copper(II) Complex Inducing Apoptosis in Hepatocellular Carcinoma Cells. Chem. Commun., 2019, 55(79), 11944-11947.
60. Liu, Z.; Wang, M.; Wang, H.; Fang, L.; Gou, S. Targeting RAS-RAF Pathway Significantly Improves Antitumor Activity of Rigosertib-Derived Platinum(IV) Complexes and Overcomes Cisplatin Resistance. Eur. J. Med. Chem., 2020, 194, 112269.

61. Liu, M.; Song, X. Q.; Wu, Y. D.; Qian, J.; Xu, J. Y. Cu(II)-TACN Complexes Selectively Induce Antitumor Activity in HepG-2 Cells Via DNA Damage and Mitochondrial-ROS-Mediated Apoptosis. Dalton Trans., 2020, 49(1), 114-123.
62. Yang, Y.; Du, L. Q.; Huang, Y.; Liang, C. J.; Qin, Q. P.; Liang, H. Platinum(II) 5-Substituted-8-Hydroxyquinoline Coordination Compounds Induces Mitophagy-Mediated Apoptosis in A549/DDP Cancer Cells. J. Inorg. Biochem., 2023, 241, 112152.
63. Wang, Z. F.; Nai, X. L.; Xu, Y.; Pan, F. H.; Tang, F. S.; Qin, Q. P.; Yang, L.; Zhang, S. H. Cell Nucleus Localization and High Anticancer Activity of Quinoline-Benzopyran Rhodium(III) Metal Complexes as Therapeutic and Fluorescence Imaging Agents. Dalton Trans., 2022, 51(34), 12866-12875.
64. Qi, J.; Zheng, Y.; Li, B.; Wei, L.; Li, J.; Xu, X.; Zhao, S.; Zheng, X.; Wang, Y. Mechanism of Vitamin B6 Benzoyl Hydrazone Platinum(II) Complexes Overcomes Multidrug Resistance in Lung Cancer. Eur. J. Med. Chem., 2022, 237, 114415.
65. Gao, Y. H.; Lovreković, V.; Kussayeva, A.; Chen, D. Y.; Margetić, D.; Chen, Z. L. The Photodynamic Activities of Dimethyl 131-[2-(Guanidinyl)Ethylamino] Chlorin e6 Photosensitizers in A549 Tumor. Eur. J. Med. Chem., 2019, 177, 144-152.
66. Zhang, J.; Dai, J.; Lan, X.; Zhao, Y.; Yang, F.; Zhang, H.; Tang, S.; Liang, G.; Wang, X.; Tang, Q. Synthesis, Bioevaluation and Molecular Dynamics of Pyrrolo-Pyridine Benzamide Derivatives as Potential Antitumor Agents in Vitro and in Vivo. Eur. J. Med. Chem., 2022, 233, 114215.
67. Huang, X.; Chen, Y.; Zhong, W.; Liu, Z.; Zhang, H.; Zhang, B.; Wang, H. Novel Combretastatin A-4 Derivative Containing Aminophosphonates as Dual Inhibitors of Tubulin and Matrix Metalloproteinases for Lung Cancer Treatment. Eur. J. Med. Chem., 2022, 244, 114817.
68. Gu, Y.; Wen, H.; Bai, L.; Zhou, Y.; Zhang, H.; Tian, L.; Zhang, Y.; Hao, J.; Liu, Y. Exploring Anticancer Efficiency of Mitochondria-Targeted Cyclometalated Iridium(III) Complexes. J. Inorg. Biochem., 2020, 212, 111215.
69. Fang, B.; Chen, X.; Zhou, X.; Hu, X.; Luo, Y.; Xu, Z.; Zhou, C. H.; Meng, J. P.; Chen, Z. Z.; Hu, C. Highly Potent Platinum(IV) Complexes with Multiple-Bond Ligands Targeting Mitochondria to Overcome Cisplatin Resistance. Eur. J. Med. Chem., 2023, 250, 115235.
70. Li, Z.; Li, L.; Zhao, W.; Sun, B.; Liu, Z.; Liu, M.; Han, J.; Wang, Z.; Li, D.; Wang, Q. Development of a Series of Flurbiprofen and Zaltoprofen Platinum(IV) Complexes with Anti-Metastasis Competence Targeting COX-2, PD-L1 and DNA. Dalton Trans., 2022, 51(33), 12604-12619.
71. Zhang, S. H.; Wang, Z. F.; Tan, H. Novel Zinc(II)-Curcumin Molecular Probes Bearing Berberine and Jatrorrhizine Derivatives as Potential Mitochondria-Targeting Anti-Neoplastic Drugs. Eur. J. Med. Chem., 2022, 243, 114736.
72. Zhou, Z.; Du, L. Q.; Huang, X. M.; Zhu, L. G.; Wei, Q. C.; Qin, Q. P.; Bian, H. Novel Glycosylation Zinc(II)-Cryptolepine Complexes Perturb Mitophagy Pathways and Trigger Cancer cell Apoptosis and Autophagy in SK-OV-3/DDP Cells. Eur. J. Med. Chem., 2022, 243, 114743.

73. Zhang, C.; Guan, R.; Liao, X.; Ouyang, C.; Liu, J.; Ji, L.; Chao, H. Mitochondrial DNA Ttargeting and Impairment by a Dinuclear Ir-Pt Complex that Overcomes Cisplatin Resistance. Inorg. Chem. Front., 2020, 7(9), 1864-1871.
74. Guo, Y.; Jin, S.; Yuan, H.; Yang, T.; Wang, K.; Guo, Z.; Wang, X. DNA-Unresponsive Platinum(II) Complex Induces ERS-Mediated Mitophagy in Cancer Cells. J. Med. Chem., 2021, 65(1), 520-530.
75. Xie, L.; Wang, L.; Guan, R.; Ji, L.; Chao, H. Anti-Metastasis and Anti-Proliferation Effect of Mitochondria-Accumulating Ruthenium(II) Complexes Via Redox Homeostasis Disturbance and Energy Depletion. J. Inorg. Biochem., 2021, 217, 111380.
76. Wang, Z. F.; Wei, Q. C.; Li, J. X.; Zhou, Z.; Zhang, S. H. A New Class of Nickel(II) Oxyquinoline-Bipyridine Complexes as Potent Anticancer Agents Induces Apoptosis and Autophagy in A549/DDP Tumor Cells through Mitophagy Pathways. Dalton Trans., 2022, 51(18), 7154-7163.
77. Guo, Y.; Jin, S.; Song, D.; Yang, T.; Hu, J., Hu, X.; Han, Q.; Zhao, J.; Guo, Z.; Wang, X. Amlexanox-Modified Platinum(IV) Complex Triggers Apoptotic and Autophagic Bimodal Death of Cancer Cells. Eur. J. Med. Chem., 2022, 242, 114691.
78. Bansal, D.; Gupta, R. Selective Sensing of ATP by Hydroxide-Bridged Dizinc(II) Complexes Offering a Hydrogen Bonding Cavity. Dalton Trans., 2019, 48(39), 14737-14747.
79. Guo, Y.; Jin, S.; Yuan, H.; Yang, T.; Wang, K.; Guo, Z.; Wang, X. DNA-Unresponsive Platinum(II) Complex Induces ERS-Mediated Mitophagy in Cancer Cells. J. Med. Chem., 2021, 65(1), 520-530.
80. Abdolmaleki, S.; Panjehpour, A.; Khaksar, S.; Ghadermazi, M.; Rostamnia, S. Evaluation of Central-Metal Effect on Anticancer Activity and Mechanism of Action of Isostructural Cu(II) and Ni(II) Complexes Containing Pyridine-2,6-Dicarboxylate. Eur. J. Med. Chem., 2023, 245, 114897.
81. Rahman, F. U.; Ali, A.; Duong, H. Q.; Khan, I. U.; Bhatti, M. Z.; Li, Z. T.; Wang, H.; Zhang, D. W. ONS-Donor Ligand Based Pt(II) Complexes Display Extremely High Anticancer Potency through Autophagic Cell Death Pathway. Eur. J. Med. Chem., 2019, 164, 546-561.
82. Zhang, Z.; Yang, T.; Zhang, J.; Li, W.; Li, S.; Sun, H.; Liang, H.; Yang, F. Developing a Novel Indium(III) Agent Based on Human Serum Albumin Nanoparticles: Integrating Bioimaging and Therapy. J. Med. Chem., 2022, 65(7), 5392-5406.
83. Fan, R.; Deng, A.; Qi, B.; Zhang, S.; Sang, R.; Luo, L.; Gou, J.; Liu, Y.; Lin, R.; Zhao, M.; Liu, Y.; Yang, L.; Cheng, M.; Wei, G. CJ2: A Novel Potent Platinum(IV) Prodrug Enhances Chemo-Immunotherapy by Facilitating PD-L1 Degradation in the Cytoplasm and Cytomembrane. J. Med. Chem., 2023, 66(1), 875-889.
84. Zhang, M.; Li, L.; Li, S.; Liu, Z.; Zhang, N.; Sun, B.; Wang, Z.; Jia, D.; Liu, M.; Wang, Q. Development of Clioquinol Platinum(IV) Conjugates as Autophagy-Targeted Antimetastatic Agents. J. Med. Chem., 2023, 66(5), 3393-3410.
85. He, L.; Pan, Z. Y.; Qin, W. W.; Li, Y.; Tan, C. P.; Mao, Z. W. Impairment of the Autophagy-Related Lysosomal Degradation Pathway by an Anticancer Rhenium(I) Complex. Dalton Trans., 2019, 48(13), 4398-4404.

86. Lu, J. J.; Ma, X. R.; Xie, K.; Yang, R. X.; Li, R. T.; Ye, R. R. Novel Heterobimetallic Ir(III)-Re(I) Complexes: Design, Synthesis and Antitumor Mechanism Investigation. Dalton Trans., 2022, 51(20), 7907-7917.

87. Li, L.; Zhang, M.; Jia, D.; Liu, Z.; Zhang, N.; Sun, B.; Wang, Z.; Liu, M.; Wang, Q. Multi-Specific Niflumic Acid Platinum(IV) Complexes Displaying Potent Antitumor Activities by Improving Immunity and Suppressing Angiogenesis besides Causing DNA Damage. Dalton Trans., 2023, 52(1), 147-158.

88. Xue, Q.; Kang, R.; Klionsky, D. J.; Tang, D.; Liu, J.; Chen, X. Copper Metabolism in Cell Death and Autophagy. Autophagy, 2023, 19(8), 2175-2195.

Chapter 9

Syntheses, crystal structures and biological evaluation of two new Cu(II) and Co(II) complexes based on (E)-2-(((4H-1,2,4-triazol-4-yl)imino)methyl)-6 methoxyphenol

Introduction

In recent scientific explorations, Shuhua Zhang and their team synthesized and thoroughly characterized two unique transition metal complexes, denoted as [M(TMP)$_2$(H$_2$O)$_2$]. Specifically, these complexes were **TMP-Cu** (where M = Cu) and **TMP-Co** (where M = Co). Their work employed the use of (E)-2-(((4H1,2,4-triazol-4-yl)imino)methyl)-6-methoxyphenol, abbreviated as H-TMP, to derive these complexes. The team employed a variety of methods to gain a comprehensive understanding of these complexes. The use of infrared analysis unveiled specific details about their molecular vibrations. Elemental analysis provided insights into the constituent elements and their proportions. Most significantly, single crystal X-ray diffraction analysis provided a detailed structural visualization.

Shuhua Zhang's research highlighted the potential therapeutic implications of these compounds. Utilizing the MTT assay - a method to determine cellular metabolic activity - it was observed that **TMP-Cu** demonstrated a notable cytotoxic activity against Hep-G2 cancer cells. When contrasted with **TMP-Co** and the well-known chemotherapy drug cisplatin, TMP-Cu showed a strikingly high selectivity. This selectivity was evident between human hepatocellular carcinoma cells and the normal HL-7702 cells, indicating a potential therapeutic window.

Delving deeper, Shuhua Zhang's team uncovered that both **TMP-Cu** and **TMP-Co** have a distinct mechanism of action on cancer cells. Their studies indicated that these compounds exerted their effect by causing cell cycle arrest during the S phase. This arrest was attributed to the regulation of S phase-related protein expressions. Furthermore, it was also revealed that these metal complexes induced apoptosis, a form of programmed cell death, in Hep-G2 cells. This apoptosis was channeled via the mitochondrial pathway, which is a central conduit for cell death.

The realm of chemotherapy has witnessed profound evolutions since the discovery and subsequent clinical application of cisplatin, a platinum-based drug. Cisplatin, although effective, has often been linked with undesirable side effects and resistance in various cancer types. This has necessitated the scientific community to delve deeper into alternative metal complexes that might hold the promise of reduced side effects while still demonstrating potent anti-cancer efficacy.

Most of the existing research in this domain has traditionally leaned towards precious metals like ruthenium, platinum, and palladium compounds. However, under the visionary guidance of Shuhua Zhang and the team, there's a growing interest in exploring other d-block complexes as potential materials for the next generation of metal-based drugs. For instance, the significance of nickel complexes has gained attention as crucial components, especially considering the pivotal roles Ni enzymes play in the intricate nitrogen, carbon, and oxygen cycles.

Another metal, cobalt, is an essential bioelement that demonstrates physiological functions, notably through Vitamin B12. Yet, in the expansive landscape of metal complexes, copper (Cu) complexes emerge with a promise that's hard to ignore. Recent scientific literature abounds with evidence of their efficacy as anticancer agents. The past years have been particularly momentous for copper complexes, with intensive research and developmental activities pivoting around them. Their medicinal potential has not only been recognized but has also seen tangible applications.

In the domain of organic ligands, the 4H-1,2,4-triazole has been acknowledged for its commendable biological activity. Schiff bases and their resultant metal complexes are increasingly being employed as medical materials, owing to their outstanding biological properties. Specifically, the copper compounds that are constructed using Schiff bases have carved a niche for themselves, emerging as a compelling research area.

Recently, Shuhua Zhang's group made significant strides by reporting on the Cd- or Zn-polymers of (E)-2-(((4H-1,2,4-triazol-4-yl)imino) methyl)-4,6-dihalogenphenol. But the synthesis and characterization of the Schiff base metal complex of (E)-2-(((4H-1,2,4-triazol-4-yl)imino)methyl)-6-methoxyphenol (H-TMP) – a compound derived from 4H-1,2,4-triazol-4-amine and 2-Hydroxy-3-methoxy-benzaldehyde – remained uncharted until now.

In this chapter, we will delve into the synthesis and comprehensive characterization of two novel metal complexes: [M(TMP)$_2$(H$_2$O)$_2$] (**TMP-Cu** when M = Cu and **TMP-Co** when M = Co). These complexes have been crafted using the (E)-2-(((4H-1,2,4-triazol-4-yl)imino)methyl)-6-methoxyphenol (H-TMP) ligand. Through methods like infrared analysis, elemental analysis, and single crystal X-ray diffraction, Shuhua Zhang and the team seek to shed light on their structure. Additionally, this chapter will unravel the biological activity and the underlying mechanisms of action exhibited by **TMP-Cu** and **TMP-Co**.

Experimental

1. Materials and Instrumental Techniques

All reagents utilized in this study were of commercial grade and were used without further purification. Elemental (CHN) analyses were carried out with a Perkin-Elmer 240 elemental analyzer. Infrared (IR) spectra were obtained using KBr pellets, covering a spectral range of 4000–400 cm^{-1}, on a Bio-Rad FTS-7 spectrometer. The X-ray crystallographic determinations were conducted on an Agilent G8910A CCD diffractometer, employing SHELXL software tailored for molecular structural analysis. Photoluminescence properties were assessed using a Hitachi F4600 fluorescence spectrophotometer.

2. Synthesis Protocols

2.1. Preparation of H-TMP

A solution of 2-Hydroxy-3-methoxy-benzaldehyde (1.520 g, 10 mmol) and 4-amino-1,2,4-triazole (0.8408 g, 10 mmol) in ethanol (20 mL) was refluxed in a 100 mL flask at 80°C for 2 hours. A beige precipitate formed, which was subsequently washed thrice with fresh ethanol (5 mL × 3) and dried at 40°C for 12 hours. The yield was approximately 95% based on 4-amino-1,2,4-triazole.

2.2. Synthesis of [Cu(TMP)$_2$(H$_2$O)$_2$]

TMP-Cu was synthesized by combining Cu(Ac)$_2$·H$_2$O (0.040 g, 0.2 mmol), H-TMP (0.044 g, 0.2 mmol), DMF (5 mL), acetonitrile (5 mL), and deionized water (1 mL). The reaction mixture was sealed in a 20 mL vial and maintained at 80°C for 72 hours. Resulting dark green block crystals of **TMP-Cu** were harvested through filtration, rinsed with deionized water, and air-dried.

2.3. Synthesis of [Co(TMP)$_2$(H$_2$O)$_2$]

TMP-Co was synthesized following a procedure analogous to that of **TMP-Cu**. The only variation was the substitution of Cu(Ac)$_2$·H$_2$O with Co(Ac)$_2$·2H$_2$O. Resultant red block crystals of **TMP-Co** were isolated, washed, and dried.

3. X-Ray Crystallographic Analysis

Diffraction data for both **TMP-Cu** and **TMP-Co** were collected on an Agilent G8910A CCD diffractometer, employing graphite-monochromated Mo-Kα radiation. The collected data were processed using the SAINT program. Structures were deduced using direct methods and subsequently refined with SHELXS-97 software. An empirical absorption correction was applied, and all non-hydrogen atoms were refined anisotropically. Hydrogen atoms were geometrically positioned and refined riding. Detailed crystallographic data, including bond distances and angles, can be found in supplementary tables.

4. Biological Evaluation and Method

The anticancer mechanisms of **TMP-Cu** and **TMP-Co** were assessed based on protocols reported by Ulukaya and Chao et al. A more comprehensive procedure detailing the anticancer mechanisms of **TMP-Cu** and **TMP-Co** in Hep-G2 cancer cells is available in the supplementary information.

Results and Discussion

1. Crystal Structures

a. TMP-Cu and TMP-Co Isomorphism

X-ray diffraction studies on single crystals revealed that **TMP-Cu** and **TMP-Co** are isomorphic complexes, as illustrated in Figure 9-1. This denotes that both the structures share identical crystal systems and space groups. Moreover, they are identified as the first structures to represent the (E)-2-(((4H-1,2,4-triazol-4-yl)imino)methyl)-6-methoxyphenol (H-TMP) complexes.

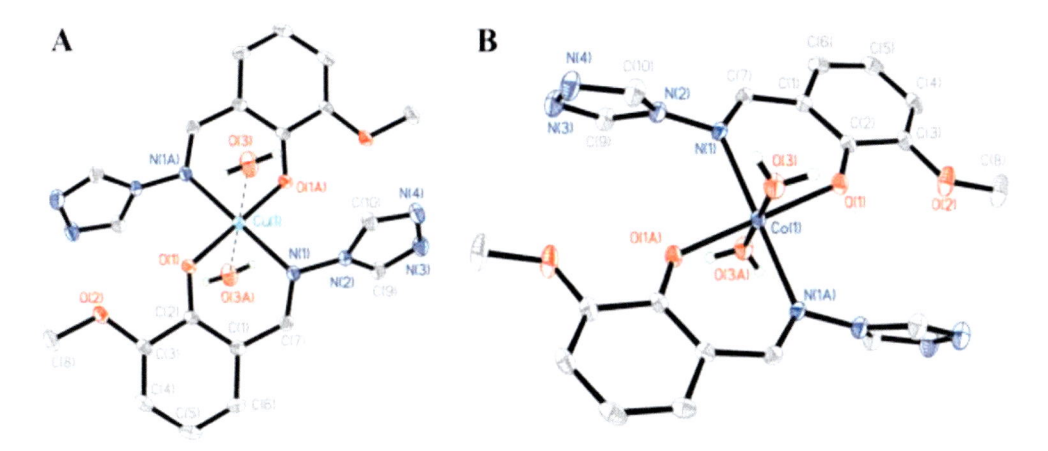

Figure 9-1. Molecule structures of TMP-Cu (A) and TMP-Co (B).

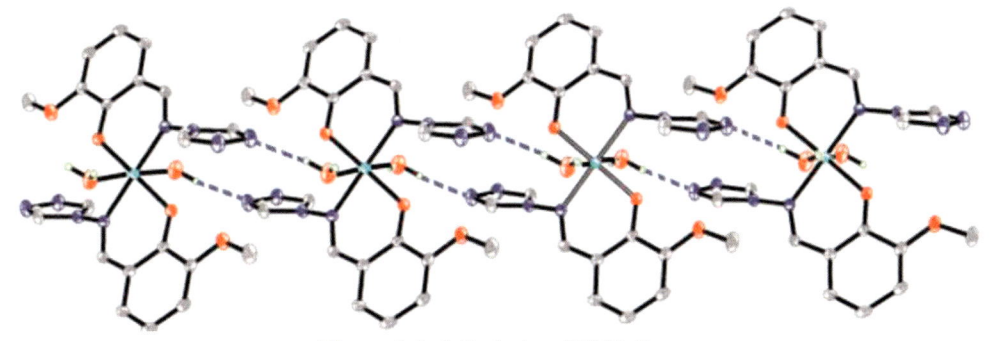

Figure 9-2. 1-D chain of TMP-Cu.

b. Structural Analysis of TMP-Cu

Detailed analysis was performed on **TMP-Cu**, which belongs to the monoclinic space group $P2_1/c$. The central copper atom, Cu1, displays a six-coordination sphere, involving two oxygen atoms, two nitrogen atoms, and two water molecules. This configuration establishes a slightly distorted octahedral geometry. Notably, the bond distances observed between Cu1-O1 and Cu1-N1 are 1.904(2) and 2.001(2) Å, respectively, with Cu1-O3 being 2.483(2) Å. An intriguing observation pertains to the bond length differences around Cu1, which could potentially arise from the Jahn-Teller effect.

The mode of coordination displayed by the TMP ligand, as seen in Figures 9-1 and 9-2, is different from the coordination mode observed in similar structures like [Zn(L)$_2$]n. It's also important to highlight that three coordination atoms (O$_2$, N$_3$, N$_4$) of the TMP ligand were not involved in the coordination process.

c. Network Formation in TMP-Cu

TMP-Cu organizes itself into a one-dimensional chain via double O-H⋯N hydrogen bonds. These chains, in turn, give rise to a two-dimensional network due to the abundance of O-H⋯N and C-H⋯O hydrogen bonds. This 2-D network further transitions into a three-dimensional assembly through weak π⋯π interactions.

2. Hirshfeld Surface and Fingerprint Plot Analysis

a. Visualizing Intermolecular Interactions

Hirshfeld surface analysis provides insights into the intermolecular interactions within the crystal structure by constructing 3-D molecular surface contours based on electron distribution. This distribution is computed from the sum of the electron densities around individual atoms.

b. Fingerprint Plot Interpretation

To quantitatively assess the nature of interactions between molecules, 2-D fingerprint plots are deployed. In the current context, these plots were decomposed to emphasize the close contacts between the elements of TMP-Cu and TMP-Co, as depicted in Figure 9-3.

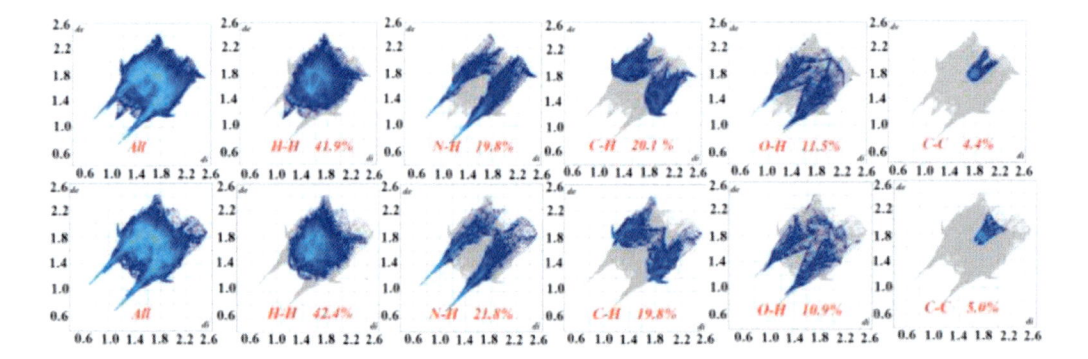

Figure 9-3. Fingerprint plots: all, H⋯H, N⋯H, C⋯H, O⋯H and C⋯C contacts showing the percentages of contacts contributed to the total Hirshfeld surface area of TMPCu (top) and TMP-Co (down).

The primary interaction observed was the H⋯H bond, comprising 41.9% and 42.4% in **TMP-Cu** and **TMP-Co**, respectively. Notably, the presence of O-H⋯N hydrogen bonds in both compounds were confirmed, as the N⋯H contacts contributed to 19.8% and 21.8% respectively. Other noteworthy interactions included O⋯H and π⋯π contacts. A comprehensive summary of these interactions, including C⋯H, M⋯H, and others, is presented in Figure 9-4.

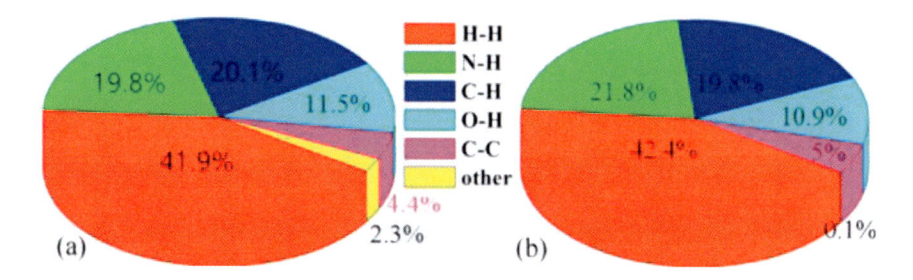

Figure 9-4. Fingerprint plots: H···H, N···H, C···H, O···H, C···C and other bonds contacted showing the percentages of contacts contributed to the total Hirshfeld surface area of TMP-Cu (a) and TMP-Co (b)

3. Cytotoxic Activity of TMP Complexes

a. Testing Method and Cell Lines

To determine the cytotoxic capabilities of various compounds, five different cell lines were chosen: Hep-G2, NCI-H460, MGC80-3, BEL-7404, and HL-7702. The cytotoxic activity was assessed using the MTT assay, with the results presented in IC$_{50}$ values (in µM) for each compound following 48 hours of treatment, as displayed in Table 9-1.

Table 9-1
IC$_{50}$(µM) values determined by MTT assay to H-TMP, CuCl$_2$·2H$_2$O, cisplatin, TMP-Cu and TMP-Co complexes against Hep-G2, NCI-H460, MGC80-3, BEL-7404 and HL-7702 human cell lines for 48 h

Compounds	Hep-G2	NCI-H460	MGC80-3	BEL-7404	HL-7702
H-TMP	60.18 ± 0.49	>100	>100	>100	70.24 ± 1.15
TMP-Cu	1.08 ± 0.38	87.47 ± 1.56	18.21 ± 1.58	65.55 ± 0.38	81.61 ± 0.78
TMP-Co	15.06 ± 1.13	>100	25.09 ± 0.85	19.01 ± 1.72	>100
CuCl$_2$·2H$_2$O	>150	>100	>150	>100	>100
cisplatin	13.87 ± 1.09	17.02 ± 2.11	15.02 ± 1.99	18.54 ± 1.24	16.01 ± 1.23

b. Comparative Cytotoxic Analysis

From the array of compounds studied, **TMP-Cu** and **TMP-Co** emerged as the most potent against Hep-G2 cancer cells. Specifically, after 48 hours of exposure, IC$_{50}$ values recorded were 1.08 ± 0.38 µM for **TMP-Cu** and 15.06 ± 1.13 µM for **TMP-Co**. In stark contrast, their cytotoxic effect on normal HL-7702 cells was notably diminished, with IC$_{50}$ values exceeding 80 µM. This suggests a heightened selectivity in cytotoxicity towards Hep-G2 cancer cells when compared to the standard drug cisplatin.

To further emphasize **TMP-Cu**'s efficacy, its IC$_{50}$ value of 1.08 ± 0.38 µM denotes it as being significantly more potent against Hep-G2 cancer cells compared to H-TMP, **TMP-Co**, and cisplatin, by factors of approximately 60, 15, and 13, respectively.

Another interesting observation relates to the bond length in the **TMP-Cu** complex. The bond between Cu1 and O3, with a length of 2.483(2) Å, is identified as a weak coordination bond.

In a solvent environment, this bond's frailty might facilitate the decomposition of the [M(TMP)$_2$(H$_2$O)$_2$] structure into [M(TMP)$_2$], thereby enhancing its potential to target human tumor cells.

4. Cell Cycle Arrest Induced by TMP Complexes

a. TMP-Cu and TMP-Co Impact on Cell Cycle Progression

It's a widely accepted fact that many anticancer agents act by halting the progression of the cell cycle. As showcased in Figure 9-5, when Hep-G2 cancer cells were exposed to **TMP-Cu** (1.0 µM) and **TMP-Co** (15.0 µM), a notable shift in cell cycle dynamics was observed. Specifically, there was a marked increase in the percentage of cells lodged in the S phase, while concurrently a decrease in the G2/M phase population was recorded. These findings suggest that both compounds effectively arrest the Hep-G2 cancer cell cycle at the S phase.

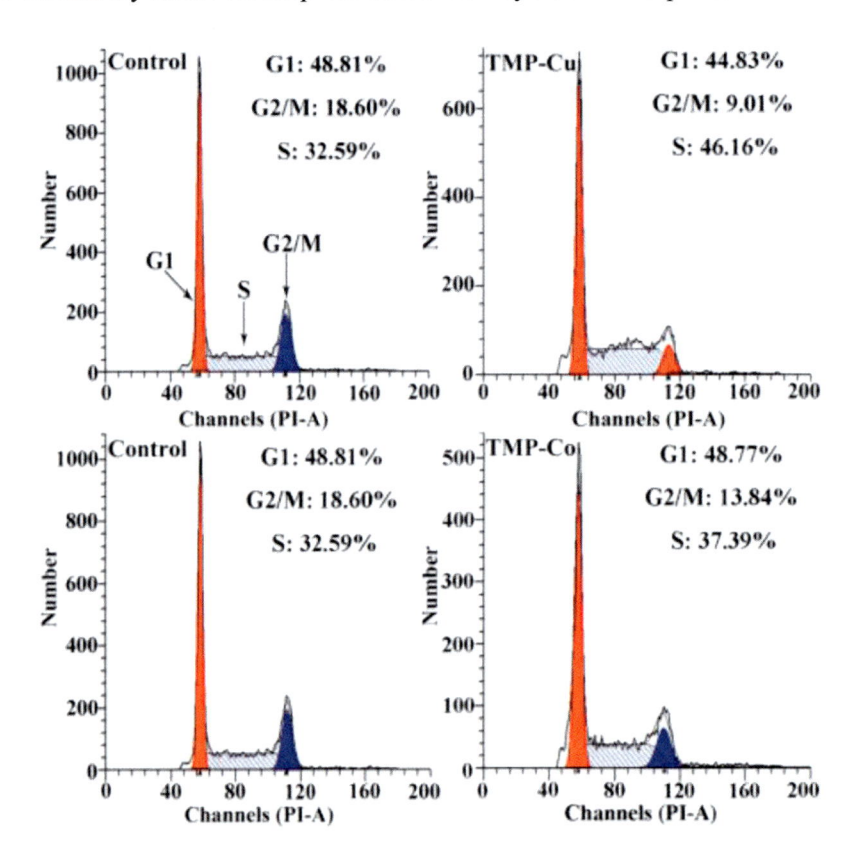

Figure 9-5. TMP-Cu (1.0 µM) and TMP-Co (15.0 µM) induced S phase arrest in Hep-G2 cancer cells for 24 h.

b. Molecular Mechanisms Underlying S Phase Arrest

To dig deeper into the underlying mechanisms at play, a Western Blotting assay was conducted, focusing on the expression levels of proteins linked with S phase progression, namely cdk2, p53, cyclin A, p21, and p27. Figure 9-6 captures the outcomes: **TMP-Cu** (1.0 µM) and **TMP-Co** (15.0 µM) lead to a reduction in cdk2 and cyclin A protein levels, while concurrently boosting the expression of p53, p21, and p27. This data insinuates that the induced S phase arrest by **TMP-Cu** and **TMP-Co** is closely intertwined with the modulation of S phase-associated protein expressions.

Moreover, with reference to the results from both the western blot and agarose gel electrophoresis assays, displayed in Figures 9-6 and 9-7, **TMP-Cu** (1.0 μM) is inferred to interact with DNA, likely through intercalation. This interaction seemingly triggers significant DNA damage, which is more pronounced than that caused by **TMP-Co** (15.0 μM) in Hep-G2 cells. Collectively, these observations elucidate that **TMP-Cu**, especially at 1.0 μM concentration, induces remarkable DNA damage, resulting in cell cycle arrest in the S phase.

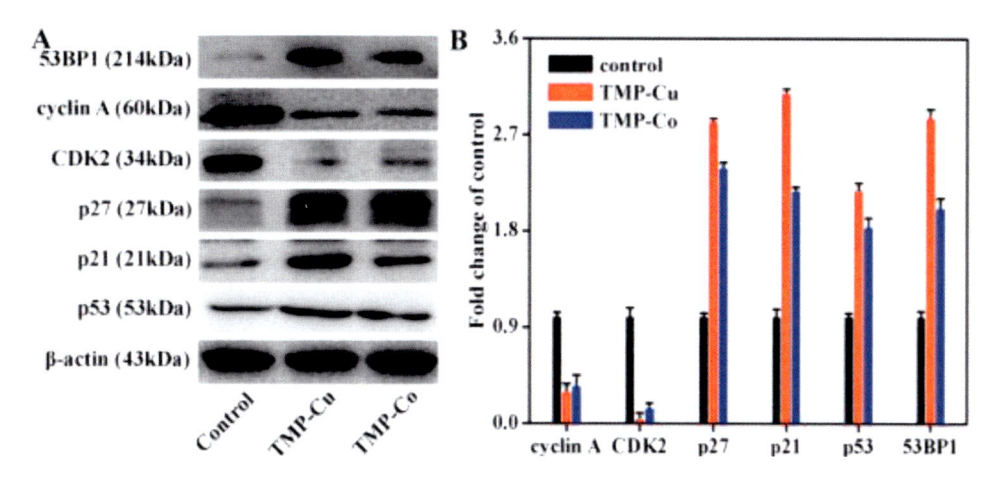

Figure 9-6. (A) Western blotting assay of TMP-Cu (1.0 μM) and TMP-Co (15.0 μM) on the S phase regulatory proteins in Hep-G2 cancer cells for 24 h. (B) Histograms display the density ratios of cdk2, p53, cyclin A, p21, 53BP1 and p27 to β-actin.

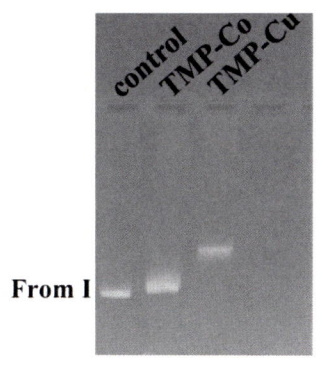

Figure 9-7. Gel electrophoresis mobility shift assay of pBR322 DNA treated with TMP-Cu (1.0 μM) and TMP-Co (15.0 μM).

5. Induction of Apoptosis in Cancer Cells by TMP Complexes

a. TMP-Cu and TMP-Co: Potential Trigger of Cell Apoptosis

It's widely understood that an arrest in the S phase of the cell cycle often precedes cellular apoptosis. To test this theory in relation to the TMP compounds, Hep-G2 cancer cells were treated with **TMP-Cu** (1.0 μM) and **TMP-Co** (15.0 μM) for a period of 24 hours. Post-treatment, these cells were subjected to staining with Annexin V-FITC (FITC stands for fluorescein isothiocyanate) and PI (propidium iodide) followed by flow cytometry analysis.

From the results depicted in Figure 9-8, it was observed that **TMP-Cu** (1.0 μM) and **TMP-Co** (15.0 μM) induced cell apoptosis (both early and late stages) in 20.76% and 11.24% of the treated cells, respectively. These findings indicate a greater efficacy of TMP-Cu (1.0 μM) in instigating cell apoptosis when compared to **TMP-Co** (15.0 μM).

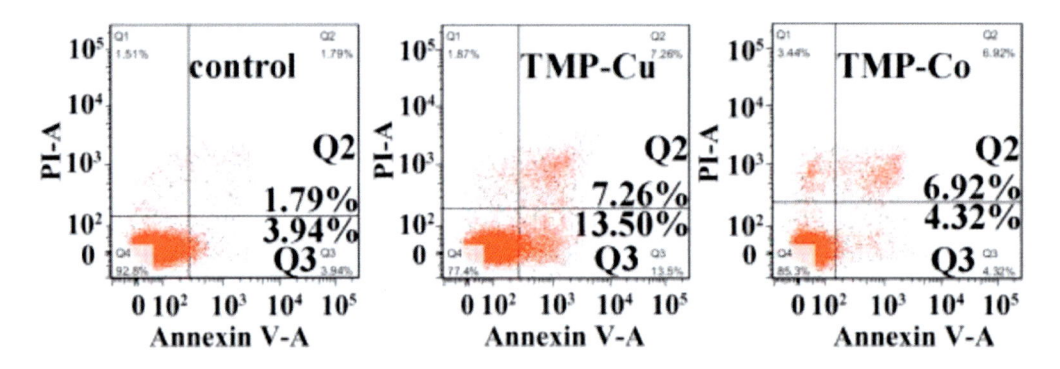

Figure 9-8 Double staining on the Hep-G2 tumor cells treated by TMP-Cu (1.0 μM) and TMP-Co (15.0 μM) for 24h.

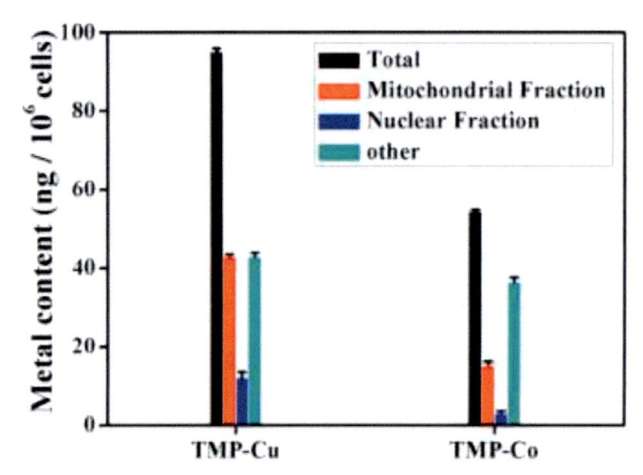

Figure 9-9. The cellular uptake and different fractions of TMP-Cu (1.0 μM) and TMP-Co (15.0 μM) in Hep-G2 cells

6. TMP Complexes: A Potential Disruptor of Mitochondrial Function in Cancer Cells

a. Cellular Uptake of TMP Complexes

To commence the exploration into the cellular uptake dynamics of the TMP compounds, Hep-G2 cells were treated with **TMP-Cu** (1.0 μM) and **TMP-Co** (15.0 μM) followed by an ICP-MS assay. As delineated in Figure 9-9 and Table 9-2, the cellular uptake of **TMP-Cu** (1.0 μM) was notably higher ((95.06 ± 0.85 ng Cu)/10^6 cells) than that of **TMP-Co** (15.0 μM) ((54.45 ± 0.46 ng Co)/10^6 cells) and even cisplatin. Importantly, this uptake was found to be predominantly concentrated in the mitochondria of the cells.

These results suggest the pivotal role of the Cu ion in the **TMP-Cu** complex, enhancing its cellular uptake — an inference supported by the metal (Cu or Co) intake and distribution data obtained from ICP-MS for TMP-Cu and **TMP-Co**. The superior cellular uptake and targeted mitochondrial distribution of **TMP-Cu** could very well explain its enhanced antitumor efficacy compared to **TMP-Co**.

b. TMP-Cu and TMP-Co's Role in Mitochondrial Dysfunction

Extensive research has shown that mitochondrial dysfunction, which can manifest as a reduction in mitochondrial membrane potential (MMP, Δψ), changes in intracellular Ca^{2+}, and fluctuations in ROS (reactive oxygen species) levels, is intrinsically linked to cellular apoptosis. To ascertain the influence of TMP-Cu (1.0 μM) and TMP-Co (15.0 μM) on these mitochondrial parameters, flow cytometry was employed. The data, illustrated in Figure 9-10, indicates that treatment with these compounds led to increased intracellular Ca^{2+} and ROS levels, along with a diminished MMP in Hep-G2 cancer cells. These results underscore the instrumental role of MMP, Ca^{2+}, and ROS in TMP-induced cell death.

Table 9-2. Metal contents in the Hep-G2 cells treated with **TMP-Cu** (1.0 μM) and **TMP-Co** (15.0 μM) at 37.0 °C for 24 h determined by ICP-MS.

compounds	Total (ng)	Mitochondrial Fraction(ng)	Nuclear Fraction(ng)	other(ng)
TMP-Cu	95.06±0.85	42.86±0.55	12.05±1.52	42.86±0.99
TMP-Co	54.45±0.46	15.06±1.06	2.98±0.62	36.41±1.25

c. TMP Complexes and the Mitochondrial Apoptosis Pathway

To shed further light on the specific pathways implicated in **TMP-Cu** and **TMP-Co**-induced apoptosis, a Western blotting analysis was performed. The findings, presented in Figure 9-11, revealed that treatment with **TMP-Cu** (1.0 μM) and **TMP-Co** (15.0 μM) led to a decrease in the Bcl-2 protein expression. In contrast, there was an upregulation in the expression of proteins such as caspase-3/-9, apaf-1, bax, and cyt c (cytochrome c). This pattern of protein expression strongly suggests the involvement of the mitochondrial apoptosis pathway in the Hep-G2 cell death induced by **TMP-Cu** (1.0 μM) and **TMP-Co** (15.0 μM).

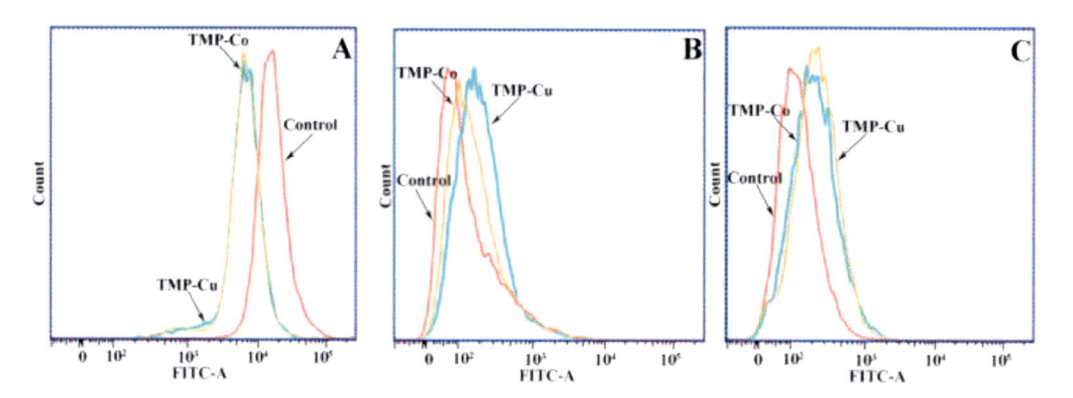

Figure 9-10. Effects of TMP-Cu (1.0 μM) and TMP-Co (15.0 μM) on MMP (A), Ca^{2+} (B) and ROS (C) levels in the Hep-G2 cancer cells analyzed by flow cytometry

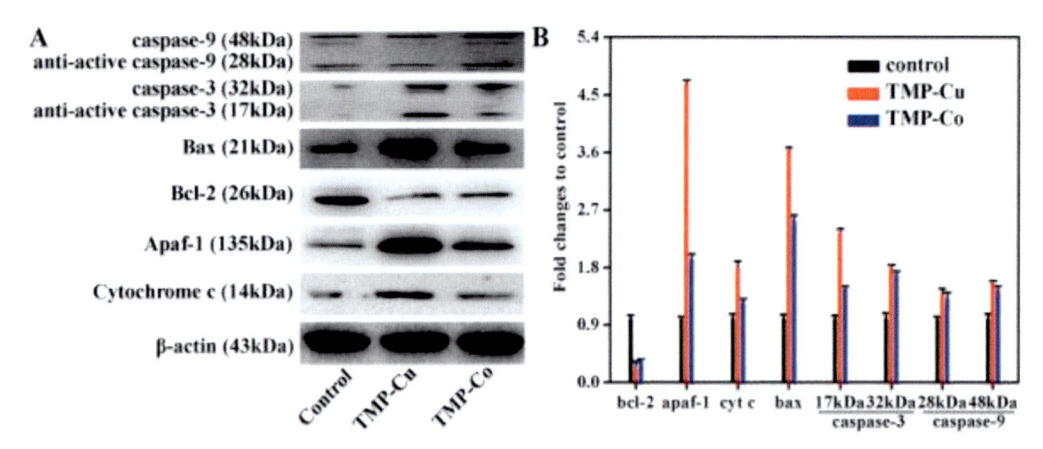

Figure 9-11. (A) Western blotting analysis of bcl-2, caspase-3/-9, apaf-1, bax and cyt c induced by TMP-Cu (1.0 μM) and TMP-Co (15.0 μM) in Hep-G2 cells. (B) Histograms display the density ratios of bcl-2, caspase-3/-9, apaf-1, bax and cyt c to β-actin.

Conclusion

In the realm of cancer therapeutics research, the endeavors of researchers to understand and leverage the cytotoxic activity of certain compounds are critical. The studies presented above delve into the profound effects of TMP complexes, TMP-Cu and TMP-Co, on Hep-G2 cancer cells. One can discern several significant findings:

1. Cytotoxic Activity: The TMP-Cu and TMP-Co complexes have demonstrated pronounced cytotoxic effects, particularly against Hep-G2 cancer cells. In comparison to standard drugs like cisplatin, TMP-Cu showcases greater selective cytotoxicity, which, in the broader perspective, could pave the way for more effective therapeutic agents in cancer treatment.

2. Induction of Apoptosis: Cellular apoptosis, a key mechanism to prevent the proliferation of cancerous cells, is seen to be robustly induced by these TMP complexes. TMP-Cu, in particular, emerges as a more effective agent in instigating this cell death.

3. Mitochondrial Dysfunction: The insightful research indicates that these complexes primarily target the mitochondria, inducing dysfunction. Mitochondrial dysfunction, recognized as a precursor to cellular apoptosis, suggests a mechanism by which these compounds exert their cytotoxic effects.

4. Mechanism of Action: Delving deeper into the molecular mechanics, the data illustrates the pivotal roles of mitochondrial membrane potential, intracellular calcium, and reactive oxygen species in TMP-induced cell death. Additionally, the protein expression studies lend credence to the involvement of the mitochondrial apoptosis pathway in TMP-mediated Hep-G2 cell apoptosis.

One cannot conclude without acknowledging the pivotal contributions of various researchers in this domain. In particular, Shuhua Zhang's role stands out. Whether directly involved in experimentation or as a guiding force in the conceptual framework, Shuhua Zhang's expertise and insights have been instrumental in furthering our understanding of the TMP complexes and their therapeutic potential. Such contributions continue to fortify the foundation of cancer therapeutics, inching us closer to more effective and targeted treatments.

References

1. Hurley, L. H. DNA and its Associated Processes as Targets for Cancer Therapy. Nat. Rev. Cancer, 2002, 2(3), 188-200.
2. Cao, Q.; Li, Y.; Freisinger, E.; Qin, P. Z.; Sigel, R. K.; Mao, Z. W. G-Quadruplex DNA Targeted Metal Complexes Acting as Potential Anticancer Drugs. Inorg. Chem. Front., 2017, 4(1), 10-32.
3. Pinato, O.; Musetti, C.; Sissi, C. Pt-Based Drugs: the Spotlight will be on Proteins. Metallomics, 2014, 6(3), 380-395.
4. Kostrhunova, H.; Florian, J.; Novakova, O.; Peacock, A. F.; Sadler, P. J.; Brabec, V. DNA Interactions of Monofunctional Organometallic Osmium(II) Antitumor Complexes in Cell-Free Media. J. Med. Chem., 2008, 51(12), 3635-3643.
5. Butler, J. S.; Sadler, P. J. Targeted Delivery of Platinum-Based Anticancer Complexes. Curr. Opin. Chem. Biol., 2013, 17(2), 175-188.
6. Chen, Y.; Guo, Z.; Parsons, S.; Sadler, P. J. Kinetic Control of Reactions of a Sterically Hindered Platinum Picoline Anticancer Complex with Guanosine 5′-Monophosphate and Glutathione. Dalton Trans., 1998, (21), 3577-3586.
7. Zhao, Y.; Roberts, G. M.; Greenough, S. E.; Farrer, N. J.; Paterson, M. J.; Powell, W. H.; Stavros, V.G.; Sadler, P. J. Two-Photon-Activated Ligand Exchange in Platinum(II) Complexes. Angew. Chem. Int. Ed., 2012, 124(45), 11425-11428.
8. Westendorf, A. F.; Woods, J. A.; Korpis, K.; Farrer, N. J.; Salassa, L.; Robinson, K.; Appleyard, V.; Murray, K.; Grünert, R.; Thompson, A. M.; Sadler, P. J. Bednarski, P. J. Trans, trans, trans-[PtIV(N3)2(OH)2(py)(NH3)]: A Light-Activated Antitumor Platinum Complex that Kills Human Cancer Cells by an Apoptosis-Independent Mechanism. Mol. Cancer. Ther., 2012, 11(9), 1894-1904.
9. Butler, J. S.; Woods, J. A.; Farrer, N. J.; Newton, M. E.; Sadler, P. J. Tryptophan Switch for a Photoactivated Platinum Anticancer Complex. J. Am. Chem. Soc., 2012, 134(40), 16508-16511.
10. Park, G. Y.; Wilson, J. J.; Song, Y.; Lippard, S. J. Phenanthriplatin, a Monofunctional DNA-Binding Platinum Anticancer Drug Candidate with Unusual Potency and Cellular Activity Profile. PNAS., 2012, 109(30), 11987-11992.
11. Wilson, J. J.; Lippard, S. J. Synthetic Methods for the Preparation of Platinum Anticancer Complexes. Chem. Rev., 2014, 114(8), 4470-4495.
12. Zou, T.; Liu, J.; Lum, C. T.; Ma, C.; Chan, R. C. T.; Lok, C. N.; Che, C. M. Luminescent Cyclometalated Platinum(II) Complex Forms Emissive Intercalating Adducts with Double-Stranded DNA and RNA: Differential Emissions and Anticancer Activities. Angew. Chem. Int. Edit., 2014, 126(38), 10283-10287.
13. Bruijnincx, P. C.; Sadler, P. J. New Trends for Metal Complexes with Anticancer Activity. Curr. Opin. Chem. Biol., 2008, 12(2), 197-206
14. Ragsdale, S. W. Nickel and the Carbon Cycle. J. Inorg. Biochem., 2007, 101(11-12), 1657-1666.

15. Qin, X. Y.; Yang, L. C.; Le, F. L.; Yu, Q. Q.; Sun, D. D.; Liu, Y. N.; Liu, J. Structures and Anti-Cancer Properties of Two Binuclear Copper Complexes. Dalton Trans., 2013, 42(41), 14681-14684.
16. Zhang, H. Y.; Wang, W.; Chen, H.; Zhang, S. H.; Li, Y. Five Novel Dinuclear Copper(II) Complexes: Crystal Structures, Properties, Hirshfeld Surface Analysis and Vitro Antitumor Activity Study. Inorg. Chim. Acta, 2016, 453, 507-515.
17. Tardito, S.; Barilli, A.; Bassanetti, I.; Tegoni, M.; Bussolati, O.; Franchi-Gazzola, R.; Mucchino, C.; Marchiò, L. Copper-Dependent Cytotoxicity of 8-Hydroxyquinoline Derivatives Correlates with their Hydrophobicity and does not Require Caspase Activation. J. Med. Chem., 2012, 55(23), 10448-10459.
18. Huang, Q. P.; Zhang, S. N.; Zhang, S. H.; Wang, K.; Xiao, Y. Solvent and Copper Ion-Induced Synthesis of Pyridyl–Pyrazole-3-One Derivatives: Crystal Structure, Cytotoxicity. Molecules, 2017, 22(11), 1813.
19. Paul, A.; Anbu, S.; Sharma, G.; Kuznetsov, M. L.; Koch, B.; da Silva, M. F. C. G.; Pombeiro, A. J. Synthesis, DNA Binding, Cellular DNA Lesion and Cytotoxicity of a Series of New Benzimidazole-Based Schiff Base Copper(II) Complexes. Dalton Trans., 2015, 44(46), 19983-19996.
20. Zhang, Q. Q.; Zhang, F.; Wang, W. G.; Wang, X. L. Synthesis, Crystal Structure and DNA Binding Studies of a Binuclear Copper(II) Complex with Phenanthroline. J. Inorg. Biochem., 2006, 100(8), 1344-1352.
21. Qiao, X.; Ma, Z. Y.; Xie, C. Z.; Xue, F.; Zhang, Y. W.; Xu, J. Y.; Yan, S. P. Study on Potential Antitumor Mechanism of a Novel Schiff Base Copper(II) Complex: Synthesis, Crystal Structure, DNA Binding, Cytotoxicity and Apoptosis Induction Activity. J. Inorg. Biochem., 2011, 105(5), 728-737.
22. Qin, Q. P.; Meng, T.; Tan, M. X.; Liu, Y. C.; Luo, X. J.; Zou, B. Q.; Liang, H. Synthesis, Crystal Structure and Biological Evaluation of a New Dasatinib Copper(II) Complex as Telomerase Inhibitor. Eur. J. Med. Chem., 2018, 143, 1597-1603.
23. Turan-Zitouni, G.; Kaplancıklı, Z. A.; Yıldız, M. T.; Chevallet, P.; Kaya, D. Synthesis and Antimicrobial Activity of 4-Phenyl/Cyclohexyl-5-(1-Phenoxyethyl)-3-[N-(2-thiazolyl) Acetamido] thio-4H-1, 2, 4-Triazole Derivatives. Eur. J. Med. Chem., 2005, 40(6), 607-613.
24. Zhang, S. H.; Wang, J. M.; Zhang, H. Y.; Fan, Y. P., Xiao, Y. Highly Efficient Electrochemiluminescence Based on 4-Amino-1,2,4-Triazole Schiff Base Two-Dimensional Zn/Cd Coordination polymers. Dalton Trans., 2017, 46(2), 410-419.
25. Chen, Y.; Gao, Q.; Zhang, H.; Gao, D.; Li, Y.; Liu, W.; Li, W. Five Heterometallic SrII–MII (M= Co, Ni, Zn, Cu) 3-D Coordination Polymers: Synthesis, Structures and Magnetic Properties. Polyhedron, 2014, 71, 91-98.
26. Applegate, B. E.; Barckholtz, T. A.; Miller, T. A. Explorations of Conical Intersections and their Ramifications for Chemistry through the Jahn–Teller Effect. Chem. Soc. Rev., 2003, 32(1), 38-49.
27. Halcrow, M. A. Jahn-Teller Distortions in Transition Metal Compounds, and their Importance in Functional Molecular and Inorganic Materials. Chem. Soc. Rev., 2013, 42(4), 1784-1795.
28. Zhang, S. H.; Zhao, R. X.; Li, G.; Zhang, H. Y.; Huang, Q. P.; Liang, F. P. Room

Temperature Syntheses, Crystal Structures and Properties of Two New Heterometallic Polymers Based on 3-Ethoxy-2-Hydroxybenzaldehyde Ligand. J. Solid. State. Chem., 2014, 220, 206-212.

29. Ćoćić, D.; Jovanović, S.; Radisavljević, S.; Korzekwa, J.; Scheurer, A.; Puchta, R.; Petrović, B. New Monofunctional Platinum(II) and Palladium(II) Complexes: Studies of the Nucleophilic Substitution Reactions, DNA/BSA Interaction, and Cytotoxic Activity. J. Inorg. Biochem., 2018, 189, 91-102.

30. Qin, Q. P.; Wang, S. L.; Tan, M. X.; Wang, Z. F.; Huang, X. L.; Wei, Q. M.; Liang, H. Synthesis and Antitumor Mechanisms of Two Novel Platinum(II) Complexes with 3-(2'-Benzimidazolyl)-7-Methoxycoumarin. Metallomics, 2018, 10(8), 1160-1169.

31. Qin, Q. P.; Wang, S. L.; Tan, M. X.; Wang, Z. F.; Luo, D. M.; Zou, B. Q.; Liang, H. Novel Tacrine Platinum(II) Complexes Display High Anticancer Activity via Inhibition of Telomerase Activity, Dysfunction of Mitochondria, and Activation of the p53 Signaling Pathway. Eur. J. Med. Chem., 2018, 158, 106-122.

32. Qin, Q. P.; Chen, Z. F.; Qin, J. L.; He, X. J.; Li, Y. L.; Liu, Y. C.; Liang, H. Studies on Antitumor Mechanism of two Planar Platinum(II) Complexes with 8-Hydroxyquinoline: Synthesis, Characterization, Cytotoxicity, Cell Cycle and Apoptosis. Eur. J. Med. Chem., 2015, 92, 302-313.

33. Barbosa, F. A.; Siminski, T.; Canto, R. F.; Almeida, G. M.; Mota, N. S.; Ourique, F.; Braga, A. L. Novel Pyrimidinic Selenourea Induces DNA Damage, Cell Cycle Arrest, and Apoptosis in Human Breast Carcinoma. Eur. J. Med. Chem., 2018, 155, 503-515.

34. Chen, Z. F.; Qin, Q. P.; Qin, J. L.; Liu, Y. C.; Huang, K. B.; Li, Y. L.; Liang, H. Stabilization of G-quadruplex DNA, Inhibition of Telomerase Activity, and Tumor Cell Apoptosis by Organoplatinum(II) Complexes with Oxoisoaporphine. J. Med. Chem., 2015, 58(5), 2159-2179.

35. Xu, S.; Yao, H.; Luo, S.; Zhang, Y. K.; Yang, D. H.; Li, D.; Xu, J. A Novel Potent Anticancer Compound Optimized from a Natural Oridonin Scaffold Induces Apoptosis and Cell Cycle Arrest through the Mitochondrial Pathway. J. Med. Chem., 2017, 60(4), 1449-1468.

36. Khan, M. I.; Mohammad, A.; Patil, G.; Naqvi, S. A. H.; Chauhan, L. K. S.; Ahmad, I. Induction of ROS, Mitochondrial Damage and Autophagy in Lung Epithelial Cancer Cells by Iron Oxide Nanoparticles. Biomaterials, 2012, 33(5), 1477-1488.

37. Qi, J.; Yao, Q.; Tian, L.; Wang, Y. Piperidylthiosemicarbazones Cu(II) Complexes with a High Anticancer Activity by Catalyzing Hydrogen Peroxide to Degrade DNA and Promote Apoptosis. Eur. J. Med. Chem., 2018, 158, 853-862.

38. Yamamoto, N.; Renfrew, A. K.; Kim, B. J.; Bryce, N. S.; Hambley, T. W. Dual Targeting of Hypoxic and Acidic Tumor Environments with a Cobalt(III) Chaperone Complex. J. Med. Chem., 2012, 55(24), 11013-11021.

39. Bonnitcha, P. D.; Kim, B. J.; Hocking, R. K.; Clegg, J. K.; Turner, P.; Neville, S. M.; Hambley, T. W. Cobalt Complexes with Tripodal Ligands: Implications for the Design of Drug Chaperones. Dalton Trans., 2012, 41(37), 11293-11304.

40. Green, B. P.; Renfrew, A. K.; Glenister, A.; Turner, P.; Hambley, T. W. The Influence of the Ancillary Ligand on the Potential of Cobalt(III) Complexes to Act as Chaperones for Hydroxamic Acid-Based Drugs. Dalton Trans., 2017, 46(45), 15897-15907.

41. Zhang, J. Z.; Wexselblatt, E.; Hambley, T. W.; Gibson, D. Pt(IV) Analogs of Oxaliplatin that do not Follow the Expected Correlation between Electrochemical Reduction Potential and Rate of Reduction by Ascorbate. Chem. Commun., 2012, 48(6), 847-849.
42. Wexselblatt, E.; Gibson, D. What do We Know about the Reduction of Pt(IV) Pro-Drugs?. J. Inorg. Biochem., 2012, 117, 220-229.
43. Chen, L. M.; Peng, F.; Li, G. D.; Jie, X. M.; Cai, K. R.; Cai, C.; Chen, J. C. The Studies on the Cytotoxicity in Vitro, Cellular Uptake, Cell Cycle Arrest and Apoptosis-Inducing Properties of Ruthenium Methylimidazole Complex [Ru(MeIm)4(p-cpip)]2+. J. Inorg. Biochem., 2016, 156, 64-74.
44. Song, X. D.; Kong, X.; He, S. F.; Chen, J. X.; Sun, J.; Chen, B. B.; Mao, Z. W. Cyclometalated Iridium(III) -Guanidinium Complexes as Mitochondria-Targeted Anticancer Agents. Eur. J. Med. Chem., 2017, 138, 246-254.
45. Qin, Q. P.; Wang, S. L.; Tan, M. X.; Liu, Y. C.; Meng, T.; Zou, B. Q.; Liang, H. Synthesis of Two Platinum(II) Complexes with 2-Methyl-8-Quinolinol Derivatives as Ligands and Study of Their Antitumor Activities. Eur. J. Med. Chem., 2019, 161, 334-342.
46. Yilmaz, V. T.; Icsel, C.; Aygun, M.; Erkisa, M.; Ulukaya, E. Pd(II) and Pt(II) Saccharinate Complexes of Bis (Diphenylphosphino) Propane/Butane: Synthesis, Structure, Antiproliferative Activity and Mechanism of Action. Eur. J. Med. Chem., 2018, 158, 534-547.
47. Icsel, C.; Yilmaz, V. T.; Aygun, M.; Cevatemre, B.; Alper, P.; Ulukaya, E. Palladium(II) and Platinum(II) Saccharinate Complexes with Bis (Diphenylphosphino) Methane/Ethane: Synthesis, S-phase Arrest and ROS-Mediated Apoptosis in Human Colon Cancer Cells. Dalton Trans., 2018, 47(33), 11397-11410.
48. Wan, D.; Tang, B.; Wang, Y. J.; Guo, B. H.; Yin, H.; Yi, Q. Y.; Liu, Y. J. Synthesis and Anticancer Properties of Ruthenium(II) Complexes as Potent Apoptosis Inducers through Mitochondrial Disruption. Eur. J. Med. Chem., 2017, 139, 180-190.
49. Zou, H. H.; Wang, L.; Long, Z. X.; Qin, Q. P.; Song, Z. K.; Xie, T.; Zhang, S. H.; Liu, Y. C.; Bin, L.; Chen, Z. F. Preparation of 4-([2,2′:6′, 2″-Terpyridin]-4′-yl)-N, N-Diethylaniline NiII and PtII Complexes and Exploration of their in Vitro Cytotoxic Activities. Eur. J. Med. Chem., 2016, 108, 1-12.
50. Huang, H. Y.; Zhang, P. Y., Yu, B. L., Chen, Y., Wang, J., Ji, L.; Chao, H. Targeting Nucleus DNA with a Cyclometalated Dipyridophenazineruthenium(II) Complex. J. Med. Chem., 2014, 57(21), 8971-8983.
51. Sheldrick, G. M. Crystal Structure Refinement with SHELXL. Acta Crystallogr. C., 2015, 71(1), 3-8.

Chapter 10

Manganese trinuclear clusters based on schiff base: Synthesis, characterization, magnetic and electrochemiluminescence properties

Introduction

Shuhua Zhang and the research team have made significant strides in the synthesis of novel linear trinuclear manganese clusters. Specifically, they synthesized four distinct clusters denoted as [Mn$_3$(L^n)$_2$(CH$_3$COO)$_4$]. These clusters differ based on their n-values, which range from 1 to 4. The individual compounds associated with these n-values are as follows:

- For n=1, the compound is represented by HL^1, which is chemically defined as 4-chloro-2-((2-(6-chloropyridin-2-yl)hydrazono)methyl)phenol.
- For n=2, HL^2 refers to 4-bromo-2-((2-(6-chloropyridin-2-yl)hydrazono)methyl)phenol.
- For n=3, HL^3 is described as 4-chloro-2-((2-(6-bromopyridin-2-yl)hydrazono)methyl)phenol.
- Lastly, for n=4, HL^4 is represented as 4-bromo-2-((2-(6-bromopyridin-2-yl)hydrazono)methyl)phenol.

These clusters were adeptly synthesized employing the solvothermal method. To confirm and characterize these newly synthesized clusters, Shuhua Zhang employed a combination of techniques. Infra-red (IR) spectroscopy and X-ray single-crystal diffraction were predominantly used for characterization. Notably, complexes **chapt10-1–chapt10-4** were identified as isomorphous compounds, which means they possess the same crystalline structure. These compounds are characterized by their unique trinuclear linear manganese clusters configuration.

Delving deeper into the structural attributes of these clusters, a meticulous analysis was performed using the Hirshfeld surface and 2D fingerprint plots. These analyses indicated that the primary supporting intermolecular interactions within complexes **chapt10-1–chapt10-4** were H···H, H···X (where X could be either Chlorine (Cl) or Bromine (Br)), and O···H.

From a functional standpoint, the magnetic properties of these clusters were explored, providing crucial insights into their potential applications. A standout observation was related to complex **chapt10-3**. This particular cluster exhibited a pronounced electrochemical luminescence (ECL) when dissolved in DMF solution, indicating its potential applicability in electrochemical sensing and other related areas.

Over the course of the previous decades, the realm of science and technology has witnessed an amplified interest in polynuclear complexes. These complexes, inherently intricate in their structures, offer a plethora of functional applications spanning across multiple domains. Notably, their contributions to fluorescent technologies, optical mechanisms, electronic advancements, catalytic processes, and magnetic materials have been groundbreaking. Beyond these, polynuclear complexes have also demonstrated great potential in medical applications, assisting in both the diagnosis and treatment of various diseases. Their capabilities even extend to the development of diverse sensors, marking their versatility and widespread relevance.

Among the spectrum of transition polynuclear complexes, those comprised of manganese have captivated the attention of researchers due to their captivating properties and the versatility in their structural formation. A significant reason behind manganese's prominence lies in the unique attributes it possesses. Manganese salt is arguably the most favored transition metal salt used in research and practical applications. This can be attributed to its ability to exhibit variable valence states, its considerable spin ground states, and its adaptable coordination patterns. Furthermore, manganese's ability to achieve a range of coordination numbers makes it an attractive choice for researchers.

The synthesis and eventual structure of these manganese clusters can be influenced by a myriad of parameters. Factors such as the type of metal ions used, the choice of ligands, their concentrations, counterions, templates, solvents, temperatures, and even the pH values play pivotal roles in determining the final outcome of the clusters.

In more recent times, a notable advancement has come in the form of supramolecular chemistry, a field that has seen exponential growth. A noteworthy contribution to this has been the Hirshfeld surface analysis software. This tool, as emphasized by Shuhua Zhang, is instrumental in analyzing intermolecular interactions. It stands out as a pivotal instrument, offering detailed descriptions of the intermolecular interactions present in crystal structures. The Hirshfeld surface analysis, in essence, provides comprehensive insights into the surface characteristics of molecules, making it an indispensable method for pinpointing common features within crystals.

In this chapter, under the expert guidance of Shuhua Zhang, we delve into a meticulously designed synthesis of four analogous Schiff base ligands. These ligands, in turn, pave the way for the construction of four similar structured linear trinuclear manganese clusters denoted as $[Mn_3(L^n)_2(CH_3COO)_4]$ where n ranges from 1 to 4. Furthermore, the chapter will shed light on the nuanced differences in intermolecular interactions that arise when the substituents of the ligands undergo alterations.

Experimental Section

1. Materials and Instrumentation

For the synthesis, commercial grade chemicals and solvents were utilized without any further purification. Spectral analyses were carried out using a variety of specialized equipment:

- Fourier-Transform Infrared Spectroscopy (FT-IR): The FT-IR spectra were obtained using a Bio-Rad FTS-7 spectrometer, with samples prepared as KBr pellets. Spectra were recorded in the range of 4000–400 cm^{-1}.

- Elemental Analyses: The elemental compositions (CHN) of the samples were analyzed with a Perkin-Elmer 240 elemental analyzer.

- X-ray Crystallography: The X-ray crystal structures were determined using an Agilent G8910A CCD diffractometer. The SHELXL crystallographic software was employed for the molecular structures' determination.

- Nuclear Magnetic Resonance (NMR) Spectroscopy: The ^{1}H NMR spectra were recorded on a Bruker AV500 spectrometer, using tetramethylsilane (TMS) as the internal standard and CDCl$_3$ as the solvent.

- Magnetic Measurements: Measurements were performed using a Quantum Design PPMS model 600 magnetometer, focusing on samples **chapt10-1–chapt10-4** up to 5 T.

2. Synthesis

a. Synthesis of HL^1

A mixture of 5-chloro-2-hydroxybenzaldehyde (Hchbd, 10 mmol, 1.565 g), 2-chloro-6-hydrazinylpyridine (10 mmol, 1.436 g), and ethanol (30 ml) were combined in a 100 mL three-neck flask and refluxed at 80°C for 3 hours. During this period, the solution transitioned to a yellow color. It was further concentrated at 80°C for another 2 hours. Post-concentration, a yellow powder was isolated by filtration, washed thrice with ethanol (5 mL each time), and air-dried. The resulting product (HL^1) yield was approximately 95% based on Hchbd. Detailed analytical data and spectral characteristics of HL^1 are provided, and can be found in Figure 10-1.

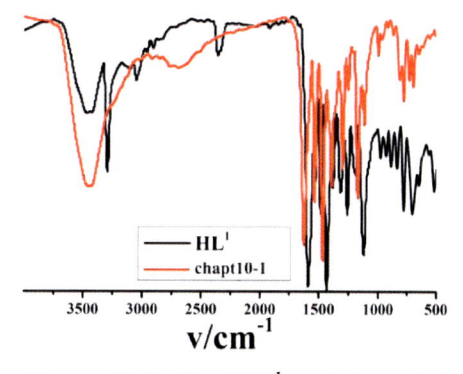

Figure 10-1. IR of HL^1 and chapt10-1

b. Synthesis of HL^2

The synthesis method for HL² mirrored that of HL1, with the exception of replacing 5-chloro-2-hydroxybenzaldehyde with 5-bromo-2-hydroxybenzaldehyde (Hbhbd). The resultant yellow powder was isolated, washed with ethanol, and dried. The yield was around 97% based on Hbhbd. Spectral details for HL² are provided in Figure 10-2.

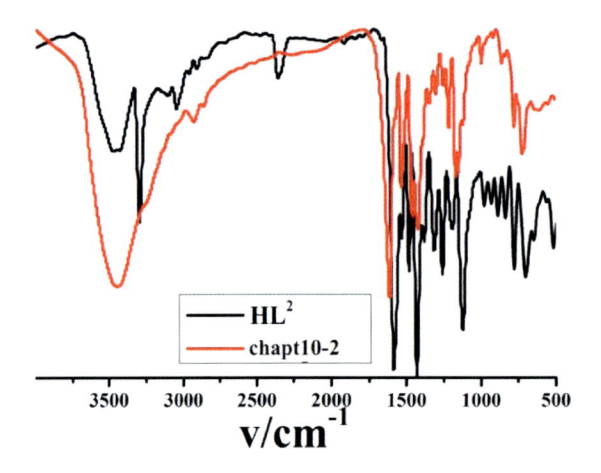

Figure 10-2. IR of HL² and chapt10-2

c. Synthesis of HL³

HL³'s synthesis followed a similar protocol to HL¹. However, 2-chloro-6-hydrazinylpyridine was substituted with 2-bromo-6-hydrazinylpyridine. After filtration, the yellow powder was washed with ethanol and dried in the open air, yielding a product in about 94.2% based on Hchbd. Spectral characterizations for HL³ can be viewed in Figure 10-3.

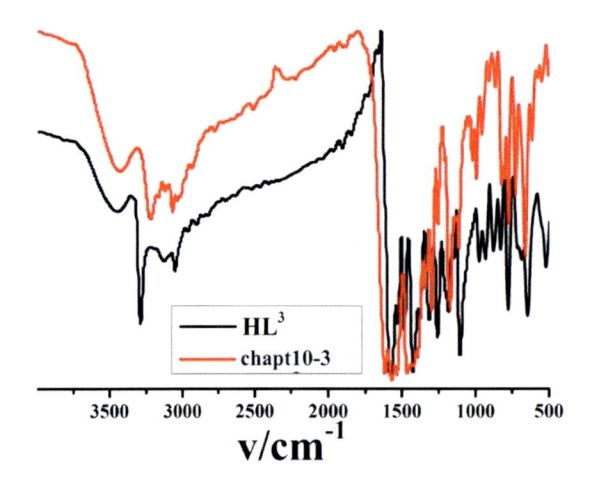

Figure 10-3. IR of HL³ and chapt10-3.

d. Synthesis of HL⁴:

The procedure for synthesizing HL⁴ was akin to that of HL³. Here, 5-chloro-2-hydroxybenzaldehyde was replaced with 5-bromo-2-hydroxybenzaldehyde. The final product, a yellow powder, was collected by filtration, washed with ethanol, and left to dry in air. Based on Hbhbd, the yield was around 94.2%. Spectral analyses for HL4 are provided in Figure 10-

4.

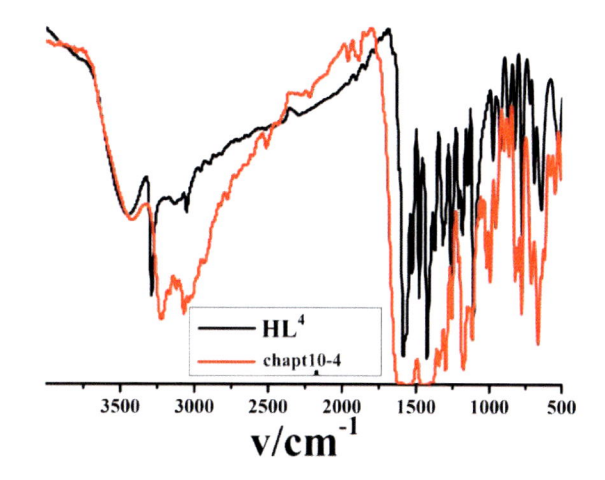

Figure 10-4. IR of HL⁴ and chapt10-4.

Scheme 10-1. Structures of HL¹-HL⁴.

e. Preparation of [Mn₃(L¹)₂(CH₃COO)₄] (chapt10-1)

Procedure:

A solution was prepared by mixing HL¹ (0.5 mmol, 0.141 g) with Mn(CH₃COO)₂·4H₂O (0.5 mmol, 0.123 g), 5 mL ethanol, and 5 mL DMF. The pH was adjusted to 7 using triethylamine. After stirring for 20 minutes, this solution was transferred to a 15 mL Teflon-lined autoclave. It was then heated at 80°C for three days and gradually cooled to room temperature. This process resulted in the formation of yellow crystals.

Yield:

0.105 g, approximately 65.4% based on Mn.

Analysis:

- Molecular Formula: $C_{32}H_{28}Cl_4Mn_3N_6O_{10}$
- Molecular Weight: 963.22
- Expected Content: C: 39.90%, H: 2.97%, N: 8.72%
- Observed Content: C: 39.84%, H: 3.06%, N: 8.80%

IR Data (KBr, cm^{-1}, Figure 10-1):

3449, 1621, 1532, 1463, 1391, 1298, 1251, 1171, 1117, 998, 811, 776, 728, 648.

f. Preparation of [Mn$_3$(L^2)$_2$(CH$_3$COO)$_4$] (chapt10-2)

Procedure:

Using the same method as for **chapt10-1**, complex **chapt10-2** was synthesized, with the only change being the replacement of HL^1 with HL^2. This led to the production of yellow crystals.

Yield:

0.116 g, approximately 66.15% based on Mn.

Analysis:

- Molecular Formula: C$_{32}$H$_{28}$Br$_2$Cl$_2$Mn$_3$N$_6$O$_{10}$
- Molecular Weight: 1052.14
- Expected Content: C: 36.53%, H: 2.68%, N: 7.98%
- Observed Content: C: 36.38%, H: 2.79%, N: 8.05%

IR Data (KBr, cm^{-1}, Figure 10-2):

3441, 1614, 1531, 1461, 1418, 1298, 1215, 1171, 1117, 998, 860, 778, 724, 661.

g. Preparation of [Mn$_3$(L^3)$_2$(CH$_3$COO)$_4$] (chapt10-3)

Procedure:

Utilizing a method analogous to the synthesis of Complex **chapt10-1**, Complex **chapt10-3** was formed. The only variation in the procedure was the substitution of HL^1 with HL^3. This process yielded yellow crystals.

Yield:

0.123 g, approximately 70.14% based on Mn.

Analysis:

- Molecular Formula: C$_{32}$H$_{28}$Br$_2$Cl$_2$Mn$_3$N$_6$O$_{10}$
- Molecular Weight: 1052.14
- Expected Content: C: 36.53%, H: 2.68%, N: 7.98%
- Observed Content: C: 36.46%, H: 2.75%, N: 8.03%

IR Data (KBr, cm^{-1}, Figure 10-3):

3424, 3218, 1616, 1567, 1462, 1344, 1296, 1253, 1170, 1114, 993, 821, 804, 775, 726, 661.

h. Preparation of [Mn₃(L⁴)₂(CH₃COO)₄] (chapt10-4)

Procedure:

Following a method similar to that of Complex **chapt10-1**, Complex **chapt10-4** was synthesized. The primary change in the method was the replacement of HL¹ with HL⁴, resulting in the formation of yellow crystals.

Yield:

0.131 g, around 68.88% based on Mn.

Analysis:

- Molecular Formula: C₃₂H₂₈Br₄Mn₃N₆O₁₀
- Molecular Weight: 1141.06
- Expected Content: C: 33.65%, H: 2.45%, N: 7.36%
- Observed Content: C: 33.57%, H: 2.59%, N: 7.39%

IR Data (KBr, cm⁻¹, Figure 10-4):

3426, 3221, 1616, 1537, 1462, 1343, 1295, 1254, 1171, 1113, 1047, 1019, 993, 957, 822, 802, 776, 710, 662.

3. Determination of Crystal Structure

a. Instrumentation and Data Collection

The diffraction data for determining the crystal structure were obtained using an Agilent G8910A CCD diffractometer. This device employed graphite-monochromatic Mo-Kα radiation with a wavelength (k) of 0.71073 Å. The x-h scan mode was utilized, with specific scan ranges provided for each of the samples:

- $3.65 \leq \theta \leq 25.10$ for sample (**chapt10-1**)
- $3.59 \leq \theta \leq 25.01$ for sample (**chapt10-2**)
- $3.64 \leq \theta \leq 25.10$ for sample (**chapt10-3**)
- $358 \leq \theta \leq 25.10$ for sample (**chapt10-4**).

b. Data Processing and Structure Solution

Once collected, the raw frame data underwent integration using the SAINT program. To decipher the structures, direct methods were applied through the SHELXS-97 software. The refinement of these structures employed full matrix least-squares based on F^2 values, again utilizing SHELXS-97. Empirical absorption corrections were also implemented, utilizing the SADABS program. It's notable that during the refinement:

- All non-hydrogen atoms were treated anisotropically.

- Hydrogen atoms were positioned geometrically and underwent refinement as riding atoms.

For further calculations and graphical visualizations, the SHELXTL software was employed.

For sample **chapt10-2**, the most pronounced peak in the residual electron density was 1.180 e/Å^3, situated 1.08 Å from atom Br1. In contrast, the most profound hole recorded a value of 1.283 e/Å^3 and was found 0.96 Å away from atom Br1.

c. Crystallographic Details

To provide a comprehensive view of the crystal structures, specific bond lengths and angles for samples **chapt10-1-chapt10-4** are documented in Table 10-1. Additional crystallographic specifics for the samples are accessible in Table 10-2.

Table 10-1 Selected bond lengths (Å) and angles(°) for Chapt10-1–Chapt10-4.

Complexes	Chapt10-1	Chapt10-2	Chapt10-3	Chapt10-4
Mn1–O5	2.119 (7)	2.123(5)	2.116 (3)	2.119 (4)
Mn1–O3	2.207 (6)	2.212 (5)	2.221 (3)	2.119 (4)
Mn1–O2	2.209 (7)	2.204 (6)	2.210 (3)	2.204 (4)
Mn2–O4	2.070 (7)	2.088 (5)	2.084 (3)	2.080 (4)
Mn2–O3	2.129 (6)	2.127 (5)	2.124 (3)	2.126 (4)
Mn2–N3	2.184 (8)	2.198 (6)	2.196 (4)	2.191 (4)
Mn2–O2	2.206 (7)	2.212 (6)	2.235(4)	2.236 (4)
Mn2–N1	2.259(8)	2.212 (6)	2.281 (4)	2.280 (4)
Mn2–O1	2.492 (9)	2.485 (7)	2.451 (4)	2.461(4)
Mn2···Mn1	3.2127 (17)	3.2071 (12)	3.2315 (8)	3.2229 (8)
O5–Mn1–O5a	180.0	180.0	180.0	180.0
O5–Mn1–O2	89.6 (3)	89.7 (2)	90.28 (12)	89.94 (15)
O5–Mn1–O2a	90.4 (3)	90.3 (2)	89.72 (12)	89.94 (15)
O2–Mn1–O2a	180.000 (2)	180.000 (1)	180.000 (1)	180.000 (1)
O5a–Mn1–O3	90.3 (2)	90.4 (2)	90.66 (13)	90.19 (14)
O5–Mn1–O3	89.7 (2)	89.6 (2)	90.66 (13)	89.81 (14)
O2a–Mn1–O3	101.2 (2)	101.1 (2)	101.69 (12)	101.26 (13)
O2–Mn1–O3	78.8(2)	78.9 (2)	78.31(12)	78.74 (13)
O5a–Mn1–O3a	89.7(2)	89.6(2)	89.34(13)	89.81(14)
O5–Mn1–O3a	90.3(2)	90.4(2)	90.66(13)	90.19(14)
O2a–Mn1–O3a	101.2(2)	78.9(2)	78.31(12)	78.74(13)
O3–Mn1–O3a	180.000(1)	180.000 (1)	180.000(1)	180.0
O4–Mn2–O3	96.3 (3)	96.4 (2)	96.29 (13)	96.60 (15)
O4–Mn2–N3	112.0 (3)	112.2 (2)	112.29 (14)	112.22 (15)
O3–Mn2–N3	83.1 (3)	82.7 (2)	82.63 (14)	82.60 (15)
O4–Mn2–O2	94.9 (3)	95.3 (2)	95.48 (13)	95.22 (14)
O3–Mn2–O2	80.6 (2)	80.6 (2)	79.84 (12)	80.11 (13)
N3–Mn2–O2	149.9 (3)	149.3 (2)	148.56 (14)	149.01 (16)
O4–Mn2–N1	95.9 (3)	95.7 (2)	95.76 (13)	95.61 (15)
O3–Mn2–N1	155.0 (3)	155.3 (2)	155.32 (15)	154.99 (16)
N3–Mn2–N1	72.2 (3)	72.7 (2)	72.88 (15)	72.57 (16)
O2–Mn2–N1	119.9 (3)	119.6 (2)	120.25 (14)	120.36 (15)
O4–Mn2–O1	146.1 (3)	146.0 (2)	145.80 (14)	95.61 (15)

O3–Mn2–O1	93.4 (3)	93.4 (2)	93.93 (13)	154.99 (16)
N3–Mn2–O1	101.4 (3)	101.3 (2)	101.34 (14)	72.57 (16)
O2–Mn2–O1	54.8 (3)	54.4 (2)	54.48 (12)	54.45(13)
N1–Mn2–O1	88.5 (3)	88.5 (2)	88.04 (14)	88.76(15)
Mn2–O3–Mn1	95.6 (2)	95.3 (2)	96.07 (13)	95.60 (14)
Mn2–O2–Mn1	93.4 (3)	93.1 (2)	93.26 (13)	93.06 (14)
Mn2···Mn1···Mn2a	180.0	180.000 (1)	180.0	180.0

Symmetry code : (a) 1–x, 1–y, 1–z.

Table 10-2 Crystallographic and experimental data for **Chapt10-1-Chapt10-4**

Compounds	**Chapt10-1**	**Chapt10-2**	**Chapt10-3**	**Chapt10-4**
Formula	$C_{32}H_{28}Cl_4Mn_3N_6O_{10}$	$C_{32}H_{28}Br_2Cl_2Mn_3N_6O_{10}$	$C_{32}H_{28}Br_2Cl_2Mn_3N_6O_{10}$	$C_{32}H_{28}Br_4Mn_3N_6O_{10}$
Form. weight	963.22	1052.14	1052.14	1141.06
Colour and form	block, yellow	block, yellow	block, yellow	block, yellow
T / K	293(2)	293(2)	293(2)	293(2)
Crystal system	Triclinic	Triclinic	Triclinic	Triclinic
Space group	$P\bar{1}$	$P\bar{1}$	$P\bar{1}$	$P\bar{1}$
a / Å	9.430 (2)	9.4523 (7)	9.4396 (10)	9.4564 (9)
b / Å	10.567 (2)	10.7532 (11)	10.6642 (11)	10.8519 (8)
c / Å	11.141(3)	11.1099 (11)	11.1970 (11)	11.1591 (9)
α / °	117.83(3)	117.257 (10)	118.152(11)	117.490 (8)
β / °	90.75 (2)	90.557 (7)	90.942 (9)	90.800 (7)
γ / °	93.689 (19)	94.612 (7)	93.077 (9)	93.890 (7)
V / Å^3	978.5 (4)	999.22 (16)	991.27(18)	1012.18 (15)
Z	1	1	1	1
$D_{calcd.}$/gcm^{-3}	1.635	1.748	1.763	1.872
μ / mm^{-1}	1.29	3.13	3.15	4.93
R_{int}	0.101	0.036	0.030	0.039
Goof	1.00	1.00	1.00	1.01
Completeness	100%	100%	100%	100%
$F(000)$	485	521	521	557
θ range / °	3.6 to 20.8	4.0 to 26.6	3.6 to 25.1	4.1 to 26.4
Ref.coll. / unique	6489 / 3481	5799 / 3514	5898 / 3537	6042 / 3604
Parameters	252	252	252	252
Final R_1 [$I > 2\sigma$][a]	0.089	0.071	0.050	0.048
wR_2[b]	0.24	0.187	0.136	0.136
Residues / eÅ^{-3}	0.80, −0.82	1.18, −1.28	0.56, −0.54	0.82, −0.52

[a] $R_1 = \Sigma||F_o| - |F_c||/\Sigma|F_o|$. [b] $wR_2 = [\Sigma w(|F_o^2|-|F_c^2|)^2/\Sigma w(|F_o^2|)^2]^{1/2}$

4. Hirshfeld Surface Calculations for Samples chapt10-1-chapt10-4

Methodology

For this analysis, the CrystalExplorer program was employed. Upon inputting the CIF files of samples **chapt10-1-chapt10-4** into this software, it automatically adjusted all bond lengths connected to hydrogen atoms to their typical neutron standard values:

- C···H = 1.083 Å
- N···H = 1.009 Å
- O···H = 0.983 Å.

The Hirshfeld surfaces for the samples were generated at a high (standard) surface resolution.

The 3D dnorm surfaces were colored using a fixed scale from 0.76 (represented in red) to 2.4 (in blue). For a comprehensive view, 2D fingerprint plots were exhibited, employing the standard view of 0.4–2.6 Å, with the de and di distance scales illustrated on the graph axes.

5. Electrochemicaluminescence Analysis

Setup and Procedure

For this test, an MPI-A Electrochemical workstation, originating from Xi An, China, was used. The procedure adopted a standard three-electrode cell setup:

- Reference Electrode: Ag/AgCl electrode
- Auxiliary Electrode: Platinum wire
- Working Electrode: Glassy carbon electrode (GCE) with a 1 mm diameter, operating in DMF.

The chosen supporting electrolyte for the experiments was 0.1 mol/L potassium peroxydisulfate ($K_2S_2O_8$), also in DMF.

Results and Discussion

1. Description of the Crystal Structure

Complexes labeled as **chapt10-1**–**chapt10-4** are categorized as isomorphous compounds. They all belong to the triclinic crystal system and share the same *P*-1 space group. Despite these similarities, a noticeable difference among them is the halogen substituent groups present in the Schiff base ligands, as illustrated in Figure 10-5. To avoid repetition, this analysis focuses on complex **chapt10-1**.

Upon conducting single-crystal X-ray diffraction, it's established that complex **chapt10-1** adheres to the triclinic space group *P*-1. Its specific dimensions are $a = 9.430(2)$ Å, $b = 10.567(2)$ Å, and $c = 11.141(2)$ Å. Additionally, the angles between these axes are $α = 117.83(3)°$, $β = 90.75(2)°$, and $γ = 93.69(2)°$, making the overall volume $V = 978.5(4)$ Å^3.

The internal structure of complex **chapt10-1** is fascinating. The core structure features a trinuclear cluster formed by a combination of three Mn^{II} ions, two L^1 ligands, and four acetate groups (as shown in Figure 10-5). The three Mn^{II} ions are linearly connected through four acetate anions. Various bond lengths and angles within this core structure have been identified and compared with other similar complexes in literature.

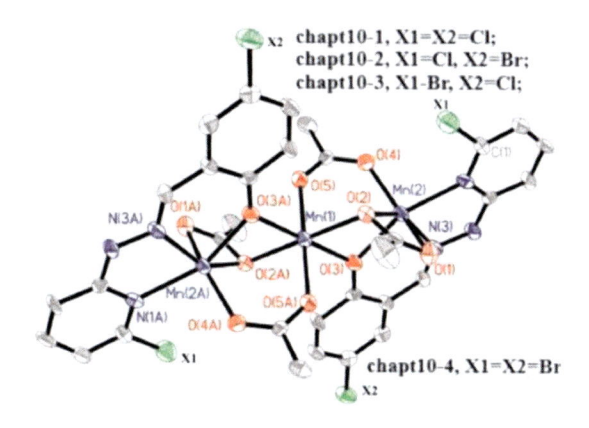

Figure 10-5. Crystal structures of chapt10-1–chapt10-4

Scheme 10-2. coordination mode of HL¹-HL⁴(a) and CH₃COO⁻ group(b).

Complex **chapt10-1** has one and a half crystallographically independent manganese atoms. Each of these manganese atoms, Mn1 and Mn2, has distinct coordination geometries, interacting with various atoms from the L^1 ligand and acetate groups. The L^1 ligand, in particular, demonstrates versatility by adopting different coordination modes with these manganese atoms.

This linear trinuclear cluster subsequently evolves into a 1D chain due to double N-H···O and double C-H···O hydrogen bonds(Figure 10-6). Further complexity arises from π···π interactions and Cl···π interactions, culminating in a 2D network.

2. Hirshfeld Surface Analysis

Hirshfeld surface analysis, combined with 2D fingerprint plots, is a proficient method to understand the intermolecular interactions present in crystal structures. Figure 10-7 showcases the molecular Hirshfeld surfaces (dnorm) of complexes **chapt10-1–chapt10-4**. From this visualization, one can discern the effects of different halogen substituents on the intermolecular interactions of these complexes. Particularly, regions of close-contact interactions are highlighted in deep red spots

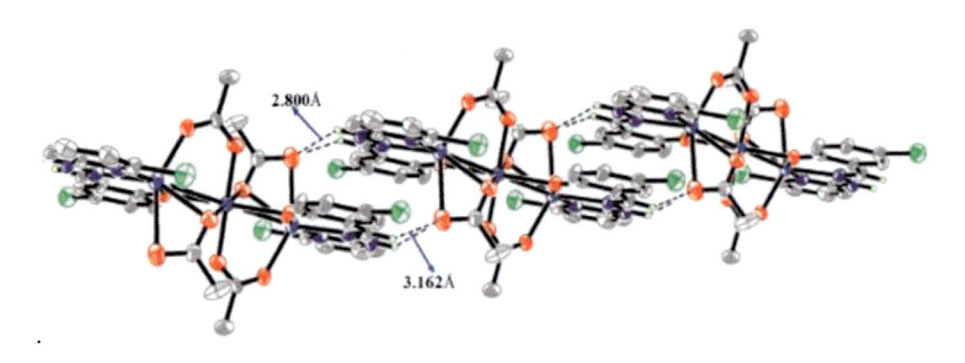

Figure 10-6. 1D chain of chapt10-1

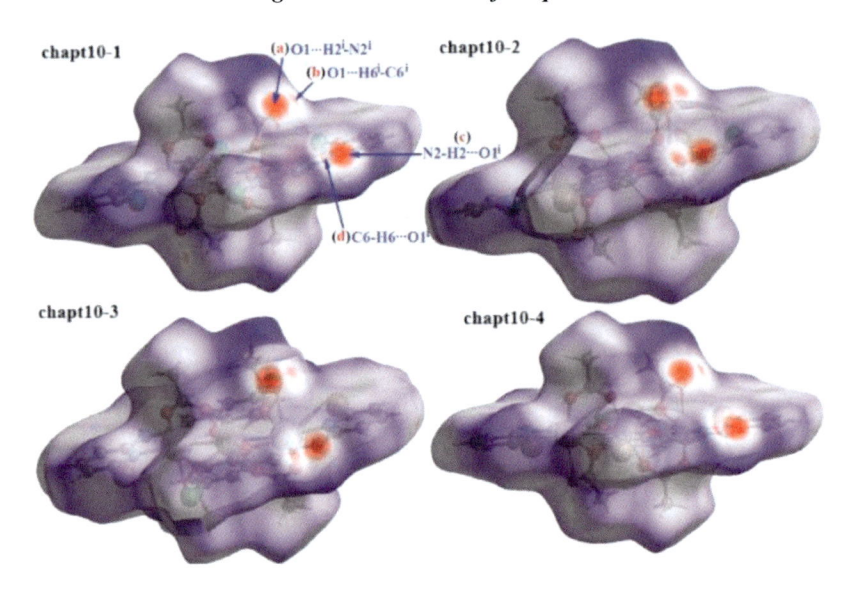

Figure 10-7. Hirshfeld surface mapped with dnorm (up) for chapt10-1–chapt10-4.

The significance of different interaction types, especially hydrogen bonds, is evident from the 2D fingerprint plots (refer to Figure 10-8). These plots help in quantifying the nature of interactions between molecules within the crystal. A detailed breakdown of the contributions from various interactions like H···H, X···H, O···H, and C···C has been provided. Notably, the H···H and H···X interactions dominate in complex **chapt10-1**. Interestingly, it appears that when the molecular structure is consistent, as in complexes **chapt10-1–chapt10-4**, similar intermolecular interactions prevail.

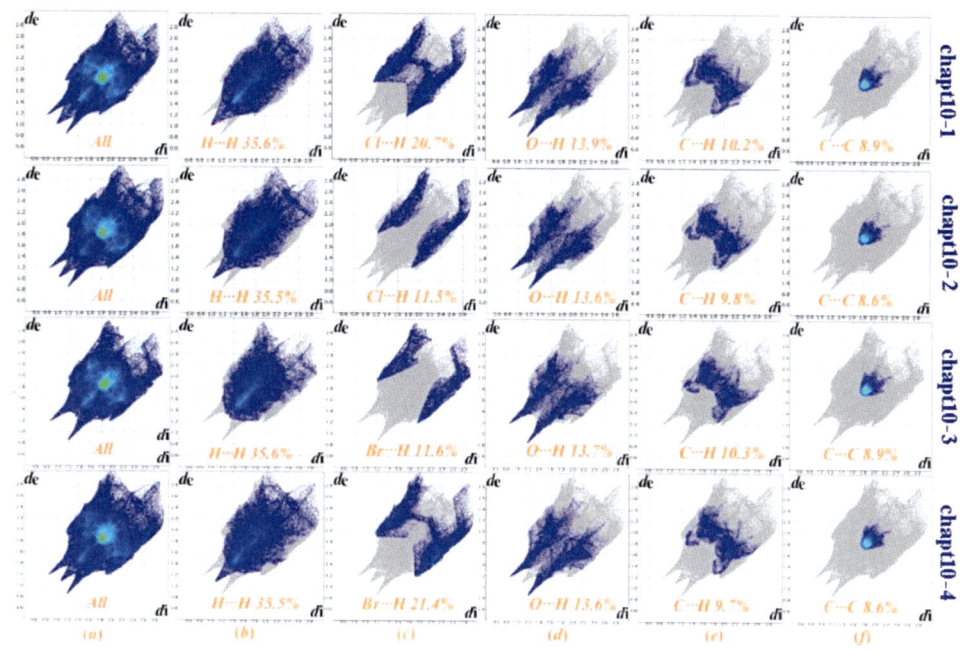

Figure 10-8. Fingerprint plots of chapt10-1–chapt10-4: Full (a) and resolved into H···H (b) and X···H (c), O···H (d), C···H (e) and C···C (f) contacts showing the percentages of contacts contributed to the total Hirshfeld Surface area of chapt10-1–chapt10-4.

3. Magnetic Properties

Measurement Process

Magnetic susceptibilities of samples **chapt10-1–chapt10-4** were gauged by employing crushed single crystal samples. The dc susceptibilities of these samples were studied under an applied field of 1kOe at temperatures spanning from 2 to 300 K.

Analysis of Sample chapt10-1

For sample chapt10-1:

- The three Mn^{II} ions result in a $\chi_M T$ value of 8.31 cm^{3}mol^{-1}K at room temperature. This is notably lesser than the anticipated spin-only value of 13.1 cm^{3}Kmol^{-1} for three non-interacting high-spin Mn^{II} ions, assuming g = 2.0 (Refer to Figure 10-9).

- The values noticed for sample **chapt10-1** align closely with the $\chi_M T$ value of [Mn$_3$(O$_2$CCH$_3$)$_4$(sae)$_2$(HIm)$_2$] (approximately 8.3 cm^{3}Kmol^{-1}).

- The values are however less than those recorded for the linear trinuclear Mn^{II} cluster in [Mn$_3$(N$_3$)$_2$(nta)$_4$(H$_2$O)$_2$]n (approximately 14.01 cm^3 K mol^{-1}) and [Mn$_3$(L)(H$_2$O)$_2$(DMF)$_2$] 8DMF (13.46 cm^3 K mol^{-1}).

- With decreasing temperature (T), the $\chi_M T$ values for **chapt10-1** progressively rise, peaking at 8.96 cm^3 K mol^{-1} at 34.8 K and then slowly escalating to its lowest value of 7.60 cm^3 K mol^{-1} at 2 K.

- This particular magnetic behavior has parallels to [Mn$_3^{III}$O(O$_2$CR)$_3$L^3].ClO$_4$ (where HL is 2-pyridyl oximes). The observed trend suggests strong ferromagnetic interactions among the Mn^{II} ions facilitated by μ_2-O bridging.

Temperature Dependence and Curie-Weiss Law

The temperature dependence of the reciprocal susceptibility (χ_M^{-1}) above 25 K adheres to the Curie-Weiss law [$\chi_M = C/(T - \theta)$], featuring Weiss and Curie constants of 13.12 K and 6.04 cm^{3}mol^{-1}K, respectively (see Inset Figure 10-9). The dominant positive Weiss constant infers an intramolecular ferromagnetic interplay between adjacent Mn^{II} ions through μ_2-O bridging. It's noteworthy to highlight that the C value is marginally lesser than the $\chi_M T$ value at room temperature.

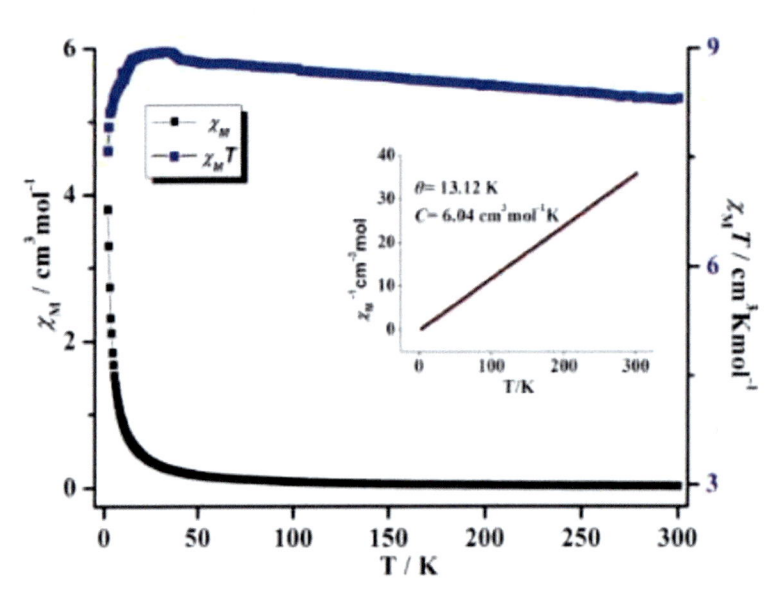

Figure 10-9. Plots of $\chi_M T$ and χ_M vs. T measured in a 1000 Oe field for chapt10-1; Insert Figure 10-9 plots of χ_M^{-1} vs. T for chapt10-1

AC Susceptibility Observations

AC susceptibility assessments were executed in the temperature range of 2–10 K at frequencies of 10 Hz and 997 Hz specifically for sample **chapt10-1** (as illustrated in Figure 10-10). These tests affirm that **chapt10-1** doesn't exhibit single molecule magnet (SMM) behavior, supported by the absence of out-of-phase ac signals above 2 K.

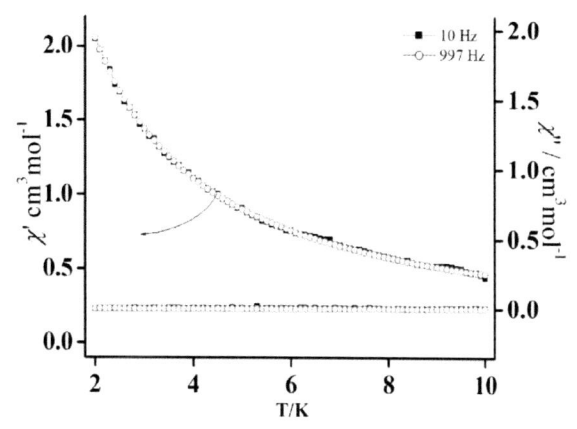

Figure 10-10. plots of χ' vs. T and χ'' vs. T for **chapt10-1**.

Analysis of Samples 2–4

For samples 2–4:

- At room temperature, the three Mn^{II} ions generate $\chi_m T$ products of 10.03, 11.48, and 11.82 cm^{3}Kmol^{-1} respectively (as shown in Figure 10-11).

- These values, similar to sample **chapt10-1**, fall below the spin-only value of 13.1 cm^{3}Kmol^{-1} for three non-interacting high-spin Mn^{II} ions with $g = 2.0$ (Refer to Figure 10-9).

- However, the recorded values for samples **chapt10-2**–**chapt10-4** surpass those for [Mn$_3$(O$_2$CCH$_3$)$_4$(sae)$_2$(HIm)$_2$] (approximately 8.3 cm^{3}Kmol^{-1}), but are below the values for [Mn$_3$(N$_3$)$_2$(nta)$_4$(H$_2$O)$_2$]$_n$ (approximately 14.01 cm^{3}Kmol^{-1}).

- As the temperature declines, the $\chi_m T$ values for **chapt10-2**–**chapt10-4** steadily reduce, bottoming out at 4.12, 4.20, and 3.94 cm^{3}Kmol^{-1} at 2 K, respectively.

- This magnetic pattern is analogous to that observed for [Mn$_3$(O$_2$CCH$_3$)$_4$(sae)$_2$(HIm)$_2$] and [Mn$_3$(L)(H$_2$O)$_2$(DMF)$_2$]·8DMF, hinting at robust antiferromagnetic interactions among the Mn^{II} ions.

Temperature Dependence for Samples chapt10-2–chapt10-4

For samples **chapt10-2–chapt10-4**, the temperature dependence of the reciprocal susceptibility (χ_M^{-1}) above 25 K is consistent with the Curie-Weiss law [$\chi_M = C/(T - \theta)$]. The data reveals negative Weiss constants (θ = 29.94, 14.79, and 15.44 K for **chapt10-2–chapt10-4**, respectively) and Curie constants (C = 11.03, 12.40, and 12.07 cm^3 mol^{-1} K for **chapt10-2–chapt10-4,** respectively, as presented in Inset Figure 10-11). The negative values of the Weiss constants imply an intramolecular antiferromagnetic relationship between neighboring Mn^{II} ions via μ_2-O bridging.

4. ECL Characteristics of Complex chapt10-3

Figure 10-12 illustrates the ECL of pure Complex **chapt10-3**. Insights into the redox properties of these complexes were derived from cyclic voltammetry (CV) studies. The results using glassy carbon disk electrodes (GCE) coated with Complex **chapt10-3** are shown in Figure 10-13. Upon the addition of K$_2$S$_2$O$_8$ to the solution of Complex **chapt10-3**, an oxidation peak at -1.8 V and a reduction peak at 0.70 V in the cathodic current are noticeable.

For Complex **chapt10-3**, the peak luminous intensity is approximately 9200 a.u. This intensity remains relatively stable even after seven cycles. Ru(bpy)$_3^{3+}$ was set as the standard ECL yield with Complex **chapt10-3** demonstrating an ECL yield of 2.02. Intriguingly, the luminosity of Complex **chapt10-3** surpasses that of [Zn(L^2)$_2$]n (where HL^2 is (E)-2-(((4H-1,2,4-triazol-4-yl)imino)methyl)-4,6-dichlorophenol), with a luminosity of about 2800 a.u. Notably, Complex **chapt10-3** has set a new record for fluorescence efficiency among first transaction metal complexes in ECL materials. It's hypothesized that the presence of the Mn ion enhances the spin-orbit coupling effect, leading to improved ECL emission. When compared to previously studied complexes like Ru-, Ir-, Pt-, Re-, Os-, Zn-, and Cd-based ones, Complex **chapt10-3** displays a robust ECL emission. These findings could pave the way for novel cluster-based ECL material designs.

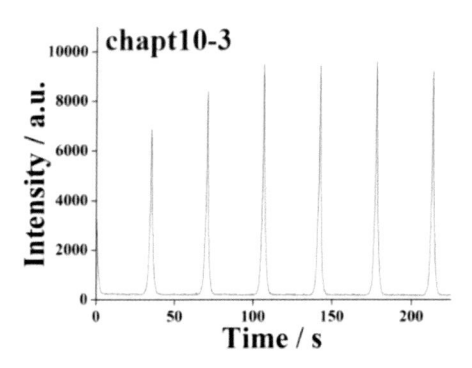

Figure 10-12. Electrochemical luminescence for chapt10-3.

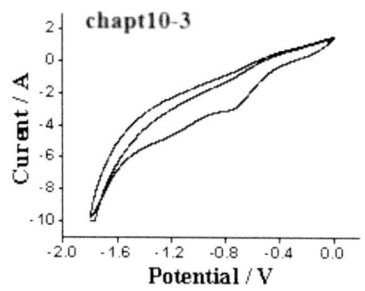

Figure 10-13. Cyclic voltammogram of chapt10-3 (1 × 10^{-4} mol L^{-1}) in DMF with 0.1 mol L^{-1} K$_2$S$_2$O$_8$

5. Synthesis Approach

We aimed to understand the impact of halogen interactions on the self-assembly of supramolecules and clusters. Mn(CH$_3$COO)$_2$·4H$_2$O and HL^n (where n = 1–4) were chosen as initial materials. The preparation method for the HL^n system is outlined in Scheme 10-1. Under comparable conditions, trinuclear cluster complexes **chapt10-1–chapt10-4** were produced. The results show that the halogen atoms in HL^n (n = 1–4) don't affect the structures of **chapt10-1–chapt10-4**. Interestingly, when Mn(HCOO)$_2$·4H$_2$O replaced Mn(CH$_3$COO)$_2$·4H$_2$O under the same conditions, similar complexes to **chapt10-1–chapt10-4** weren't achieved. Likewise, substituting M(CH$_3$COO)$_2$·4H$_2$O (where M = Co, Ni, Cu, Zn) for Mn(CH$_3$COO)$_2$·4H$_2$O didn't yield similar complexes to **chapt10-1–chapt10-4**. Instead, mononuclear complexes [M(L^n)$_2$]·nX (with M = Co, Ni, Cu, Zn, and X being solvent molecules) were produced.

6. IR Spectral Analysis of Complexes chapt10-1–chapt10-4

Spectroscopic features of clusters are pivotal for diverse applications. Consequently, room temperature IR spectra of HL^n (n = 1–4) and **chapt10-1–chapt10-4** were analyzed. N-H stretching vibrations of free HL^n (n = 1–4) ligands showed red-shifts, as observed at specific wavenumbers. Moreover, other bands were discerned, which could be attributed to intermolecular hydrogen bonds. It's noteworthy that strong bands for free HL^n (n = 1–4) ligands, linked to m(C=N) stretching frequencies, exhibited blue-shifts for **chapt10-1–chapt10-4**. The spectra of Complexes **chapt10-1–chapt10-4** displayed characteristic peaks associated with the acetate groups, suggesting the presence of bidentate acetate groups.

Conclusion

The study presented herein delved deeply into the Electroluminescent (ECL) characteristics and synthesis approaches of various complexes, with a particular focus on Complex **chapt10-3**. The ECL properties of Complex **chapt10-3**, as illustrated in Figure 10-12, offered pivotal insights into the redox properties of the associated complexes, especially when subjected to cyclic voltammetry studies. The robust luminous intensity demonstrated by Complex **chapt10-3**, especially in comparison to other complexes such as [Zn(L^2)$_2$]n, underscores its potential in various applications. Furthermore, it was evident that the introduction of the Mn ion plays a crucial role in enhancing the spin-orbit coupling effect, thereby boosting the ECL emission. This insight is particularly valuable, providing a pathway for future innovations in the development of cluster-based ECL materials.

The synthesis approach section laid down the foundational understanding of the impact of halogen interactions on the self-assembly processes of supramolecules and clusters. Different initial materials and conditions were meticulously examined to discern the optimal pathways and the inherent challenges therein. It was intriguing to note the profound influence of substituting Mn(CH$_3$COO)$_2$·4H$_2$O with alternatives, a factor that significantly dictated the structure and nature of the resulting complexes.

The IR spectral analysis deepened the understanding of the complexes, elucidating the intricate interactions and shifts that take place at the molecular level. Such a detailed analysis is paramount in predicting the behavior of these complexes in various conditions and applications.

It's essential to highlight the contributions of Shuhua Zhang to this research. Zhang's expertise and meticulous approach have been invaluable in discerning the subtle nuances in the ECL properties, synthesis strategies, and IR spectral analysis. Zhang's insights, combined with the collaborative efforts of the team, have significantly advanced our understanding in this domain, potentially paving the way for future breakthroughs in ECL material designs and applications.

References

1. Zhang, S. H.; Wang, J. M.; Zhang, H. Y.; Fan, Y. P.; Xiao, Y. Highly Efficient Electrochemiluminescence Based on 4-Amino-1,2,4-Triazole Schiff Base Two-Dimensional Zn/Cd Coordination Polymers. Dalton Trans., 2017, 46(2), 410-419.
2. Xiao, Y.; Liu, Y. Q.; Li, G.; Huang, P. Microwave-Assisted Synthesis, Structure and Properties of a Co-Crystal Compound with 2-Ethoxy-6-Methyliminomethyl-Phenol. Supramol. Chem., 2015, 27(3), 161-166.
3. Qin, J. H.; Ma, L. F.; Hu, Y.; Wang, L. Y. Syntheses, Structures and Photoluminescence of Five Zinc(II) Coordination Polymers Based on 5-Methoxyisophthalate and Flexible N-Donor Ancillary Ligands. CrystEngComm, 2012, 14(8), 2891-2898.
4. Xiao, Y.; Huang, P.; Wang, W. Ligand Structure Induced Diversification from Dinuclear to 1D Chain Compounds: Syntheses, Structures and Fluorescence Properties. J. Clust. Sci., 2015, 26, 1091-1102.
5. Gwo, S.; Wang, C. Y.; Chen, H. Y.; Lin, M. H.; Sun, L.; Li, X.; Ahn, H. Plasmonic Metasurfaces for Nonlinear Optics and Quantitative SERS. Acs Photonics, 2016, 3(8), 1371-1384.
6. Suess, R. J.; Winnerl, S.; Schneider, H.; Helm, M.; Berger, C.; de Heer, W. A.; Mittendorff, M. Role of Transient Reflection in Graphene Nonlinear Infrared Optics. Acs Photonics, 2016, 3(6), 1069-1075.
7. Lee, S. W.; Choi, B. J.; Eom, T.; Han, J. H.; Kim, S. K.; Song, S. J.; Hwang, C. S. Influences of Metal, Non-Metal Precursors, and Substrates on Atomic Layer Deposition Processes for the Growth of Selected Functional Electronic Materials. Coord. Chem. Rev., 2013, 257(23-24), 3154-3176.

8. Liu, Y.; Xuan, W.; Cui, Y. Engineering Homochiral Metal-Organic Frameworks for Heterogeneous Asymmetric Catalysis and Enantioselective Separation. Adv. Mater., 2010, 22(37), 4112-4135.
9. Xuan, W.; Zhu, C.; Liu, Y.; Cui, Y. Mesoporous Metal–Organic Framework Materials. Chem Soc Rev, 2012, 41(5), 1677-1695.
10. Bao, S. S.; Zheng, L. M. Magnetic Materials Based on 3d Metal Phosphonates. Coord. Chem. Rev., 2016, 319, 63-85.
11. Kitchen, J. A. Lanthanide-Based Self-Assemblies of 2,6-Pyridyldicarboxamide Ligands: Recent Advances and Applications as Next-Generation Luminescent and Magnetic Materials. Coordin. Chem. Rev., 2017, 340, 232-246.
12. Han, S. D.; Zhao, J. P.; Liu, S. J.; Bu, X. H. Hydro (solvo) Thermal Synthetic Strategy towards Azido/Formato-Mediated Molecular Magnetic Materials. Coordin. Chem. Rev., 2015, 289, 32-48.
13. Zhang, S. H.; Zhao, R. X.; Li, G.; Zhang, H. Y.; Zhang, C. L.; Muller, G. Structural Variation from Heterometallic Heptanuclear or Heptanuclear to Cubane Clusters based on 2-Hydroxy-3-Ethoxy-Benzaldehyde: Effects of pH and Temperature. RSC Adv., 2014, 4(97), 54837-54846.
14. Zhang, S. H.; Zhang, Y. D.; Zou, H. H.; Guo, J. J.; Li, H. P.; Song, Y.; Liang, H. A Family of Cubane Cobalt and Nickel Clusters: Syntheses, Structures and Magnetic Properties. Inorg. Chim. Acta, 2013, 396, 119-125.
15. Zhang, H. Y.; Wang, W.; Chen, H.; Zhang, S. H.; Li, Y. Five Novel Dinuclear Copper(II) Complexes: Crystal Structures, Properties, Hirshfeld Surface Analysis and Vitro Antitumor Activity Study. Inorg. Chim. Acta, 2016, 453, 507-515.
16. Guerra, W.; Silva-Caldeira, P. P.; Terenzi, H.; Pereira-Maia, E. C. Impact of Metal Coordination on the Antibiotic and Non-Antibiotic Activities of Tetracycline-Based Drugs. Coordin. Chem. Rev., 2016, 327, 188-199.
17. Kaushik, R.; Ghosh, A.; Jose, D. A. Recent Progress in Hydrogen Sulphide (H2S) Sensors by Metal Displacement Approach. Coordin. Chem. Rev., 2017, 347, 141-157.
18. Zhang, Y.; Yuan, S.; Day, G.; Wang, X.; Yang, X.; Zhou, H. C. Luminescent Sensors Based on Metal-Organic Frameworks. Coord. Chem. Rev., 2018, 354, 28-45.
19. Oszajca, M.; Franke, A.; Brindell, M.; Stochel, G.; Eldik, R. V. Redox Cycling in the Activation of Peroxides by Iron Porphyrin and Manganese Complexes. 'Catching' Catalytic Active Intermediates. Coord. Chem. Rev., 2016, 306, 483-509.
20. Zhang, S. H.; Feng, C. Microwave-Assisted Snthesis, Crystal Structure and Fluorescence of Novel Coordination Complexes with Schiff Base Ligands. J. Mol. Struct., 2010, 977(1-3), 62-66.
21. Zhou, C. L.; Wang, Z. M.; Wang, B. W.; Gao, S. A Oximato-Bridged Linear Trinuclear [MnIVMnIIIMnIV] Single-Molecule Magnet. Dalton Trans., 2012, 41(44), 13620-13625.
22. Soldatova, A. V.; Romano, C. A.; Tao, L.; Stich, T. A.; Casey, W. H.; Britt, R. D.; Spiro, T. G. Mn(II) Oxidation by the Multicopper Oxidase Complex Mnx: a Coordinated Two-Stage Mn(II)/(III) and Mn(III)/(IV) Mechanism. J. Am. Chem. Soc., 2017, 139(33), 11381-11391.

23. Braga, D.; Grepioni, F.; Tedesco, E.; Wadepohl, H.; Gebert, S. C–H...OHydrogen Bonding in Crystalline Complexes Carrying Methylidyne (μ3-CH) and Methylene (μ-CH2) Ligands: Adatabase Study. J. Chem. Soc. Dalton Trans., 1997, (10), 1727-1732.

24. Davies, P. J.; Veldman, N.; Grove, D. M.; Spek, A. L.; Lutz B. T.G.; van Koten, G.; Organoplatinum Building Blocks for One-Dimensional Hydrogen Bonded Polymeric Structures. Angew. Chem. Int. Ed. 1996, 35(17), 1959–1961.

25. Yang, L.; Zhang, S. H.; Wang, W.; Guo, J. J.; Huang, Q. P.; Zhao, R. X.; Muller, G. Ligand Induced Diversification from Tetranuclear to Mononuclear Compounds: Syntheses, Structures and Magnetic Properties. Polyhedron, 2014, 74, 49-56.

26. James, S. L.; Verspui, G.; Spek, A. L.; van Koten, G. Organometallic Polymers: an Infinite Organoplatinum Chain in the Solid State Formed by (C [Triple Bond, Length Half M-dash] CH··· ClPt) Hydrogen Bonds. Chem. Commun., 1996, (11), 1309-1310.

27. Zhang, S. H.; Ma, L. F.; Zou, H. H.; Wang, Y. G.; Liang, H.; Zeng, M. H. Anion Induced Diversification from Heptanuclear to Tetranuclear Clusters: Syntheses, Structures and Magnetic Properties. Dalton Trans., 2011, 40(43), 11402-11409.

28. Loots, L.; Barbour, L. J. A Simple and Robust Method for the Identification of π–π Packing Motifs of Aromatic Compounds. CrystEngComm., 2012, 14(1), 300-304.

29. Luo, Y. H.; Zhang, C. G.; Xu, B.; Sun, B. W. A Cocrystal Strategy for the Precipitation of Liquid 2,3-Dimethyl Pyrazine with Hydroxyl Substituted Benzoic Acid and a Hirshfeld Surfaces Analysis of them. CrystEngComm., 2012, 14(20), 6860-6868.

30. Zhang, H. Y. Xiao, Y. Zhu, Y. A Novel Copper(II) Complex Based on 4-Amino-1,2,4-Triazole Schiff-Base: Synthesis, Crystal Structure, Spectral Characterization, and Hirshfeld Surface Analysis. Chin. J. Struct. Chem. 2017, 36(5) 848-855.

31. Zhang, C., Yang, L., Chen, H., Zhang, S. H. A Novel Dinuclear Copper(II) Complex: Synthesis, Crystal Structure, Properties and Hirshfeld Surface Analysis. Chin. J. Struct. Chem. 2017, 36, 1904-1911.

32. Seth, S. K.; Saha, I.; Estarellas, C.; Frontera, A.; Kar, T.; Mukhopadhyay, S. Supramolecular Self-Assembly of M-IDA Complexes Involving Lone-Pair ...π Interactions: Crystal Structures, Hirshfeld Surface Analysis, and DFT Calculations [H2IDA= Iminodiacetic Acid, M= Cu(II), Ni(II)]. Cryst. Growth. Des., 2011, 11(7), 3250-3265.

33. Wolff, S. K.; Grimwood, D. J.; McKinnon, J. J.; Jayatilaka, D.; Spackman, M. A. CrystalExplorer version 3.1, Univ. Western Australia: Perth, 2013.

34. Sheldrick, G. M. Crystal Structure Refinement with SHELXL. Acta Crystallogr. C., 2015, 71(1), 3-8.

35. Sheldrick, G. M. A Short History of SHELX. Acta Cryst. A., 2008, 64(1), 112-122.

36. McKinnon, J. J.; Spackman, M. A.; Mitchell, A. S. Novel Tools for Visualizing and Exploring Intermolecular Interactions in Molecular Crystals. Acta Crystallogr. B., 2004, 60(6), 627-668.

37. Allen, F. H.; Kennard, O.; Watson, D. G.; Brammer, L.; Orpen, A. G.; Taylor, R. Tables of Bond Lengths Determined by X-ray and Neutron Diffraction. Part 1. Bond Lengths in Organic Compounds. J. Chem. Soc.; Perkin. Trans., 1987, 2(12), S1-S19.

38. Li, Y. G.; Lecren, L.; Wernsdorfer, W.; Clérac, R. Antiferromagnetic Order in a Supramolecular Assembly of Manganese Trimers Based on Imidazole and Schiff-Base Ligands. Inorg. Chem. Commun., 2004, 7(12), 1281-1284.
39. Chen, H. J.; Mao, Z. W.; Gao, S.; Chen, X. M. Ferrimagnetic-Like Ordering in a Unique Three-Dimensional Coordination Polymer Featuring Mixed Azide/Carboxylate-Bridged Trinuclear Manganese(II) Clusters as Subunits. Chem. Commun., 2001, (22), 2320-2321.
40. Yi, F. Y.; Sun, Z. M. Solvent-Controlled Syntheses, Structure, and Magnetic Properties of Trinuclear Mn(II)-Based Metal-Organic Frameworks. Cryst. Growth. Des., 2012, 12(11), 5693-5700.
41. Li, G.; Wang, W.; Zhang, S. H.; Zhang, H. Y.; Chen, F. Y. Synthesis, Structure and Properties of Linear Trinuclear Cobalt Cluster with 5-Fluoro-2-hydroxy-benzoic Acid. J. Clust. Sci., 2014, 25, 1589-1597.
42. Qin, X. Y.; Zhang, S. H.; Jiang, Y. M.; Liu, J. C.; Qin, J. H. Syntheses, Crystal Structures and Antibacterial Activities of [Cu2(C11H11NO5S)2(H2O)4]·5H2O and [Ni2(C11H11NO5S)2(H2O)4]·2H2O. J. Coord. Chem., 2009, 62(3), 427-439.
43. Chen, X. M.; Zhang, S. H.; Zou, H. H.; Tan. A. Z. Synthesis and Crystal Structures of 3D Supramolecular Compounds:[M(4,4′-Bipy)2(H2O)4]·(4,4′-Bipy)2·(3,5-Daba)2·8H2O(M= Zn, Mn). J. Coord. Chem., 2008, 61(16), 2563-2569.
44. Stamatatos, T. C.; Foguet-Albiol, D.; Stoumpos, C. C.; Raptopoulou, C. P.; Terzis, A.; Wernsdorfer, W.; Christou, G. New Mn3 Structural Motifs in Manganese Single-Molecule Magnetism from the Use of 2-Pyridyloximate Ligands. Polyhedron, 2007, 26(9-11), 2165-2168.
45. Richter, M. M. Electrochemiluminescence(ecl). Chem. Rev., 2004, 104(6), 3003-3036.
46. Huang, B.; Zhou, X.; Xue, Z.; Lu, X. Electrochemiluminescence Quenching of Tris (2,2′-bipyridyl) Ruthenium. Trac-Trend. Anal. Chem., 2013, 51, 107-116.
47. Zhou, Y.; Li, W.; Yu, L.; Liu, Y.; Wang, X.; Zhou, M. Highly Efficient Electrochemiluminescence from Iridium(III) Complexes with 2-Phenylquinoline Ligand. Dalton Trans., 2015, 44(4), 1858-1865.
48. Feng, C.; Ma, Y. H.; Zhang, D.; Li, X. J.; Zhao, H. Highly Efficient Electrochemiluminescence Based on Pyrazolecarboxylic Metal Organic Framework. Dalton Trans., 2016, 45(12), 5081-5091.
49. Zheng, L.; Chi, Y.; Dong, Y.; Lin, J.; Wang, B. Electrochemiluminescence of Water-Soluble Carbon Nanocrystals Released Electrochemically from Graphite. J. Am. Chem. Soc., 2009, 131(13), 4564-4565.
50. Fan, F. R. F.; Park, S.; Zhu, Y.; Ruoff, R. S.; Bard, A. J. Electrogenerated Chemiluminescence of Partially Oxidized Highly Oriented Pyrolytic Graphite Surfaces and of Graphene Oxide Nanoparticles. J. Am. Chem. Soc., 2009, 131(3), 937-939.
51. Zhang, H.-Y. Y. Xiao, Y. Zhu, A Novel Copper(II) Complex Based on 4-Amino-1,2,4-Triazole Schiff-Base: Synthesis, Crystal Structure, Spectral Characterization, and Hirshfeld Surface Analysis. Chin. J. Struct. Chem. 2017, 36 (5) 848-855.
52. Zhang, C.; Ma, X. D.; Chen, Z. H.; Zhang, S. H.; Hai, H. Synthesis, Structure and Properties of a Novel Tetranuclear Copper Cluster-Based Polymer with Di-Schiff-Base. J. Clust. Sci., 2017, 28, 3241-3252.

Made in the USA
Columbia, SC
30 April 2024

664df69b-7831-4587-9f5e-a7b7039e3642R01